THERAPEUTIC ASPECTS OF NUTRITION

Fourth Nutricia Symposium

THERAPEUTIC ASPECTS
OF NUTRITION

Groningen 9—11 May 1973

EDITORS:

J. H. P. JONXIS M.D., H. K. A. VISSER M.D. AND
J. A. TROELSTRA M.D.

1973
SPRINGER-SCIENCE+BUSINESS MEDIA, B.V.

ISBN 978-94-010-2365-8   ISBN 978-94-010-2363-4 (eBook)
DOI 10.1007/978-94-010-2363-4

Copyright 1973 Springer Science+Business Media Dordrecht
Originally published by H. E. Stenfert Kroese B.V. Leiden Holland in 1973
Softcover reprint of the hardcover 1st edition 1973

CONTENTS

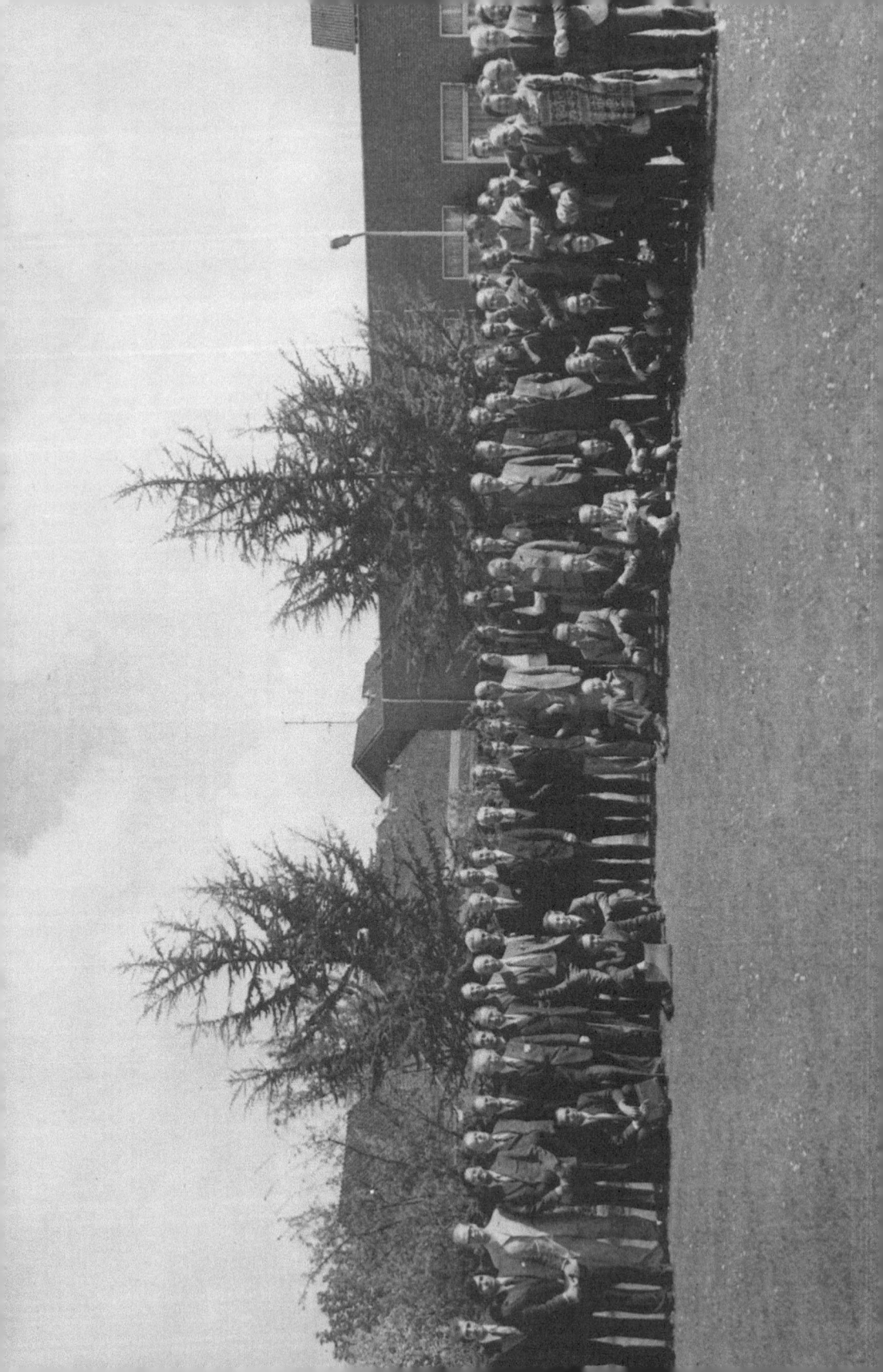

PARTICIPANTS

R. ABREU BLONDET, Paediatrician, Santiago.

ABDULLA ABDUL-AZIZ AL-RASHEID, Paediatrician, Kuwait.

K. ADRIAANSSENS, Paediatrician, Antwerpen.

H. BICKEL, University Children's Hospital, Heidelberg.

M. L. BLOK, Department of Internal Medicine, University Hospital Wilhelmina Gasthuis, Amsterdam.

J. BOLDINGH, Unilever Research, Vlaardingen.

D. CARTON, Department of Paediatrics, University Hospital, Gent.

E. CASADO DE FRIAS, Department of Paediatrics, University Hospital, Zaragoza.

C. CASSIMOS, Paediatrician, Thessaloniki.

F. H. CORSTENS, Department of Internal Medicine, University Hospital St. Radboud, Nijmegen.

J. DODION-FRANSEN, Department of Obstetrics and Gynaecology, University Hospital St. Pierre, Brussels.

N. M. DRAYER, Department of Paediatrics, University Hospital, Groningen.

R. EECKELS, Department of Paediatrics, University Hospital St. Rafaël, Louvain.

E. EGGERMONT, Department of Paediatrics, University Hospital St. Rafaël, Louvain.

J. FERNANDES, Sophia Children's Hospital and Neonatal Unit, Medical School of Rotterdam, Rotterdam.

C. FESTEN, Department of Surgery, University Hospital St. Radboud, Nijmegen.

M. GEUDEKE, Department of Paediatrics, Free University Hospital, Amsterdam.

L. GONZÁLEZ-COVIELLA DORTA, Servicio de Neonatología, Sanatoria Provincial Francisco Franco, Madrid.

J. P. GOLAERTS, Department of Paediatrics, University Hospital St. Pierre, Brussels.

J. G. A. J. HAUTVAST, Department of Nutrition, Landbouwhogeschool, Wageningen.

D. M. HEGSTED, Department of Nutrition, Harvard University, Boston.

R. HEFFINCK, Paediatrician, Aalst.

W. T. J. M. HEKKENS, Department of Gastroenterology, University Hospital, Leiden.

F. A. HOMMES, Laboratory of Developmental Biochemistry, University Hospital, Groningen.

F. ISMANGOEN, Department of Child Health, Gadja Mada University, Yogyakarta.

F. JANSSEN, Department of Paediatrics, University Hospital St. Pierre, Brussels.

S. JARNUM, Division of Gastroenterology, Rigshospitalet, Copenhagen.

J. H. P. JONXIS, Department of Paediatrics, University Hospital, Groningen.

R. K. J. KOUMANS, Department of Surgery, Zuiderziekenhuis, Rotterdam.

R. KLUTHE, Department of Internal Medicine, University Hospital, Freiburg.

P. J. KUIJJER, Department of Surgery, University Hospital, Groningen.

A. LAMBRECHTS, Department of Paediatrics, University Hospital, Liège.

R. DE LEEUW, Department of Paediatrics, University Hospital Wilhelmina Gasthuis, Amsterdam.

I. MACDONALD, Department of Physiology, Guy's Hospital Medical School, London.

K. MAMELETZIS, Paediatrician, Salonica.

L. MARTÍN SANZ, Servicio de Cirurgía Infantil, Sanatoria Provincial Francisco Franco, Madrid.

J. MATOS, Servicio de Pediatría, Hospital Infantil Ciudad, Madrid.

R. A. MCCANCE, Dunn Nutritional Laboratory, Infant Nutrition Research Division, University of Cambridge and Medical Research Council, Cambridge.

C. F. MILLS, Nutritional Biochemistry Department, The Rowett Research Institute, Bucksburn – Aberdeen.

I. MOLENAAR, Center for Medical Electron Microscopy, University Hospital, Groningen.

J. C. MOLENAAR, Department of Surgery, Free University Hospital, Amsterdam.

H. MULLER, Department of Surgery, University Hospital Dijkzigt, Rotterdam.

D. A. NICOLOPOULOS, Department of Paediatrics, University Hospital, Athens.

H. POEN, Department of Internal Medicine, University Hospital, Utrecht.

H. PRINS, Nutricia Ltd., Zoetermeer.

P. RICHARDS, Department of Internal Medicine, St. Mary's Hospital Medical School, London.

C. RICOUR, Hôpital des Enfants Malades, Paris.

J. H. RUYS, Department of Paediatrics, University Hospital, Leiden.

E. D. A. M. SCHRETLEN, Department of Paediatrics, University Hospital St. Radboud, Nijmegen.

R. C. A. SENGERS, Department of Paediatrics, University Hospital St. Radbout, Nijmegen.

J. SENTERRE, Department of Paediatrics, University of Liège.

J. C. L. SHAW, Department of Paediatrics, University College Hospital, London.

D. H. SHMERLING, Children's Hospital, Zürich.

M. SUTEDJO, Department of Child Health, University of Indonesia, Djakarta.

F. J. VAN SPRANG, Wilhelmina Children's Hospital, Utrecht.

S. W. STANBURY, Department of Medicine, University Hospital, Manchester.

U. G. STAUFFER, Children's Hospital, Zürich.

R. STEENDIJK, Department of Paediatrics, University Hospital Binnengasthuis, Amsterdam.

O. J. TEN THIJE, Department of Internal Medicine, University Hospital, Utrecht.

J. A. TROELSTRA, Department of Paediatrics, University Hospital, Groningen.

T. VALAES, Aghia Sophia Children's Hospital, Athens.

W. VEEGER, Department of Internal Medicine, University Hospital, Groningen.

VERELLEN, Department of Paediatrics, University Hospital St. Rafaël, Louvain.

A. J. VERGROESEN, Unilever Research, Vlaardingen.

D. VERVAT, Sophia Children's Hospital and Neonatal Unit, Medical School of Rotterdam, Rotterdam.

I. VILLA, Servicio de Neonatologia, Maternidad de Santa Cristina, Madrid.

H. K. A. VISSER, Sophia Children's Hospital and Neonatal Unit, Medical School of Rotterdam, Rotterdam.

E. M. WIDDOWSON, Dunn Nutritional Laboratory, Infant Nutrition Research Division, University of Cambridge and Medical Research Council, Cambridge.

A. WIERSINGA, Department of Internal Medicine, University Hospital, Utrecht.

J. H. P. WILSON, Department of Internal Medicine, University Hospital Dijkzigt, Rotterdam.

A. WRETLIND, Nutrition Unit, Karolinska Institutet, Stockholm.

GHOLAMREZA ZABOLINEJAD, Sina Hospital, Mashad, Iran.

N. ZÖLLNER, Department of Internal Medicine, University Hospital, München.

OPENING

PROF. DR. J. H. P. JONXIS

I am very happy to have the opportunity to welcome you here. I hope that you all had a good journey to Groningen. This is the fourth Nutricia Symposium. The first was held in this lecture room in 1964; the second was also here, in 1967 and the third was in Rotterdam in 1970. And now we are again here in Groningen. I hope that this symposium will proceed in the same amical fashion as the previous and that we shall have the same pleasant open discussions as we had then. There is a slight change in the subject. The earlier conferences dealt with the physiology and pathology of the newborn, especially in relation to nutrition. We had the feeling that it was time to shift the theme somewhat. On the one hand we have retained the same subject: the conference is still about nutrition. Nutrition is interwoven with the phenomenon of growth, especially infant growth, and we will deal again with this aspect. On the other hand we thought it might be good to discuss in addition nutrition in patients of other age groups.

The practice of medicine has advanced tremendously during the last two decades. Consequently the problems of the nutrition of patients of all age groups, who otherwise would have died but now survive, have become important. The hospital staffs are increasingly interested in the nutritional problems of these patients. For that reason we believe that a symposium on that part of medical treatment might be worthwhile.

In the Netherlands the situation pertaining to the science of nutrition is, I should say, a somewhat remarkable one. Early in this century Dutch scientists played an important role in nutritional science. Some of them were medical doctors, others were not. Since then, although the food industry is economically important in this country, the interests of the average doctor as well as those working in hospitals have shifted to other fields of medicine and we have neglected somewhat the nutritional problems in our clinics. This was even true of the paediatrician who at the beginning of this century was so deeply interested in these problems. Recently however there has been a change and I hope that this conference will help to increase interest in the nutritional problems of our patients.

PHYSIOLOGICAL ASPECTS OF NUTRITION

ENERGY REQUIREMENT

E. M. WIDDOWSON*

The first, now historic, Nutricia Symposium was held in this lecture hall in February 1964. It had the general title 'The adaptation of the newborn infant to extra-uterine life', and the session devoted to 'Temperature control of the newborn' was an exciting occasion, for we heard of new work that has a direct bearing on energy requirements. June HILL (1) told us about the development of thermal stability in the newborn baby, and table 1 is based on the values she

Table 1. *Basal oxygen consumption and energy expenditure of full term babies during first year* (1).

Age	Oxygen consumption ml O$_2$/kg/min	Energy expenditure kcal/kg/24 h
0–6 hours	4.8	33.0
18–36 hours	6.6	45.5
6–10 days	7.0	48.3
10 days to 1 year	7.0	48.3

gave us for the oxygen consumption of full term babies from birth to 1 year, measured in the neutral zone of environmental temperature, and expressed per kg body weight. The oxygen consumption, and with it the energy expenditure, rise between birth and 7–10 days without any important change in body weight. From about 1 week to 1 year the basal oxygen consumption remains at about 7 ml/kg/min, which is equivalent to 48 kcal/kg/24 hours. Dr. HILL, and Dr. BRÜCK who gave the next paper on 'General aspects of temperature regulation of small subjects' (2), discussed the response of the baby to a colder environment that the thermoneutral one. We heard that the oxygen consumption and energy expenditure rise and that the increase is roughly proportional to the decrease in environmental temperature.

* Dunn Nutritional Laboratory, University of Cambridge and Medical Research Council.

The amount of the increase varies from baby to baby, but a naked baby with a metabolic rate of 2 kcal/kg/h at 32° may well double this to 4 kcal/kg/h if the environmental temperature is lowered to 28°. Dr. BRÜCK suggested that this response to cold is triggered off by stimulation of the cold receptors in the skin, and one important way in which the baby's body produces heat is by the so-called non shivering thermogenesis. The next paper, by Dr. MOORE (3), dealt with this. Under the title 'Chemical regulation of heat production in the neonate', he described his work on the role of the sympathetic nervous system and particularly of noradrenaline in signalling that more fat must be oxidised to produce more heat. The session ended with a paper by the late Michael DAWKINS and David HULL (4) on brown adipose tissue. They told us of their new discoveries about the importance of the localised production of heat in the brown fat, particularly in some species such as the rabbit. The local release of noradrenaline in the brown fat leads to increased hydrolysis of triglycerides and this is followed by oxidation of fatty acids within the cell. It is mainly this localised consumption of oxygen that produces the heat.

So much for the past. Today we have come to talk about therapeutic aspects of nutrition. Our concern is with the small sick baby rather than the full term normal one. At the first Nutricia Symposium nothing was said about the energy requirements for growth. Although, generally, more of the food is used to provide for the tissues already there than to lay down new ones, the requirements for growth are important for the young baby, and far more so for the one that is underweight. Table 2 shows the calorific value of the increments of

Table 2. *Energy value of increments in protein and fat in body of baby between birth and 1 year*

Age	Energy value of increments in protein and fat		
months	Total kcal	kcal/day	kcal/kg/day
0–2	9100	149	33
2–4	6920	113	18
4–6	3580	59	7
6–8	2350	39	4
8–10	2500	41	4
10–12	1850	31	3

protein and fat in the body of a full term baby as it grows from 3.5 kg at birth to 10.5 kg at one year. The values are approximations, based on FOMON's estimates of body composition (5), but they serve to show that the calorific material added daily to each kilogram of the baby's body is much lower after the age of 4 months or so than it is soon after birth. Table 3 sets out how much this amounts to in relation to the

Table 3. *Intake and expenditure of energy kcal/kg/ 24h.*

Age	Intake	Expenditure		
months		Basal metabolism	Increment in body	Remainder, for thermogenesis, activity and energy cost of growth
0–2	126	48	33	45
2–3	116	48	18	50
3–4	106	48	18	40
4–5	100	48	7	45
5–12	100	48	4	48

total intake of energy (5) and the fraction expended on basal requirements. During the first two months about 30% of the energy intake is accounted for by increments of fat and protein in the body; from 5 months the percentage is only 4.

The small premature baby born at 28 weeks gestation weighing 1.1 kg would lay down protein and fat with an energy value of 35 kcal/kg/day if it grew to 3.5 kg in 12 weeks, and had the same body composition then as a baby born at full term. This would represent just over 25% of its energy intake, and this is close to that of the full term baby during the first 2 months after birth.

Besides the energy value of the protein and fat actually deposited in the body, energy must also be expended in depositing it – the so-called energy cost of growth. We have no quantitative information about the energy cost of tissue synthesis in the young baby, but values have been calculated for older but fast-growing rats. These are 7.5 kcal/g protein and 15.9 kcal/g fat (6). Another estimate for protein is 24 kcal/g. Whatever the correct figures, it looks as though for the rat after the suckling period it takes considerably more energy to build new body tissue than the calorific value of the tissue that is built.

During the period just after birth when the animal or baby is living on mother's milk it seems as though growth must take place with greater efficiency than this. Table 4 shows some calculations for the calorific increment in the body of the pig during the first 4 weeks after birth (7). The body weight increases by nearly 7 times, and so

Table 4. *Comparison of the gain in calories in the body of the pig with its calorie intake during the first 4 weeks after birth* (7).

Week after birth	Body wt. (kg)	Fat in body (g)	Protein in body (g)	Calorific value of body (kcal)	Gain in body calories during week (kcal)	Calorie intake during week (kcal)	Gain in body calories (% calorie intake)
0	1.5	18	174	882			
1	3.2	306	437	4640	3758	6830	55
2	5.5	796	770	10500	5860	11450	51
3	8.0	1280	1098	16380	5880	11600	50
4	10.0	1763	1427	22250	5870	12200	48

much fat is laid down that the calorific value of the body increases by more than 20 times. The amount of milk the piglet takes to achieve this provides only about twice as many calories as the energy value of the new body tissue. If half the energy intake can be accounted for by increments of protein and fat in the body, the energy cost of laying down this new tissue must be less than the energy value of the tissue itself for some energy must be expended on basal requirements and activity. The newborn rat is even more striking in this connection, for calculations on its intake of energy and body composition suggest that 80% of its energy intake from protein, fat and carbohydrate in its food can be accounted for by increments of protein and fat in its body during the first week after birth. It looks as though the energy cost of laying down new tissue by a newborn animal living on mother's milk may be less than that for the older growing animal on a different kind of diet. It may be a question of age or food, or both.

Children who are undernourished are often ravenously hungry and will take far more food than the normal child. The digestive tract, moreover, which does not lack the digestive enzymes, can deal with the food, and the weight at once begins to rise. In practice, of course, it is not always so simple, for the undernutrition may be complicated or perhaps even caused by something which will have to be treated before the refeeding will lead to a rapid gain in weight. I remember Dr. Cicily WILLIAMS, at a meeting in Cambridge on Calorie Deficiencies and Protein Deficiencies (8), describing a child who was undernourished, not because there was anything wrong with its diet, but because it had such dreadful scabies that it spent all its time scratching and never got any rest at all. All the energy it could get went on this, and consequently growth was out of the question. Clearing up the scabies put everything right.

Fig. 1 shows the growth of Agnes, an African child, who weighed only 1.3 kg when she was born and 2.5 kg at 9 months when she was admitted to the Medical Research Council's Unit in Kampala under Professor McCANCE's care (9). He based her treatment on his experience with pigs, and she was allowed to eat her fill of a diet providing 8% of its calories as protein. She had no setbacks. She took over 230 kcal/kg/day during the first 7 weeks she was in hospital and this enabled her to double her weight during this time. Fig. 2 shows the weight of another marasmic child, Kivumbi, during the first month he was in hospital. He was 14 months old when he was admitted and

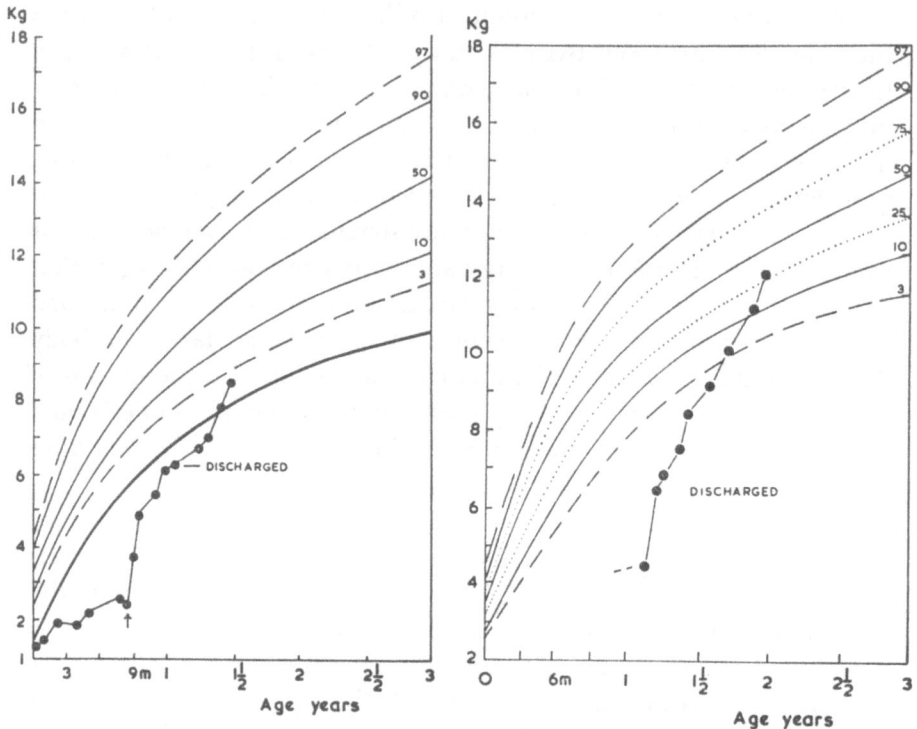

Fig. 1. Weight of Agnes during recovery from undernutrition (9).

Fig. 2. Weight of Kivumbi during recovery from undernutrition (9).

weighed 4.55 kg–45% of his expected weight for age. He had a very shaky start, with serious attacks of pyrexia and bronchitis during his first 3 weeks, but from then on did remarkably well on a high calorie diet, taking 170 kcal/kg/day and he gained 2 kg in weight in 4 weeks. He was discharged in the care of his grandmother who was intelligent enough to give him the food provided for him, in the quantities prescribed and his weight continued to go ahead.

ASHWORTH (10) has had similar experiences in Jamaica. Her marasmic children aged 10–36 months, with a mean weight of 5 kg at the beginning, took 160 kcal/kg/day over the first 8 weeks, and she believed they would have taken more had it been offered to them. Her diet, like the one used in Kampala, provided about 8% of its energy as protein. The Jamaican children gained 3.7 kg during the first 8 weeks they were in hospital. ASHWORTH reckoned that the mean rate of gain in weight of her children was 15 times as fast as the normal growth rate of children of the same age and 5 times as fast as that of younger children of the same weight.

How much the gain in weight of undernourished children depends on the energy intake is illustrated in fig. 3 (11). This shows the change

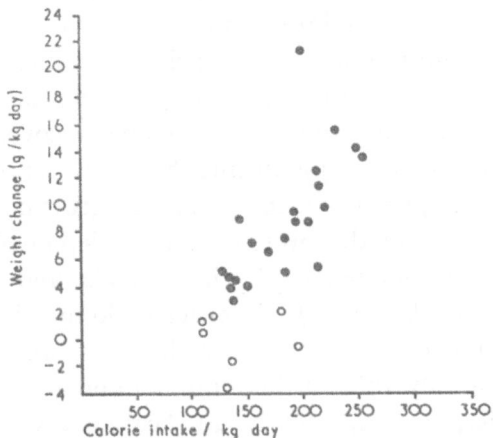

Fig. 3. Change in weight and calorie intake of undernourished children given diets providing 4 g protein/kg/day. O Weight change associated with diarrhoea or infection. ● Weight change uncomplicated by infection (11).

in weight of Ugandan children given a diet providing 8% of its energy as protein, or 4 grams of protein per kilogram/day. No advantage is to be gained by giving more protein than this. The solid circles represent children who had no infection, and the rise in the gain of weight with the increase in protein and energy intakes is clearly shown. The open circles represent children who had diarrhoea or other infection, and they gained less weight on similar energy intakes. Calorie intakes of 230, 170 or even 160/kg/day are far above those recommended for or taken by normal children. Up to five or six years ago it was thought that 100 kcal/kg/day were sufficient for undernourished children and they were given no more, but experimental work with undernourished animals, and studies on children, has made it clear how much more the severely undernourished child needs and will willingly take. Unless the diet provides more than 150 kcal/kg/day the child will not return to its proper growth curve. The child will grow on fewer calories, but not catch up, and it will necessarily, therefore, remain underweight for a long time, and possibly for the rest of its life. The younger the child and the more underweight it is, the more energy and protein per kg it will need. A really marasmic baby will take 300 kcal/kg/day, but by 4 years of age an equally wasted child can take no more than about 150 kcal/kg/day.

Once the child has recovered its weight and is approaching its proper growth curve its appetite begins to fall off (10). The reduction in food intake, after the children had reached their expected weight for height, was substantial and surprisingly uniform. The mean intake, which had been 160 kcal/kg/day during the early part of rehabilitation dropped to 116 kcal/kg/day after recovery.

Although growth is very rapid during the first weeks of rehabilitation the energy intake required to bring about this growth is well in excess of the calorific value of the protein and fat deposited in the body. Agnes, for example, gained 2.5 kg in 7 weeks and consumed 230 kcal/kg/day – 42,000 kcal in all – in order to do so. The increments of protein and fat in her body could hardly have amounted to more than 7000 kcal. This is only 17% of the total amount she ate, and the fate of the remainder, 35,200, (nearly 200 kcal/kg/day) remains to be considered. This is nearly twice as many as a normal child of the same age needs for maintenance and growth. Where does all this extra energy go? ASHWORTH (12) and BROOKE and ASHWORTH (13) measured the oxygen consumption of 12 malnourished children 3–20 months old whose weights on admission averaged 66% of that expected for their heights. Measurements were made before and at intervals after food while the child was still undernourished, during the period of rapid growth, and after recovery. Fig. 4 shows the results. The undernourished children on admission had lower metabolic rates before the meal than they had during or after recovery. After the test meal, however, which provided 27 kcal and 0.7 g protein/kg/body weight, the metabolic rate rose more and stayed high longer while the children were growing rapidly during the active stages of recovery than it did while they were still undernourished, or after they had completely recovered. The authors attribute this to the energy cost of growth, and postulate consequently that children who are gaining weight rapidly must synthesise tissue most rapidly after a meal. They said that the amount synthesised may not be closely related to the size of the meal, but it requires a lot of energy to synthesise it. When the undernourished children were first admitted they did not respond to their first meal with more than a trifling rise in metabolic rate. However, we know

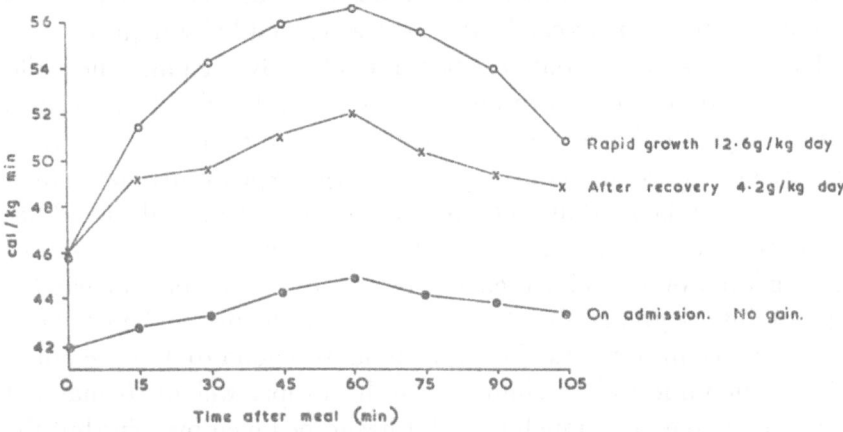

Fig. 4. Metabolic rate (MR) before and after a meal. Children studied before, during and after recovery from malnutrition. o—o on admission; ●—● during rapid growth; x—x after recovery (13).

that malnourished children and animals do increase their oxygen consumption and resting metabolic rate very soon after treatment begins, perhaps not after one meal, but certainly before any change in body weight is demonstrable (14) (15). It seems likely that the intital response to food is rapid protein synthesis in the liver, and studies on undernourished rats have shown that the liver doubles in size within 3 days after rehabilitation has begun. Protein synthesis in the liver may account for the rise in the metabolic rate after meals, but the so-called thermic affect of food is only a small part of the total energy required for a rapid rate of growth. These children being rehabilitated after severe undernutrition may not be able to lay down tissue as efficiently as younger children or animals on mother's milk. Everything involved in a fast gain in weight requires energy; a large quantity of food is being eaten; the swallowing, digesting and absorbing of all this requires energy; the conversion of carbohydrate to glycogen and the reconversion of it to glucose requires more, and so does the conversion of carbohydrate to fat and the conversion of amino acids to protein. This is going on all round the 24 hours, and it is this high rate of metabolism all the time in all the tissues that requires so much oxygen and uses up so much energy.

The normal baby, and the baby that is undernourished because of a shortage of food, have a considerable capacity to adjust their intakes of food to their requirements for all purposes, and this adjustment is far more complicated than it is for an adult who has merely to maintain himself in energy balance. As it grows a normal baby requires more food in total amount, but less per unit of body weight. The child recovering from undernutrition requires and takes much more food than a normal child of the same age, or of the same weight. As he recovers he requires – and takes – less. Energy expenditure comes first, and energy intake is adjusted to meet it. When, however, the child has no control over the amount of food he gets because he is being fed by stomach tube or by vein, then the person in charge of him has the responsibility of giving him the amount of food he needs. This is when it is so important to realise the large amounts of food that are required to bring the underweight child back to his proper weight. It may not be very easy to give so much food if it has to be given by vein; but the child being fed in this way needs it as much as the one being fed by mouth – and this is the challenge.

I shall finish by looking at the other side of the picture – the over-weight child. Much has been said and written in the past few years about the number of fat cells in the body. The danger of overfeeding children during the first year has been emphasised, because this is when the fat cells are dividing and expanding most rapidly, and the process can be speeded up by giving calories in excess of the number needed to satisfy the requirements for maintenance, activity and growth (16). The fat baby is likely to become the fat child and the obese a-dult. Juts as the sensors that regulate energy intake will always make the undernourished child eat enough food to bring his body weight and body composition back to what they ought to have been had he grown normally, so these same sensors make the overnourished child who has been 'slimmed' take more food when given the chance so that he again becomes obese. The appetite regulators always work upwards, never downwards, and there seems to be no regulating mechanism which would make an overweight individual eat less food so that he loses weight. The body jealously guards its substance, even when it has far too much of it, and it is just as important to prevent a young child getting caught up in the obesity cycle today as it was when I spoke about it at the 3rd International Congress of Nutrition in Amsterdam 19 years ago (17).

REFERENCES

1. HILL, J. R. (1964), The development of thermal stability in the newborn baby. In: *The adaptation of the newborn infant to extra-uterine life*, J. H. P. Jonxis, H. K. A. Visser and V. J. A. Troelstra (eds), Stenfert Kroese, Leiden, p. 223.
2. BRÜCK, K. (1964), General aspects of temperature regulation of small subjects. In: *The adaptation of the newborn infant to extra-uterine life*, J. H. P. Jonxis, H. K. A. Visser and V. J. A. Troelstra (eds.), Stenfert Kroese, Leiden, p. 229.
3. MOORE, R. E. (1964), Chemical regulation of heat production in the neonate. In: *The adaptation of the newborn infant to extra-uterine life*, J. H. P. Jonxis, H. K. A. Visser and V. J. A. Troelstra (eds.), Stenfert Kroese, Leiden, p. 248.
4. DAWKINS, M. J. R. and HULL, D. (1964), Brown adipose tissue and non-shivering thermogenesis in newborn animals. In: *The adaptation of the newborn infant to extra-uterine life*, J. H. P. Jonxis, H. K. A. Visser and V. J. A. Troelstra (eds.), Stenfert Kroese, Leiden, p. 269.
5. FOMON, S. J. (1967), *Infant nutrition*, Saunders, Philadelphia and London.
6. MCCRACKEN, K. (1968), Energy metabolism of young rats fed different levels of protein and/or calories. 1. The partition of the metabolizable energy intake of pair-gained and pair-fed littermates. *Proc. Nutr. Soc.* 27, 40A.
7. WIDDOWSON, E. M. (1971), Food intake and growth in the newly-born. *Proc. Nutr. Soc.* 30, 127.
8. WILLIAMS, C. D. (1968), Discussion in: *Calorie deficiencies and protein deficiencies*, R. A. McCance and E. M. Widdowson (eds.), Churchill, London, p. 315.
9. MCCANCE, R. A. (1971), Malnutrition in Uganda, *Proc. Nutr. Soc. India* 10, 132.
10. ASHWORTH, A. (1969), Growth rates of children recovering from protein-calorie malnutrition. *Brit. J. Nutr.* 23, 835.
11. RUTISHAUSER, I. H. E. and MCCANCE, R. A. (1968), Calorie requirements for growth after severe undernutrition. *Arch. Dis. Childh.* 43, 252.
12. ASHWORTH, A. (1969), Metabolic rates during recovery from protein-calorie malnutrition; the need for a new concept of specific dynamic action. *Nature* London, 223, 407.
13. BROOKE, O. G. and ASHWORTH, A. (1972), The influence of malnutrition on the postprandial metabolic rate and respiratory quotient. *Brit. J. Nutr.* 27, 407.
14. MOUNT, L. E., LISTER, D. and MCCANCE, R. A. (1963), Severe undernutrition in growing and adult animals. 11. The first effects of rehabilitation on the metabolic rate and body temperature. *Brit. J. Nutr.* 17, 407.
15. ABLETT, J. G. and MCCANCE, R. A. (1971), Energy expenditure of children with kwashiorkor. *Lancet* 2, 517.
16. BROOK, C. G. D. (1972), Evidence for a sensitive period in adipose-cell replication in man. Lancet 2, 624.
17. WIDDOWSON, E. M. (1955), Reproduction and obesity. *Voeding* 16, 94.

TRACE ELEMENT NUTRITION

C. F. MILLS*

INTRODUCTION

Clinical syndromes attributable to deficiences of the elements iron, copper, cobalt, zinc, chromium, manganese, iodine and possibly selenium have now been identified in a wide variety of mammalian species. In addition, recent studies with small laboratory animals suggest that the elements molybdenum, vanadium, tin, nickel, silicon and possibly boron may be essential nutrients for mammals. Although the essentiality of many of these elements for man has not been demonstrated there are no good grounds for suggesting that man, may be unique in having a less extensive range of requirements.

Rather than broadly but superficially surveying the evidence which indicates essential roles for these elements this paper will examine the arguments which suggest that deficiences of the elements copper or zinc may be of significance in the aetiology of human disease and will pay particular attention to the circumstances which lead to clinical manifestations of deficiences of these two elements. The examples chosen will illustrate both the diversity of situations which may promote deficiency and will indicate the complexity of the task of assessing the adequacy of the trace element content of the diet or of the tissue trace element status of human subjects.

In this paper attention will be drawn repeatedly to deficiency syndromes in species other than man. Such comparisons are particularly warrantable in view of the scarcity of studies in man and the fact that, from the more extensive study of the clinical and biochemical consequences of deficiency in non-human species have emerged pointers to the nature and sequence of development of clinical and

* Department of Nutritional Biochemistry, Rowett Research Institute, Bucksburn, Aberdeen, Scotland.

metabolic lesions which are decidedly relevant to the furtherance of human studies in this field.

COPPER DEFICIENCY IN INFANTS

The earliest studies demonstrating the essentiality of copper as a nutrient were carried out with the rat and all centred around the role of this element in haematopoiesis. From this work developed the attitude held until comparatively recently that anaemia must be an accompaniment of clinical cases of copper deficiency. Thus the failure of WILSON & LAHEY to demonstrate a copper deficiency anaemia in the small number of experimentally depleted human infants during a short term study (1) has led to the tacit assumption that copper deficiency in man is extremely unlikely.

This view persisted despite a growing knowledge of the involvement of copper in processes of connective and elastic tissue formation, skeletal matrix formation, amine metabolism, myelin synthesis, keratinization and oxidative phosphorylation and the appreciation that disturbances to iron metabolism and haemopoiesis are comparatively late manifestations of deficiency.

Considerable progress has been made during the last 10 years towards the definition of the marked changes in tissue copper concentration and copper enzyme activity that occur in man during foetal development and from birth to adulthood. Fig. 1, drawn from data

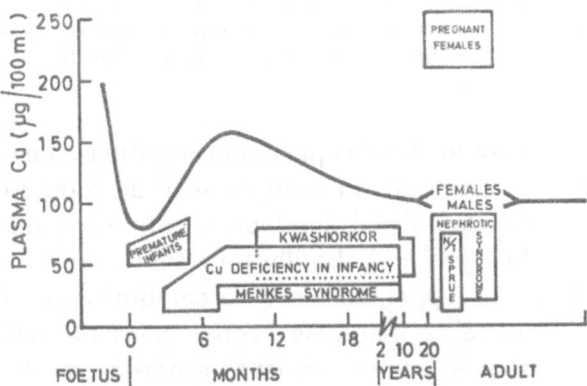

Fig. 1. Diagrammatic representation of changes with age in the plasma copper concentration of normal human subjects (—), in pregnancy and in various pathological states. Details of the original literature sources used in constructing this diagram may be obtained from the author.

contained in 17 publications, illustrates changes with age in the serum copper concentration of normal subjects while the block diagrams also incorporated in this figure encompass the plasma copper concentrations found in subjects suffering a range of disorders often associated with a low copper status. Fig. 2, derived from 11 published sources,

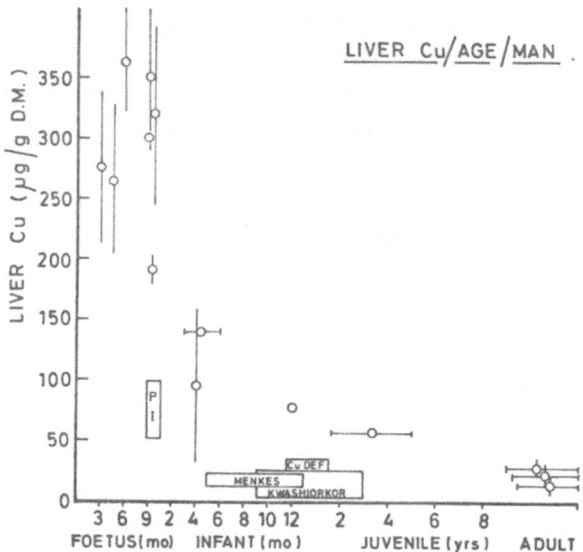

Fig. 2. Changes with age in the concentration of copper in the liver of normal human subjects with indication of age range and standard deviation of mean) and in various pathological states. (PI = premature infants; MENKES' = MENKES' syndrome in infant; Cu def. = copper deficiency in infants during hospital therapy). Details of the original literature sources used in constructing this diagram may be obtained from the author.

presents similar data for liver copper concentrations. These diagrams clearly emphasise the profound changes in tissue copper distribution which occur during late foetal development and early infancy in the clinically normal subject and also illustrate that most of the disorders now attributable to copper deficiency occur during or shortly after these changes have taken place. As a consequence of such studies the following categories of copper deficiency syndrome in the infant are now recognised:-

(a) *Anaemias responsive to combined iron and copper therapy*

A typical report describing this situation deals with case histories in children six and a half months to two and a half years old (2). All had periorbital oedema, pallor, a moderate anaemia (haemoglobin 5.2–7.5 g/100 ml) with microcytosis and marked reduction in the concentrations of serum iron (4–18 μg/100 ml) and serum copper (24–68 μg/100 ml). No evidence of renal or hepatic dysfunction was apparent nor was there evidence of a prolonged disturbance of gastrointestinal tract function. A feature common to all subjects was the prolonged administration of liquid diets based upon homogenized or evaporated milk with only a limited acceptance of solid foods. Satisfactory recovery was obtained either by combined iron and copper therapy or by the gradual introduction of 'meat-based formula' diets without the use of copper supplements. Blood, iron and copper concentrations rapidly returned to their normal levels. It should be noted that the latter treatment produced results similar to that obtained by CARTWRIGHT and his colleagues in earlier studies where blood copper concentrations rose to normal levels merely following the administration of iron supplements; a situation which led these workers to conclude that copper deficiency was a secondary consequence of the situation (3). A similar situation has been described in work with experimental animals maintained on simultaneously suboptimal concentrations of dietary iron and copper in which a haemopoietic response was obtained by each of these elements individually (4). There is obviously a mutual inter-dependence of iron and copper. The point of involvement of copper in iron metabolism and its release from ferritin for haemoglobin formation is now fairly well established; a role of iron in mediating copper release for similar purposes has yet to be established.

(b) *Hypocupraemia in the infant associated with neutropenia, skeletal demineralization and granulocytic maturation arrest in bone marrow*

Features of this syndrome are a decline in serum, copper and caeruloplasmin concentrations followed at variable intervals by a failure of iron absorption, neutropenia, leukopenia, demineralization of bone and defective erythrocyte production and survival. Diarrhoea is a common feature. Common to all the situations reported is a history of

weaning from maternal milk on to infant formulas based on homogenized or evaporated cows milk, sometimes supplemented with
cottonseed oil and sugar. In some cases the syndrome was apparent
before for hospitalization; in others it arose following hospitalization
for the treatment of kwashiorkor or marasmus and treatment of these
conditions using preparations based upon cows milk. In a study of
173 malnourished infants GRAHAM et al. (5) using neutropenia, leukopenia and hypocupraemia as diagnostic criteria of copper deficiency,
reported that 8.1% of the patients were copper deficient on admission,
and a further 11%, 18%, 22% and 63% developed a copper deficiency
syndrome during the periods 1–15 days, 16–30 days, 31–60 days and
61–100 days respectively if copper supplements were withheld from
the supplemented infant formula based upon cows milk with added
cane sugar and cottonseed oil (providing 28 to 42 μg copper/kg/day).
The highly variable characteristics of the anaemia developing in many
of these cases (and in 22 of 62 cases studied, no anaemia developed at
all) limited the value of haematological indices as diagnostic criteria,
particularly since indications were that a true copper deficiency
anaemia only occurred late in the development of the syndrome.

Several studies in this field suggest that prolonged diarrhoea causing
excessive copper depletion may play a significant part in the aetiology
of this condition. While agreeing that this is a possibility it is nevertheless quite feasible that the diarrhoea observed may itself be an
early consequence of sub-optimal copper status. Studies with the rat
and other species suggest that the water and electrolyte balance of the
gastrointestinal tract may become seriously disturbed during copper
depletion and, furthermore, indicate that normal gastrointestinal tract
function is restored very rapidly (usually within 24 hours) after
increasing the dietary intake of copper. (MILLS and DALGARNO (1973),
unpublished observation).

(c) Menkes' syndrome in the infant

DANKS and his colleagues, in an extremely comprehensive study (6),
produced convincing evidence that the progressive degenerative
cerebral lesions, skeletal lesions, hypothermia, 'pili torti' (kinky hair)
and degenerative changes in aortic elastin are all probably associated
with a low tissue copper status in the syndrome described by MENKES.
After establishing the existence of extremely low serum and liver

copper concentrations, low caeruloplasim activity and a ninefold increase in the free-sulphydryl content of hair and demonstrating the existence of widespread degeneration of arterial elastic laminae, DANKS et al. obtained a transient clinical improvement from oral copper therapy and carried out one study whcih suggested that the syndrome is associated with a defect in copper absorption from the gastrointestinal tract. While there are clear indications of an X-linked recessive inheritance of this disorder, there are also suggestions that a high proportion of the clinical cases arise following premature birth. Other recent studies (7) have shown that some premature infants may be particularly susceptible to absorptive defects influencing copper metabolism because of low tissue copper reserves at birth and a marked negative copper balance for at least 3 weeks thereafter.

COPPER IN FOODS: RELATIONSHIP TO DIETARY COPPER REQUIREMENTS

A recent estimate suggests that the minimum requirement of the human infant for dietary copper may be approximately 50 μg/kg/day (8) (or approximately 42 μg/100 kcals) and although this estimate is widely accepted it is becoming apparent that this figure must provide only a small 'margin of safety' in view of the studies of GRAHAM and his colleagues which indicate that copper deficiency can supervene following prolonged exposure to diets providing up to 42 μg copper/kg/day. A recent survey of the copper content of human foods (9) illustrated that dietary components such as rice, sugar, cornflakes, most dairy products, some cooked meats, and white or brown breads (from U.S. analyses) contain less than 40 μg copper/100 kcals and thus, if forming a major proportion of the total daily food intake, may provide insufficient copper to maintain equilibrium. With other foodstuffs providing up to 300 μg copper/100 kcals it is immediately apparent that the greatest protection against copper depletion is provided by a varied diet. In these circumstances it is not surprising that those cases of copper deficiency that have so far been described have nearly all been associated with the prolonged consumption of simplified diets composed largely of the components low in copper content referred to above. The primary cause of the appearance of copper deficiency syndromes in the infant is the use of modified milk formula diets without appropriate attention to the need for copper supplementation. Many such preparations are supplemented with iron but few with copper. HUGHES et al., (10) surveying the copper content of tinned infant foods illustrated situations where, even with an apparently complex diet supplemented with milk formula, the copper intake can be as low as 27 μg/100 kcals. These authors emphasise the hazard which may be introduced by the prolonged reliance upon low copper cereal supplements to 'milk formula' diets and stress the necessity of selecting high protein cereal or other foods containing high contents of copper if minimal requirements are to be met when the milk component of the diet contains a low concentration of copper. Their conclusions have been borne out both in clinical practice and in situations where the dilution of predominantly milk formula diets have been necessitated by economic circumstances in impoverished communities.

ZINC DEFICIENCY IN MAN

Pathological conditions in man that are believed to be associated with a sub-optimal zinc status include growth failure and delayed sexual maturity in teenage individuals (11) and young children (12), anorexia often accompanied by decreased perception of taste and smell (13), alopecia and lesions in a variety of epidermal tissues. It has also been suggested that zinc deficiency may be involved in the pathogenesis of oesophageal cancer in some Middle-Eastern population groups (14).

The results of an extensive programme of studies on the relationships of zinc to growth failure and hypogonadism in the Middle-East now leave no room for doubt that a sub-optimal zinc status is associated with this condition. It is perhaps true to say however that claims that zinc deficiency in man is associated with the other syndromes mentioned above are still the subject of discussion. The claims that zinc status markedly influences the rate of wound healing are, frankly, a subject of major controversy. The growth of interest in zinc in the nutrition of man has been recent and rapid and, accordingly, the opportunities for evaluating zinc therapy in the control of the above syndromes has not been extensive. The point has however emerged that it is extremely difficult to predict which subjects will be zinc responsive both because of the non-specific nature of the clinical signs of deficiency and because of the lack of suitable criteria for assessing either the zinc adequacy of diets or the zinc status of man. Because of this it is particularly useful to consider the extent to which studies of zinc deficiency in species other than man have revealed clinical and biochemical lesions which may ultimately be of assistance in assessing the importance of zinc in human nutrition and brief consideration will now be given to such points.

Studies with several species indicate that the consumption of diets low in zinc content is almost immediately reflected by an abrupt fall in the concentration of zinc in plasma. In the young growing animal this situation is closely followed by a marked decrease in food intake and, in non-ruminant species, by the development of an extremely erratic pattern of food consumption and an abrupt decline in the rate of growth (15) (see figures 3a and b). The lesions responsible for the

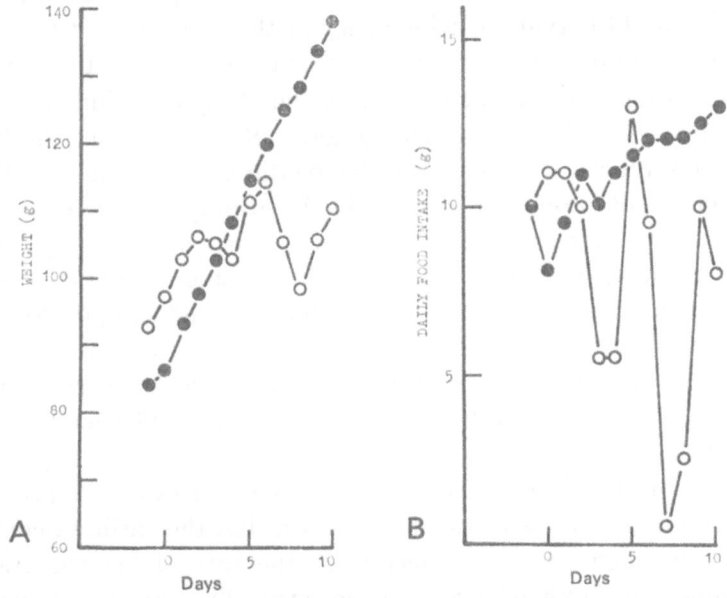

Fig. 3. Rapid cessation of weight gain (A) and development of erratic and poor food intake (B) of a rat given zinc deficient diet (o—o) compared with that of a litter-mate given zinc supplemented diet.

development of a poor and erratic pattern of food consumption have not been identified but it has recently become clear that the variability of daily food intake is positively related to the protein or essential amino acid content of the diet (16) and that the protein content of the diet substantially modifies the concentration of zinc circulating in

Table 1. *Changes during 24 hours in the plasma zinc concentration of the zinc deficient rat in response to changes in dietary protein concentration.*

Group A	Dietary protein	20%	Reduced to	5%
(n=5)	Plasma Zn	0.52 ±.08	*	0.79 ±.07
Group B	Dietary protein	5%	Increased to	20%
(n=5)	Plasma Zn	0.71 ±.05	**	0.29 ±.01

* P <0.05
** P <0.001

plasma (table 1). Such studies suggests that it is plausible to expect that periods of sub-optimal zinc intake in man, even if only brief, may have a similar effect upon food consumption and thus upon growth rate. Observations which suggest that a decreased facility for the perception of taste and smell in humans may be rectified by zinc administration (13) may be relevant to the above experimental studies but it appears unlikely that such a lesion could be solely responsible for the effects observed in view of the modifying influence of dietary protein content upon the pattern of food consumption in zinc deficient experimental subjects. Lastly, such studies with experimental animals clearly indicate that the concentration of zinc in plasma can be markedly influenced both by the total quantity and composition of the diet consumed before blood sampling takes place and they illustrate one of the problems encountered in attempting to assess the zinc status of a subject merely by determination of plasma zinc concentration.

Zinc is intimately concerned with the control of events preceding cell division. Studies with rats have shown that the earliest detectable sign of zinc deficiency is a decline in the rate of incorporation of thymidine into DNA of several tissues (17). This effect is discernible after zinc depletion for only two days and precedes the development of gross clinical lesions and effects upon food consumption and growth. Studies with lymphocyte tissue cultures show that zinc exerts a close control on events preceding DNA synthesis and that the range of concentrations within which zinc exerts this effect is comparatively narrow; above and below this range inhibitory effects are observed (18). It is thus not surprising that other studies have indicated that the mitotic response to zinc depletion is tissue specific with, for example, a decline in the mitotic index occurring in the epidermis and testis, an increase occurring in the pancreas and a very marked increase occurring in the oesophagus even following brief periods of zinc depletion (19). This last observation is of particular interest in view of suggestions that zinc deficiency may be associated with a high incidence of oesophageal cancer in some areas. The relationship of the role of zinc in cell division to the lesions leading to dwarfism and delayed sexual development in zinc deficient human subjects remains to be determined.

Experimental animal studies on the role of zinc in wound healing have given disappointingly confusing results with strongly positive indications of an acceleration in healing rate obtained in some studies but no effects attributable to differences in zinc status appearing in others. The weight of evidence suggests that an unknown variable in such studies may modify the response to zinc and, typifying this situation, are the results of recent work at this Institute demonstrating a strongly positive effect of doubling the daily intake of zinc upon the rate of tissue repair in young male cattle suffering a severe outbreak of infectious pododermatitis. Such responses were obtained even though analysis of the diet and blood plasma gave no indications that the zinc status of affected animals was inadequate to promote active tissue repair (20).

From these comments it is apparent that many close parallels exist between results obtained from studies of zinc deficiency in experimental animals and the clinical effects believed to be caused by zinc deficiency in man. Thus, despite the comparative scarcity of clinical trials with man the strong probability exists that zinc responsive situations may exist in man even following comparatively brief periods of exposure to diets low in their content of available zinc.

LOW AVAILABILITY OF DIETARY ZINC AND INCREASED ENDOGENOUS LOSSES

Experimental work with rats and practical agricultural experience with pigs and poultry has clearly shown that phytic acid in diets has a powerful effect in reducing the availability of dietary zinc. A survey of such studies suggests that when the ratio of phytic acid phosphorus/zinc (on a weight basis) exceeds 30 a very substantial risk exists that the availability of dietary zinc will be adversely affected. In making this generalisation it must however be emphasised that the effect of phytic acid is potentiated by high dietary concentrations of calcium and that in such circumstances lower PAP/Zn ratios may be associated with zinc depletion. Recent studies on the pathogenesis of dwarfism and hypogonadism in some Iranian subjects suggest that this generalisation may also be applicable to human diets. From data presented in reports of these studies (21) it can be calculated that diets with PAP/Zn ratios of between 26 and 32 frequently prevented zinc retention or promoted negative zinc balance. Although only a limited number of human foods have been analysed for both phytic acid and zinc contents it is already apparent that PAP/Zn ratios substantially in excess of 30 may not be uncommon as is suggested by the following values:- peas, 60; wheaten breakfast cereal, 72; oatmeal, 93; soya flour, 100; bread, white, 100; bread, brown, 170. In the face of such analytical data it is unreasonable to assume that a poor availability of dietary zinc is a problem solely confined to Middle-Eastern communities.

Although the initial response to a brief deprivation of food appears to be an increase in plasma zinc concentration, prolonged deprivation of human subjects promotes a subsequent decline to about one fifth of the normal and well within the range encountered in clinical cases of zinc deficiency in experimental animals. This change is accompanied by a massive increase in urinary zinc output (22) presumably occurring as a consequence of the catabolism of muscle. A similar enhancement of urinary zinc output occurs following tissue trauma in man; one typical study (23) illustrates that the daily zinc output may rise to four times the normal value during an 18 day period after the occurrence of tissue damage. Whether, in these situations, the increased endogenous losses of zinc have clinical significance remains to be determined.

CONCLUDING REMARKS

Using zinc and copper as examples, the preceding discussion has illustrated that trace element deficiency in man can arise either from the inadvertent selection of dietary components low in these elements or from the presence of dietary components which reduce availability. No mention has been made of the effect of trace element imbalance in the aetiology of deficiency disorders because our knowledge of the significance of such interactions in human nutrition is as yet very incomplete. It is however worth mention that work with the laboratory rat (CAMPBELL, J. and C. F. MILLS, to be published) and the sheep clearly indicates that the tolerance of mammals to the element cadmium is very markedly decreased if the dietary content of copper provides no margin of safety above normal requirements. A study at present in progress indicates that as little as 1 μg cadmium/g diet promotes, in such circumstances, a decline in caeruloplasmin activity to values commonly encountered only in clinically copper deficient animals. Similar studies with sheep illustrate adverse effects of cadmium upon liver copper storage and from these and other studies carried out elsewhere it is becoming apparent that the tolerance to several of the heavy metals regarded as environmental contaminants is markedly influenced by the essential trace element status of the organism.

It has been emphasised that protection against trace element depletion in human subjects is usually achieved through the variety of components used in human diets. When, through therapeutic necessity, individual preference or poverty such variety is lost the risks that clinical deficiency may supervene through accident or ignorance correspondingly increase. That such accidents led to clinical cases of copper deficiency in infants during rehabilitation from kwashiorkor or marasmus has been emphasised by GRAHAM and his colleagues. Two recent reports indicate that zinc responsive syndromes can develop in infants or adults maintained on semi-synthetic therapeutic diets containing no supplementary zinc. (25, 26) Common to both situations was the substitution of mixtures of synthetic amino acids for the usual protein component of the diet and a consequent decline in the dietary content of zinc in a highly available form normally associated with dietary proteins of animal origin.

With these indications of the need for care in the formulation of therapeutic diets it is particularly regrettable, that with the exception of the elements iron, iodine and copper, the trace element requirements of man are so inadequately defined. Until such time as an adequate definition is obtained or until better clinical and biochemical parameters for the detection of sub-optimal trace element status are available progress towards an understanding of the significance of trace elements in human disease is going to be slow. Lastly, it must be emphasised that there is a particular need for better biochemical indicators of trace element status to permit accurate monitoring to the response to therapeutic or prophylactic procedures. The need is most urgent in situations where abnormally high intakes of an element are used to promote a response as for example in the use of zinc to promote wound healing where the quantities of zinc administered during a 10 day period are often equal to, or exceed, the total body burden of this element. Such quantities administered to rats undoubtedly provoke antagonistic effects upon copper utilisation and it is highly desirable that this possibility should be monitored in human subjects that may be at risk through a marginal copper intake.

REFERENCES

1. WILSON, J. F. and LAHEY, M. E. (1960), Failure to induce dietary deficiency of copper in premature infants. *Pediatrics* 25, 40.
2. STURGEON, P. and BRUBAKER, C. (1956), Copper deficiency in infants. A syndrome characterized by hypocupraemia, iron deficiency anaemia and hypoproteinaemia. *Amer. J. Dis. Child.* 92, 254.
3. CARTWRIGHT, G. E. and WINTROBE, M. M. (1964), The question of copper deficiency in man. *Amer. J. clin. Nutr.* 15, 94.
4. MATRONE, G. (1960), Interrelationships of iron & copper in the nutrition and metabolism of animals. *Fed. Proc.* 19, 659.
5. GRAHAM, G. G. and CORDANO, A. (1969), Copper depletion and deficiency in the malnourished infant. *Johns Hopkins Med. J.* 124, 139.
6. DANKS, D. M., CAMPBELL, P. E., WALKER-SMITH, J., STEVENS, B. J., GILLESPIE, J. M., BLOMFIELD, J. and TURNER, B. (1972), Menkes' kinky-hair syndrome, *Lancet* (May 20, 1972), 1100.
7. SULTANOVA, G. F. (1970), Peculiarities in copper metabolism in prematurely born infants during the first months of life, *Pediatrics* 10, 14.
   TKACHENKO, S. K. (1970), Ingestion & excretion of some trace elements by prematurely born infants. *Pediatrics* 10, 10.
8. NATIONAL RESEARCH COUNCIL (1968), *Recommended dietary allowances.* Publn. No. 1694, National Academy of Sciences, Washington.
9. MILLS, C. F. (1973), Some aspects of trace element nutrition in man. In: *Nutritional deficiences in modern society*, Howard A. N. and I. McLean Baird eds., Newman, London, p. 56.
10. HUGHES, G., KELLY, V. J. and STEWART, R. A. (1960), The copper content of infant foods. *Pediatrics* 25, 477.
11. HALSTEAD, J. A., RONAGHY, H. A., ABADI, P., HAGHSHENASS, M., AMIRHAKEMI, G. H., BAKARAT, R. M. and REINHOLD, J. G. (1972), Zinc deficiency in man: The Shiraz experiment. *Amer. J. Med.* 53, 277.
12. HAMBIDGE, K. M., HAMBIDGE, C., JACOBS, M. and BAUM, J. D. (1972), Low level of zinc in hair, anorexia, poor growth and hypogeusia in children. *Pediat. Res.* 6, 868.
13. HENKIN, R. I. (1971), Newer aspects of copper and zinc metabolism. In: *Newer trace elements in nutrition*, Mertz, W. and Cornatzer, W. E. eds., Dekker, New York, p. 256.

14. KMET, J. and MAHBOUBI, E. (1972), Esophageal cancer in the Caspian littoral of Iran. *Science* 175, 846.
15. WILLIAMS, R. B. and MILLS, C. F. (1970), The experimental production of zinc deficiency in the rat. *Brit. J. Nutr.* 24, 989.
    CHESTERS, J. K. and QUARTERMAN, J. (1970), Effects of zinc deficiency on food intake and feeding patterns of rats. *Brit. J. Nutr.* 24, 1061.
16. CHESTERS, J. K. (1972), The role of zinc in the transformation of lymphocytes by phytohaemagglutinin. *Biochem. J.* 130, 133.
17. WILLIAMS, R. B. and CHESTERS, J. K. (1970), The effects of early zinc deficiency on DNA and protein synthesis in rats. *Brit. J. Nutr.* 24, 1053.
18. CHESTERS, J. K. (1973), Some factors controlling food intake by zinc deficient rats. *Brit. J. Nutr.* (in press).
19. FELL, B. F., LEIGH, L. C. and WILLIAMS, R. B. (1973), The cytology of various organs in zinc deficient rats with particular reference to the frequency of cell division. *Res. vet. Sci.* (in press).
20. DEMERTZIS, P. N. and MILLS, C. F. (1973), Oral zinc therapy in the control of infectious pododermatitis in young bulls. *Vet. Rec.* 93, 219.
21. REINHOLD, J. G., LAHIMGARZADEH, A., NASR, K. and HEYDAYETI, H. (1973), Effects of purified phytate and phytate-rich bread upon metabolism of zinc, calcium, phosphorus & nitrogen in man. *Lancet* (Feb. 10, 1973), 283.
22. SPENCER, H. and SAMACHSON, J. (1970), Studies of zinc metabolism in man. In: *Trace element metabolism in animals*, Mills, C. F. ed., Livingstone, Edinburgh, p. 312.
23. CUTHBERTSON, D. P., FELL, G. S., SMITH, C. S. and TILSTONE, W. J. (1972), Metabolism after injury: Effects of severity, nutrition and environmental temperature on protein, potassium, zinc & creatine. *Brit. J. Surg.* 59, 68.
24. MILLS, C. F. and DALGARNO, A. C. (1972), Copper and zinc status of ewes & lambs receiving increased dietary concentrations of cadmium. *Nature* 239, 171.
25. HOWARD, A. N. and McLEAN BAIRD, I. (1973), Personal communication.
26. BARNES, P. M. and MOYNAHAN, E. J. (1973), Zinc deficiency in acrodermatitis enteropathica with multiple dietary intolerances treated with synthetic diet. *Proc. roy. Soc. Med.* 66, 327.

VITAMIN D: APPARENT NUTRIENT, HORMONE AND THERAPEUTIC AGENT

S. W. STANBURY*

Although it has long been appreciated that cholecalciferol (vitamin D_3) is produced photochemically in the skin from 7-dehydrocholesterol, we have become habituated to the concept that 'vitamin D' is an essential nutrient. This idea was fostered by the phenomenal success with which supplementation of the diet with vitamin D preparations eliminated the pandemic of rickets that prevailed in our cities in the earlier part of this century. But there is a tendency to overlook two facts: firstly, that the tradition of supplementing the diet of children has largely lapsed; secondly, that the dietary intake of some children and more adults in Britain may be less than 40–60 I.U. of 'vitamin D' per day (1). Despite this, we have witnessed no resurgence of rickets or osteomalacia in our native population, except among the secluded elderly. This suggests that casual exposure to sunshine in the course of everyday activities may be adequate to meet requirements for vitamin D, even in our northern European cities. Indeed, evidence has recently been produced for the causal importance of lack of sunshine in the genesis of osteomalacia in the elderly (2).

The lessons of history and even the results of epidemiological studies in their country of origin (3) have been forgotten in the flurry of clinical excitement caused by the re-appearance of rickets and osteomalacia amongst our immigrant Asian population; and super-fluous hypotheses have proliferated in attempts to explain this pheno-menon. In a survey of apparently healthy Asians in a northern British town, we found a very high incidence of clinical and biochemical evidence of vitamin D deficiency (4); but in a later survey of an ethnically comparable population with the same dietary and social customs, but living in the open and sunny Punjab town of Ludhiana in Northern India, we detected no such widespread vitamin D

* Division of Metabolism, University Department of Medicine, The Royal Infirmary, Manchester.

deficiency (5). As had been implied earlier by WILSON and WIDDOWSON (3), this suggests that when rickets and osteomalacia develop in Asians – at home or in Europe – this is due to lack of sunshine. Direct evidence that these diseases in Asians in Britain are due to an absolute deficiency of vitamin D has been provided very recently by the finding of very low or unmeasurable concentrations of 25 hydroxycholecalciferol in their sera (6). Thus, if vitamin D is to be considered a nutrient at all, it is not one of a respectable biological lineage but a bastard nutrient born of social and economic conditions. None the less, such conditions persist in certain situations and they can be circumvented easily only by regarding vitamin D as a 'therapeutic nutrient' and by providing the needy with an appropriate oral supplement.

For more than a decade before cases of Asian rickets and osteomalacia began to appear in our outpatient clinics, I was encountering many cases of rickets and osteomalacia in patients with chronic renal failure (7). Once it was proved that the bone lesions in this form of renal osteodystrophy were virtually the same as those of simple vitamin D deficiency, a long programme of research into the pathogenesis of the condition was initiated. The results of these studies have been reviewed extensively in recent publications (8, 9, 10, 11, 12, 13). In essence, they showed that the uraemic patient was relatively insensitive to the effects of administered vitamin D; that the intact kidney was in some way involved in determining the expression of vitamin D activity; and that the patient with renal insufficiency required a greater intake of vitamin D and higher serum levels of antiricketic activity, to promote calcium absorption, than does the normal individual (14). It could not be determined whether the uraemic state as such affected the mechanisms of calcium transport in the target organs or if, as we now know to be the case, loss of renal tissue interfered with the biological activation of vitamin D.

Progress with this problem became possible only after the pioneering studies of DeLUCA, firstly in producing radioactive cholecalciferol of high specific activity and subsequently with his demonstration that cholecalciferol must undergo metabolic transformation before it is capable of exerting its biological effects. It is now known that cholecalciferol entering the circulating blood from the skin or from the diet first undergoes hydroxylation in the liver, at C_{25} in the side chain (15); and 25 hydroxycholecalciferol is further hydroxylated in the kidney to form 1,25 dihydroxycholecalciferol (16), which is the metabolite of cholecalciferol active in the target organs (fig. 1). The kidney is the only tissue capable of effecting this second hydroxylation (16) and this

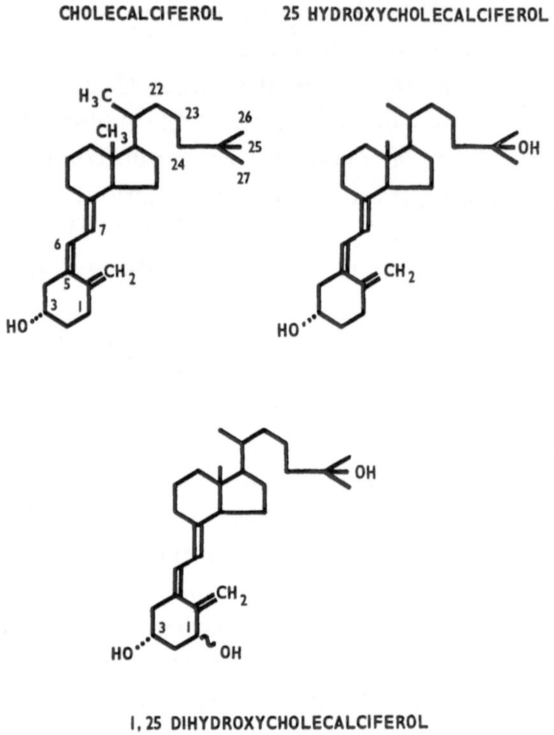

CHOLECALCIFEROL   25 HYDROXYCHOLECALCIFEROL

I, 25 DIHYDROXYCHOLECALCIFEROL

Fig. 1. The vitamin D hormones. Cholecalciferol is produced photochemically in the skin; 25 hydroxycholecalciferol is synthesized in the liver and 1,25 dihydroxy-cholecalciferol in the kidney.

fact seemed to solve the problem of apparent vitamin D resistance in renal insufficiency, at least by analogy with the results of animal experiments. We were able to demonstrate that 1,25 dihydroxy-cholecalciferol is also produced in man (17) and subsequently that the patient with advanced renal insufficiency produces effectively none of this metabolite (18). En route, it was possible to show that the uraemic patient produces 25 hydroxycholecalciferol normally (19), and it is inferred that the beneficial therapeutic effects of large doses of ergo-calciferol or cholecalciferol in renal rickets are due to the metabolic production of large amounts of their respective 25 hydroxylated derivatives (11). This has been a fascinating story and our own studies with radioactive cholecalciferol in man have taught us much about the role of adipose tissue and voluntary muscle as sites of storage of cholecalciferol and 25 hydroxycholecalciferol, and of the various mechanisms involved in limiting toxicity under conditions of high therapeutic dosage with these sterols (20, 21, 22).

But the most important development has been the recognition that the synthesis of 1,25 dihydroxycholecalciferol is subject to feed-back regulation (23), a finding which puts this triol into the category of a hormone with a central role in the control of bone turnover and calcium metabolism. It therefore seems appropriate to illustrate this function, with especial reference to experiments undertaken in our own laboratory concerning adaptation of calcium absorption by the intestine.

ADAMS, HILL and WAIN (24, 25) have produced calorie deficiency and retarded growth in the rat, and used the everted duodenal sac (26) to measure the intestinal transport of calcium in these animals *in vitro* (27). Optimally nourished, rapidly growing control animals were breast fed in litters of 3 or 4 and, after weaning at 24 days, they received a pellet diet ad libitum. The undernourished animals were fed in litters of 12 to 14 and received only a small fixed ration of the same pellet diet after weaning. In the control group of animals, the calcium transport ratio was highest at weaning and diminished exponentially with age. Also, there were significant inverse correlations between calcium transport and both the length of the femur and, as found by MORRISSEY and WASSERMAN (28), the mineral content of the whole femur. None of these relationships held in the undernourished group; calcium transport was inappropriately low for the animal's age, and for the length and mineral composition of the femur. Under-nutrition was thus associated with intestinal malabsorption of calcium despite an adequate intake of vitamin D; and this malabsorption was 'resistant' to a large dose of cholecalciferol (2.5 μg) given 24h before sacrifice of the animal.

LE ROITH and PIMSTONE (29) have reported analogous studies of the effects of protein-deprivation on the composition and turnover of bone, and on the intestinal absorption of calcium, in weanling rats. As in the study of ADAMS et al (24, 25), deprivation of protein caused retarded growth, with the production of bones that were shorter and lighter than those of age-matched controls but which had a normal concentration of mineral. These changes were accompanied by the expected reduced formation of bone collagen, reduced accretion of calcium into the bone, and also by a reduced intestinal absorption of calcium. LE ROITH and PIMSTONE (29) speculate that impaired calcium transport in the gut, conceivably due to effects of protein deficiency on the synthesis of intestinal calcium binding protein, could be the primary abnormality leading to the observed metabolic abnormalities in the bone. This is unlikely, since it would imply that the osteoporosis, or reduced bone mass, in protein deficiency is equivalent to that caused by a simple deprivation of calcium. EL-MARAGHI, PLATT and STEWART (30) have shown that the latter state, which is essentially a form of nutritional secondary hyper-parathyroidism, is histologically distinct from the 'matrix-osteoporosis' of protein deficiency.

A more logical explanation for the reduced intestinal absorption of calcium, in both calorie-deficiency and protein-deficiency, is that it is an adaptive or physiologically regulated mechanism, whereby net absorption is adjusted to correspond with the rate of bone matrix formation. Continued absorption of calcium in the face of arrested or greatly reduced formation of bone matrix would inevitably tend to cause the development of hypercalcaemia.

Indirect evidence for this hypothesis has been produced by ADAMS, HILL, MAWER and WAIN (31). They find that intravenous doses of 1,25 dihydroxycholecalciferol that are sufficient to increase intestinal transport of calcium in the vitamin D deficient rat will also increase transport of calcium in the calorie-deficient animal. It would, of course, be more satisfactory to demonstrate directly that under-nutrition causes inhibition of the synthesis of 1,25 dihydroxychole-calciferol; preliminary studies in the rat and chick suggest that this is the case.

ADAMS et al. (24, 25) made the further important observation that rehabilitation of their undernourished rats by unlimited feeding produced an increased rate of growth, accompanied by increased intestinal transport of calcium. Most significantly, it was found that calcium transport ratios in individual animals correlated closely with their relative rates of growth – and a single regression fitted the data from optimally nourished, malnourished and rehabilitated animals.

A logical extension of this relationship is to the elderly rat, in which growth is negligible and the transport and absorption of calcium are known to be low. In a group of elderly male rats (350 to 450 g), the calcium transport ratio measured in everted duodenal sacs was as low as is found in vitamin D deficient weanlings; treatment with 1,25 dihydroxycholecalciferol was equally effective in increasing calcium transport in the elderly and the D-deficient animals (31).

It is reasonable to infer from these observations that the various adaptation mechanisms in the absorption of calcium, studied by NICOLAYSEN and considered by him to reflect the operation of some 'endogenous factor' (32), are determined finally by the hormone, 1,25 dihydroxycholecalciferol. But one cannot assume that identical factors control the renal biosynthesis and secretion of this hormone when calcium absorption is adapted to a change of dietary calcium, and when calcium absorption is adjusted to the requirements of growth.

BOYLE, GRAY and DeLUCA (23) showed that a high dietary intake and raised serum concentration of calcium inhibited the synthesis of 1,25 dihydroxycholecalciferol, whereas a low calcium intake and hypocalcaemia facilitated its formation. Subsequently, DeLUCA and his collaborators produced evidence that these effects were mediated through the action of changes in serum calcium on the secretion of parathyroid hormone (33); and several groups of workers have now shown that parathyroid hormone stimulates the formation on 1,25 dihydroxycholecalciferol, at least when the serum calcium is low or normal (34, 35).

There can be no doubt that the growth-dependent changes in calcium transport and absorption (24, 25) reflect the requirement for mineralization of growing bone; and, as already suggested, continued calcium absorption with arrest of bone growth would produce alimentary hypercalcaemia. It might then be speculated that inhibition of parathyroid secretion by such hypercalcaemia could account for reduced formation of 1,25 dihydroxycholecalciferol and reduced calcium absorption in undernourished animals. We have no evidence bearing directly on this problem but we can demonstrate an analogous phenomenon in rats treated with the crystal poison disodium ethane-1-hydroxy-1, 1-diphosphonate (EHDP) (27). Animals treated with EHDP continue to grow but, because of the inhibitory effects of the drug on crystal deposition, they fail to mineralize newly formed bone matrix and develop a form of vitamin D resistant rickets or osteomalacia. In treated animals receiving a normal pellet diet there is also a vitamin D resistant failure of intestinal absorption of calcium. We have been able to demonstrate that this latter abnormality is due to inhibited synthesis of 1,25 dihydroxycholecalciferol and it can be overcome by intravenous administration of small doses of this hormone (27). If, however, vitamin D deficient animals are given continued treatment with EHDP, it is found that administration of small doses of intravenous cholecalciferol (75 ng to 2.5 μg) is followed initially by a normal synthesis of 1,25 dihydroxycholecalciferol and a normal increase of calcium transport. But, whereas the various components in this physiological response are sustained in the vitamin D deficient control animals for more than a week, synthesis of the renal hormone diminishes in EHDP treated animals from the second day after injecting vitamin D and no 1,25 dihydroxycholecalciferol is detectable in the body after seven days. At this time, intestinal calcium transport is characteristic of vitamin D deficiency *and* no increase in transport follows a further injection of cholecalciferol. The answer to this apparent paradox appears to lie in the events initiated during the first two days after injecting vitamin D, when the responses in terms of 1,25 dihydroxycholecalciferol formation are the same in control and EHDP treated vitamin D deficient animals. It is inferred that both groups of animals will respond at this time by increasing intestinal absorption of dietary calcium (and phosphorus); but, presumably because the EHDP treated animals are unable to deposit absorbed minerals into bone, they are observed (27) to develop a relative hypercalcaemia (and hyperphosphataemia). One might argue that this hypercalcaemia, like the effects of a high calcium diet in a normal animal (23), arrest the renal formation of 1,25 dihydroxycholecalciferol through inhibition of parathyroid secretion (33).

However, at this stage the situation becomes more complicated for this relative hypercalcaemia is of short duration, and the inhibition of 1,25 dihydroxycholecalciferol formation in EHDP treated rats continues when the serum concentrations of calcium and phosphorus have returned to control values (27). Similarly, ADAMS et al (24, 25) failed to detect the development of hypercalcaemia in their weanlings with retarded growth produced by deprivation of calories; the serum calcium in these animals was marginally *lower* than in their rapidly growing litter mates. All one can safely conclude is that some homeostatic mechanism(s) inhibits the synthesis of 1,25 dihydroxycholecalciferol in EHDP treated and in growth retarded rats, and thereby protects them from the development of alimentary hypercalcaemia. Without available means for measuring parathyroid hormone in the serum of the animals used, it is not finally possible to assess the role of the parathyroid glands in these experiments; but the data suggest that mechanisms other than suppression of parathyroid secretion may be involved in the observed inhibition of 1,25 dihydroxycholecalciferol synthesis.

There is accumulating evidence that the renal 1-hydroxylation of 25 hydroxycholecalciferol is an extremely complicated process, and there is confusion and debate concerning the intimate cellular mechanisms of its control. One fascinating and unexplained aspect of this process is that when 1-hydroxylation is inhibited, 25 hydroxycholecalciferol is alternatively hydroxylated in the kidney to the biologically less potent triol, 24, 25 dihydroxycholecalciferol. This can be seen to occur after parathyroidectomy (33) and in the EHDP treated rat and chick (27, 36). It is not known if this triol has a specific function or whether its formation represents an initial step in the biological inactivation of 25 hydroxycholecalciferol. Like the 1,25 derivative, 24, 25 dihydroxycholecalciferol is produced in the renal cortical mitochondria (37) and it is evident that 25 hydroxycholecalciferol converted into this metabolite will no longer be available for 1-hydroxylation. Thus the formation of 24, 25 dihydroxycholecalciferol might conceivably mitigate the intoxicating effects of an excess of 25 hydroxycholecalciferol and tend to reduce the body burden of 25-hydroxycholecalciferol.

DeLuca has now modified his original view that parathyroid hormone acts as a direct tropic influence on the renal synthesis of 1,25 dihydroxycholecalciferol itself or of the 1-hydroxylating enzyme (33). This revised opinion is based on his demonstration that the parathyroidectomized rat can produce 1,25 dihydroxycholecalciferol normally so long as elevation of the serum phosphorus is prevented by dietary or other means (38). It is proposed that inhibition of 1-hydroxylation results from an increase in the renal cortical concentration of inorganic phosphorus, and that parathyroid hormone stimulates formation of 1,25 dihydroxycholecalciferol by reducing this concentration (38).

Conversely, MacIntyre and his collaborators have inferred that the formation of 1,25 dihydroxycholecalciferol is inhibited by an increase of calcium concentration within the renal cell. This suggestion is based on two considerations. Firstly, on their demonstration in hyper-calcaemic rats that administration of parathyroid hormone inhibited (39) and of calcitonin stimulated (40) the formation of 1,25 dihydroxy-cholecalciferol; secondly on the known opposing actions of these two hormones on the entry of calcium into the cell. There is some alter-native support for this proposition, since an increase of calcium ion concentration is highly effective in inhibiting the *in vitro* biosynthesis of 1,25 dihydroxycholecalciferol by homogenates of vitamin D deficient chick kidney (41, 34), while an increase of orthophosphate con-centration is apparently without effect (41).

One has no reason to doubt the validity of the observations of either of these groups of workers, and it seems obvious that their conflicting interpretations will be resolved satisfactorily when more is known of the precise intracellular sites and the complete biochemical sequence of the processes of 1- and 24-hydroxylation. Observations we have made in primary hyperparathyroidism are relevant here. Such patients produced 1,25 dihydroxycholecalciferol normally but the amounts appearing in the serum were quantitatively less than in a control group of patients with vitamin D deficiency. Moreover, no 24, 25 dihydroxycholecalciferol was detectable in the serum of the latter patients, whereas significant amounts accumulated in the patients with primary hyperparathyroidism (42). In both groups of patients there were increased concentrations of circulating parathyroid hor-mone and also relative hypophosphataemia; but in the vitamin D deficient subjects the mean serum calcium was subnormal, whereas the patients with primary hyperparathyroidisms were, of course, hyper-calcaemic. This suggests that it is the combination of hyperparathyroi-dism and hypercalcaemia which is responsible for the reduced synthesis of the 1,25 derivative and for the formation of 24, 25 dihydroxychole-calciferol. The situation in primary hyperparathyroidism is thus qualitatively reminiscent of MacIntyre's observations on the effects of parathyroid hormone in the hypercalcaemic rat.

I have had a long personal interest in the pattern of calcium metabolism in primary hyperparathyroidism. More especially, I have been fascinated to observe in this disease that no matter how high the urinary output of calcium this tends to be matched by a commensurate increase of the intestinal net absorption of calcium, so that the external balance in most patients is maintained close to equilibrium (43). There is now little doubt that the increased intestinal absorption of calcium

in primary hyperparathyroidism is mediated by 1,25 dihydroxycholecalciferol (44); but there has remained the problem of explaining how
the kidney might monitor and signal appropriately to the intestine, the
rate of calcium excretion in the urine. I still have no completely
satisfactory working hypothesis to account for this phenomenon; but,
as evidence accumulates that one or both of two ions, calcium and
orthophosphate, reabsorbed in the renal tubule are capable of modu-
lating the renal biosynthesis of 1,25 dihydroxycholecalciferol, one can
envisage that this may prove to be another of the remarkable homeostatic feats achieved by the kidney. There are, however, other
problems associated with primary hyperparathyroidism, since intestinal
absorption of calcium may remain high after the responsible parathyroid tumour has been removed surgically (43, 44). There is now
neither hypercalcaemia nor hypercalciuria and one is faced with a
need to assess the contribution made by post-operative hypocalcaemia,
hypophosphataemia, secondary hyperparathyroidism, increased new
formation of bone and a general increase in protein anabolism to the
post-operative adaptation of calcium absorption (STANBURY, unpublished observations).

It is evidently premature to erect any definitive hypothesis for the
control of formation of 1,25 dihydroxycholecalciferol and for its role in
controlling calcium absorption. Thus, for example in rats treated with
prednisolone we have found evidence of increased formation of
1,25 dihydroxycholecalciferol but there is a failure of calcium absorption, despite the presence of normal amounts of this metabolite in
the intestinal mucosa (45). It has been claimed that the cytosol of
intestinal cells contains a specific binding protein for this metabolite
(46) and, if verified, this could obviously have some functional significance. There is certainly a soluble kidney protein with a specific,
high affinity for 25 hydroxycholecalciferol (47) and also evidence that
some soluble cytoplasmic factor is required for the mitochondrial
1-hydroxylation of 25 hydroxycholecalciferol (41, 48). The further
suggestion, that 25 hydroxycholecalciferol bound to this specific
cytosol protein may be the actual substrate of the renal 1-hydroxylase
(41), opens the potential for another factor in the regulation of
1,25 dihydroxycholecalciferol synthesis. Finally, FROLIK and DELUCA
(49) have produced evidence that the continued oral administration of
1,25 dihydroxycholecalciferol may activate mechanisms in the intestinal
mucosal cell for the degradation and biological inactivation of this sterol.

Thus, after masquerading for decades as a vitamin, 'vitamin D' has been promoted to the stature of an elaborate hormonal system with a central role in the control of mineral metabolism. Perhaps we are only beginning to understand its function and its integration with other factors maintaining calcium homeostasis.

ACKNOWLEDGEMENTS

The author is grateful to his colleagues for permission to cite various unpublished observations.

Researches on vitamin D metabolism were supported by a grant to S. W. STANBURY from the British Medical Research Council.

REFERENCES

1. STANBURY, S. W., MAWER, E. B., LUMB, G. A., HILL, L. F., HOLMAN, C. A. JONES, M. and VAN DEN BERG, C. J. (1972), Some aspects of vitamin D metabolism in man. In: *Endocrinology, 1971, Proceedings of the Third International Symposium*, p. 487, S. Taylor (ed.), Heinemann, London.

2. HODGKINSON, H. M., STANTON, B. R., ROUND, P. and MORGAN, C. (1973), Sunlight, vitamin D and osteomalacia in the elderly. *Lancet* i, 910.

3. WILSON, D. C. and WIDDOWSON, E. M. (1942), A comparative nutritional survey of various Indian communities. *Indian Med. Res. Mem.* no. 34.

4. HOLMES, A. M., ENOCH, B. A., TAYLOR, J. L. and JONES, M. E. (1973), Occult rickets and osteomalacia amongst the Asian immigrant population. *Quart. J. Med.* 42, 125.

5. HODGKIN, P., KAY, G. H., HINE, P. M., LUMB, G. A. and STANBURY S. W. (1973), Vitamin D deficiency in the Asian – at home and in Britain. *Lancet* ii, 167.

6. PREECE, M. A., FORD, J. A., McINTOSH, W. B., DUNNIGAN, M. G., TOMLINSON, S. and O'RIORDAN, J. L. H. (1973), Vitamin-D deficiency among Asian immigrants in Britain. *Lancet* i, 907.

7. STANBURY, S. W. (1957), Azotaemic renal osteodystrophy. *Brit. Med. Bull.* 13, 57.

8. STANBURY, S. W. (1967), Bony complications of renal disease In: *Renal disease*, ch. 26, D. A. K. Black (ed.), Blackwell, Oxford.

9. STANBURY, S. W. (1968), Bone disease in uremia. *Amer. J. Med.* 44, 714.

10. STANBURY, S. W. (1971), Changes in bone and in calcium and phosphorus metabolism resulting from chronic renal failure. In: *Diseases of the kidney*, 2nd edition, Ch. 8, M. B. Strauss and L. G. Welt (eds.), Little, Brown, Boston.

11. STANBURY, S. W. (1972), Azotaemic renal osteodystrophy. *Clin. Endocrinol. Metabol.* 1, 267.

12. STANBURY, S. W. and LUMB, G. A. (1962), Metabolic studies of renal osteodystrophy, 1. Calcium, phosphorus and nitrogen metabolism in rickets, osteomalacia and hyperparathyroidism complicating chronic uraemia and in the osteomalacia of the Fanconi syndrome. *Medicine, Baltimore* 41, 1.

13. STANBURY, S. W. and LUMB, G. A. (1967), The osteomalacia of renal insufficiency. In: *L'osteomalacie*, p. 367, D. J. Hioco (ed.), Masson, Paris.

14. LUMB, G. A., MAWER, E. B. and STANBURY, S. W. (1971), The apparent vitamin D resistance of chronic renal failure. A study of the physiology of vitamin D in man. *Amer. J. Med.* 50, 421.

15. PONCHON, G., KENNAN, A. L. and DELUCA, H. F. (1969), 'Activation' of vitamin D by the liver. *J. clin. Invest.* 48, 2032.

16. FRASER, D. R. and KODICEK, E. (1970), Unique biosynthesis by kidney of a biologically active vitamin D metabolite, *Nature* 228, 764.

17. MAWER, E. B., BACKHOUSE, J., LUMB, G. A. and STANBURY, S. W. (1971), Evidence for the formation of 1,25-dihydroxycholecalciferol in man. *Nature, New Biology* 232.

18. MAWER, E. B., BACKHOUSE, J., TAYLOR, C., LUMB, G. A. and STANBURY, S. W. (1973), Failure of formation of 1,25-dihydroxycholecalciferol in chronic renal insufficiency. *Lancet* i, 626.

19. MAWER, E. B., LUMB, G. A., SCHAEFER, K. and STANBURY, S. W. (1971), The metabolism of isotopically labelled vitamin D_3 in man: the influence of the state of vitamin D nutrition. *Clin. Sci.* 40, 39.

20. MAWER, E. B., BACKHOUSE, J. HOLMAN, C. A., LUMB, G. A. and STANBURY, S. W. (1973), The distribution and storage of vitamin D and its metabolites in human tissues. *Clin. Sci.* 43, 413.

21. STANBURY, S. W., HILL, L. F. and MAWER, E. B. (1973), Renal and skeletal interaction: the role of vitamin D. In: *Hard tissue growth, repair and remineralization* Ciba Foundation Symposium 11 (new series), p. 391. Elsevier-Excerpta Medica – North-Holland, Amsterdam.

22. STANBURY, S. W., MAWER, E. B., LUMB, G. A., HILL, L. F., HOLMAN, C. A., TAYLOR, C. M. and TORKINGTON, P. (1973), Vitamin D metabolism and renal bone disease. In: *International symposium on metabolic bone disease Detroit 1972*. Excerpta Medica, Amsterdam.

23. BOYLE, I. T., GRAY, R. W. and DELUCA, H. F. (1971), Regulation by calcium of the *in vivo* synthesis of 1,25-dihydroxycholecalciferol and 21,25 dihydroxycholecalciferol. *Proc. nat. Acad. Sci.* (Wash.) 68, 2131.

24. ADAMS, P. H., HILL, L. F. and WAIN, D. (1973), The control of intestinal calcium absorption in accelerated and retarded growth. *Proc. med. Res. Soc. Clin. Sci.* 44, 4P.

25. ADAMS, P. H., HILL, L. F. and WAIN, D. (1973), Intestinal calcium transport during accelerated and retarded growth. (submitted to *Clin. Sci.*).

26. SCHACHTER, D. and ROSEN, S. M. (1959), Active transport of [45]Ca by the small intestine and its dependence on vitamin D. *Amer. J. Physiol.* 196, 357.

27. HILL, L. F., LUMB, G. A., MAWER, E. B. and STANBURY, S. W. (1973), Indirect inhibition of the biosynthesis of 1,25 dihydroxycholecalciferol in rats treated with a diphosphonate. *Clin. Sci.* 44, 335.

28. MORRISSEY, R. L. and WASSERMAN, R. H. (1971), Calcium absorption and calcium-binding protein in chicks on differing calcium and phosphorus intakes. *Amer. J. Physiol.* 220, 1509.

29. LE ROITH, D. and PIMSTONE, B. L. (1973), Bone metabolism and composition in the protein-deprived rat. *Clin. Sci.* 44, 305.

30. EL-MARAGHI, N. R., PLATT, B. S. and STEWART, R. J. C. (1965), The effect of the interaction of dietary protein and calcium on the growth and maintenance of the bones of young, adult and aged rats. *Brit. J. Nutr.* 19, 491.

31. ADAMS, P. H., HILL, L. F., MAWER, E. B. and WAIN, D. (1973), Unpublished observations.

32. NICOLAYSEN, R., EEG-LARSEN, N. and MALM, O. J. (1953), Physiology of calcium metabolism. *Physiol. Rev.* 33, 424.
33. GARABEDIAN, M., HOLICK, M. F., DeLUCA, H. F. and BOYLE, I. T. (1972), Control of 25-hydroxycholecalciferol metabolism by parathyroid glands. *Proc. nat. Acad. Sci.* (Wash.) 69, 1673.
34. FRASER, D. R. and KODICEK, E. (1973), Regulation of 25-hydroxycholecalciferol-1-hydroxylase by parathyroid hormone. *Nature, New Biology* 241, 163.
35. HILL, L. F. and MAWER, E. B. (1973), The interrelationships between vitamin D, parathyroid hormone and calcitonin. *Proc. Med. Res. Soc. Clin. Sci.* 44, 4P.
36. TAYLOR, C. M., MAWER, E. B. and REEVE, A. (1973), The metabolism of cholecalciferol (vitamin D_3) in diphosphonate treated chicks. *Proc. Biochem. Soc. Bioch. J.* (in the press).
37. OMDAHL, J. L. GRAY, R. W., BOYLE, I. T., KNUTSON, J. and DeLUCA, H. F. (1972), Regulation of the Metabolism of 25-hydroxycholecalciferol by kidney tissue *in vitro* by dietary calcium. *Nature, New Biology* 237, 63.
38. TANAKA, Y. and DeLUCA, H. F. (1973), The control of 25-hydroxyvitamin D metabolism by inorganic phosphorus. *Arch. Biochem. Biophys.* 154, 566.
39. GALANTE, L., MACAULEY, S. J., COLSTON, K. W. and MACINTYRE, I. (1972), Effect of parathyroid extract on vitamin D metabolism. *Lancet* i, 985.
40. GALANTE, L., COLSTON, K. W., MACAULEY, S. J. and MACINTYRE, I. (1972), Effect of calcitonin on vitamin D metabolism. *Nature* 238, 271.
41. COLSTON, K. W., EVANS, I. M. A., GALANTE, I., MACINTYRE, I. and MOSS, D. W. (1973), Regulation of vitamin D metabolism: factors influencing the rate of formation of 1,25 dihydroxycholecalciferol by kidney homogenates. *Biochem. J.* (in the press).
42. MAWER, E. B., TAYLOR, C. M., LUMB, G. A. and STANBURY, S. W. (1973), Vitamin D metabolism in primary hyperparathyroidism. (In preparation).
43. STANBURY, S. W. (1968), The intestinal absorption of calcium in normal adults, primary hyperparathyroidism and renal failure. In: *Nutrition in renal disease*, p. 118, G. M. Berlyne (ed.), Livingstone, Edinburgh.
44. STANBURY, S. W. (1973), Parathyroid hormone and the intestinal absorption of calcium in man. In: *Symposium on electrolyte metabolism*. Sienna.
45. LUKERT, B. P., STANBURY, S. W. and MAWER, E. B. (1973), Vitamin D and intestinal transport of calcium: effect of prednisolone. *Endocrinology*, in the press.
46. HOSOYA, N. and OKU, T. (1971), Specific binding protein for active metabolites of vitamin D_3. *J. Vitaminol.* 17, 119.
47. HADDAD, J. G. and BIRGE, S. J. (1971), 25-hydroxycholecalciferol: specific binding by rachitic tissue extracts. *Biochemical and Biophysical Research Communications*, 45, no. 4.
48. KODICEK, E. (1973), Vitamin D and the skeleton. In: *Hard tissue growth, repair and remineralization*. Ciba Foundation Symposium 11 (new series), p. 359. Elsevier-Excerpta Medica-North Holland, Amsterdam.
49. FROLIK, C. A. and DeLUCA, H. F. (1973), The stimulation of 1,25 dihydroxycholecalciferol metabolism in vitamin D-deficient rats by 1,25-dihydroxycholecalciferol treatment. *J. clin. Invest.* 52, 543.

THE IMPLICATIONS OF THE MEMBRANE LOCALIZATION OF VITAMIN E FOR ITS FUNCTION, UPTAKE AND ABSORPTION

I. MOLENAAR*, C. E. HULSTAERT*, J. VOS* and F. A. HOMMES**

INTRODUCTION

Why can't we live without vitamin E? This question has impelled research forward since its discovery by EVANS and BISHOP half a century ago (1). In the first sentence 'we' illustrates that vitamin E is of importance to humans; it is also of importance to other mammals and to birds, which raises the possibility of using them as experimental animals; 'why' points up the question of the still unknown function of the vitamin, which is so important for life that the term 'can't live' is not exaggerated: those who once have seen the course of illness and death of a vitamin E deficient animal do not need to be convinced of this statement.

Research on vitamin E has made extensive use of the possibility of inducing such a deficiency. As with other vitamins, it is a major tool in studies on the function of the vitamin. Such studies can provide important knowledge of the consequences of the absence of the vitamin for the organism, its tissues, cells and organella. It must be noted however that for pure logical reasons experiments with deficient organisms, however important they may be, must fail to produce a complete and clear insight into the functional mechanism of this vitamin in the cellular metabolism of a non-deficient organism.

Nevertheless research on deficient animals has produced valuable information on the effects of depletion and repletion of the vitamin on the organism. However much of the effort has been in vain: vitamin E is a research subject where nutritionists, food technologists, oil chemists, pharmacologists, biochemists, pathologists, physicians, pediatricians, dermatologists, obstetricians and gerontologists meet, all speaking their

* Centre for Medical Electron Microscopy University of Groningen, The Netherlands.
** Department of Pediatrics, University of Groningen, The Netherlands.

own language. This makes an evaluation of their research difficult, the more so because they study not only humans but also different experimental animals such as rats, rabbits, chicks, quails, turkeys, cows, ewes, guinea pigs, hamsters, monkeys, minks, pigs, ducks, mice, lambs and calves. The matter becomes even more confused because of the large variety of macroscopical and microscopical lesions in different organs of different deficient animals. The structural integrity of muscle, reproductive organs, nervous system, vascular system, bone marrow and glandular tissues can be impaired. Furthermore it has been clearly established that the course of the illness is influenced by other nutrients, for instance polyunsaturated fatty acids, selenium, sulfur-containing amino acids and synthetic antioxidants and that these factors determine the lesion to a certain extent (2). The above-mentioned conditions have made the interpretation and integration of the results of vitamin E research difficult and it is no wonder that this has given rise to a spectacular growth of therapeutic claims, which shall not be repeated here in detail. The use of vitamin E as a panacea in therapeutics and the resulting disagreements afterwards persuaded GORDON in 1958 to call vitamin E 'a shady lady to be approached gingerly by respectable or discreet investigators in human nutrition' (3). In 1961 HORWITT noted that the lady was regaining her social position (4). In 1973 we can state that her position is fully government-supported.

To unravel this tangled network of fact and fiction, and given the fact that cell biology provides a sound basis for the study of medicine, it seems warranted to tackle the problem from the viewpoint of a cell biologist and for that purpose to choose the cellular membrane as a starting point.

CELLULAR MEMBRANES

The membrane concept emerged after sixty years of research in cell physiology when DANIELLI and DAVSON in 1935 summarized the relevant experimental data and constructed the first hypothetical model for the architecture of the cell membrane (5). This model (fig. 1) showed the membranes as a lipid bilayer with a hydrophobic centre, strengthened by the apposition of electrostatically bound protein layers on both hydrophilic sides. This postulate of a diffusion barrier, based on non-morphological evidence, was confirmed by the

EXTERIOR

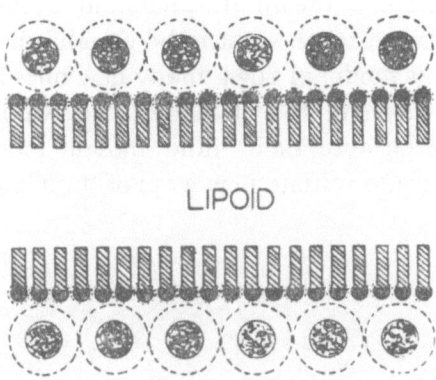

LIPOID

INTERIOR

Fig. 1. The DANIELLI-DAVSON membrane model.

visualization of the limiting cell membrane (or plasma membrane) with the electron microscope. However, more importantly, the supreme resolving power of this instrument also disclosed the existence of a hitherto unexpected multitude of membranous elements in the cytoplasm surrounding the cell nucleus (6) (fig. 2). Thus the cytoplasm turned out to be a space subdivided into compartments by membrane systems, rather than one filled with a gel-like substance as had been supposed by generations of cytologists. The nucleus is encircled by an outer and an inner nuclear membrane, the former being connected to the membranes of the endoplasmic reticulum, compartmentalizing the cytoplasm where organelles such as mitochondria, Golgi apparatus, lysosomes, etc. can be found – all with their specific membranes. Thus it is clear that cells can maintain the organization of their cytoplasmic space thanks to cellular membranes and to these structural entities only. In fact, they are one of the basic structural elements of cells. No life without DNA, but also no life without membranes.

What does the membrane look like in the electron microscope? Does this image contribute to our knowledge of the chemical anatomy of the membrane, i.e. the gross organization and structure of its proteins and lipids? After fixation in osmium tetroxide, it appears as a black line when sectioned perpendicular to its surface. At high

magnification this line appears to be double (fig. 3), which is assumed
to be caused by a binding of heavy osmium atoms to the double bonds
of the fatty acyl chains of the unsaturated lipids in the membrane. Thus
DANIELLI's lipid bilayer is thought to be visualized. However since the
presentation of this model in 1935, many new ones have been brought
forward and the newest, that of SINGER and NICOLSON (7), deserves
special attention because their 'fluid mosaic model' of membrane
structure (fig. 4) could initiate new ways of thinking about membrane

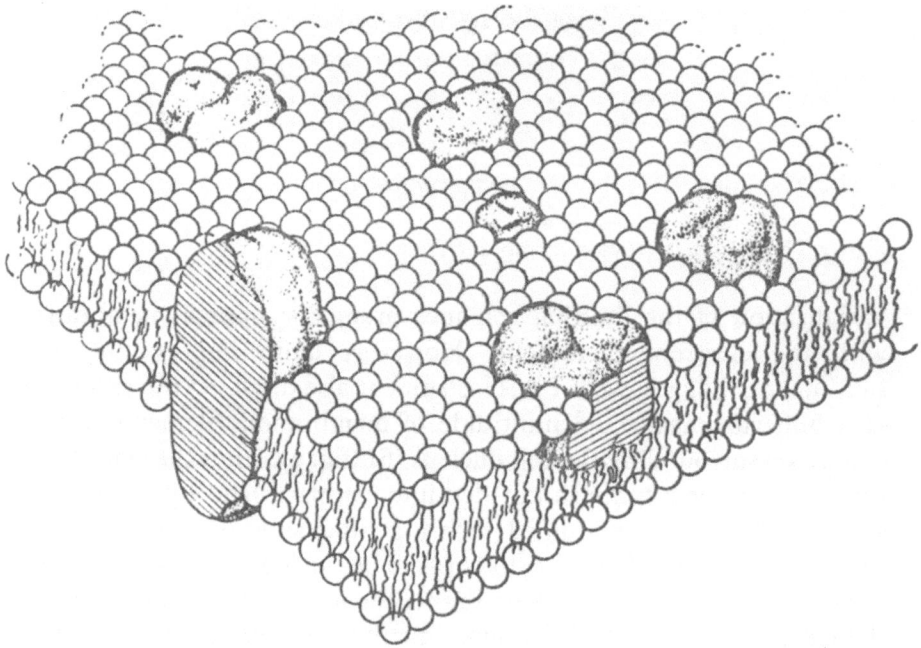

Fig. 4. The lipid-globular protein mosaic model with a lipid matrix (the fluid
mosaic model); schematic three-dimensional and cross-sectional views. The solid
bodies with stippled surfaces represent the globular integral proteins, which at long
range are randomly distributed in the plane of the membrane. From: SINGER, S. J.
and NICOLSON, G. L., (1972) ref. (7). (Copyright 1973 by the American Association
for the Advancement of Science).

functions. It is important to recognize that their model is consistent
with the restrictions imposed by thermodynamics. The proteins
belonging in sensu strictu to the membrane (integral proteins) are a
heterogenous set of globular molecules, each arranged in an amphipa-

thic structure, i.e. with the ionic and highly polar groups protruding from the membrane into the aqueous phase and the non-polar groups largely buried in the hydrophobic interior of the membrane. These globular molecules are partially embedded in a matrix of phospholipid, the latter being organised mainly as a discontinuous fluid bilayer although a small fraction of the lipid may interact specifically with the membrane proteins. Formally therefore the fluid mosaic structure is analogous to a two-dimensionally oriented solution of integral proteins (or lipoproteins) in the viscous phospholipid bilayer solvent. (7).

Now let us see if, with this membrane concept in mind, we can find a cause for the previously mentioned embarrassing diversity in the histopathology of vitamin E deficiency. If we should succeed, we could try to use this concept to attain a better understanding of the findings on vitamin E and its behavior during uptake and absorption and as a nutrient.

As stated above, cellular membranes divide tissues into cells and cells into compartments, each with its own micromilieu. Such a milieu is particularly determined and controlled by specific properties of the membrane. Otherwise stated: membrane properties define to a large extent cellular and tissue properties. Pathological changes in membrane properties introduce functional and morphological aberrations, depending in character upon the kind of membrane affected. Now, if we postulate the presence of vitamin E in the membrane and an effect of the vitamin on the membrane composition (see following paragraphs), it follows that the symptoms of a vitamin E deficiency are primarily determined by the kind of membrane affected, i.e. by the composition of the membrane. In view of these considerations, cellular membranes with their highly varied composition of lipids, proteins and carbohydrates (8) can only give rise to a bewildering multitude of histopathological lesions.

VITAMIN E AND CELLULAR MEMBRANES

As to the question of whether vitamin E is present in cellular membranes, it can be stated that its presence has been proven in the inner membrane of mitochondria and in the plasma membrane of erythrocytes (9, 10). Moreover, it was found that membrane-bound vitamin E plays a role in certain enzymatic reactions and is degraded during these reactions (11, 12). Morphological evidence for the postulate that vitamin E fulfills a function in the membrane will be presented in the next paragraph.

How is vitamin E thought to function in the membrane? There are several hypotheses on the function of vitamin E relevant to cellular membranes:

1. Vitamin E controls membrane stability and permeability (LUCY and DIPLOCK, 13, 14).
2. Vitamin E protects membrane lipids against peroxidation during electron transport functions (McCAY et al., 11, 12).
3. Vitamin E functions as an overall biological lipid antioxidant, preventing the formation of peroxides (TAPPEL, 15, 16).

The first hypothesis is the most general one and is based on studies of molecular models. The phytyl side chain of vitamin E is thought to form a stable complex with the polyunsaturated fatty acids (particularly arachidonic acid) of phospholipids, thus facilitating the packing of these phospholipids in the membrane (fig. 5). Without vitamin E, packing of polyunsaturated phospholipids in the membrane would be disorderly because the polyunsaturated fatty acid chain has either a curled or an α-helical configuration. In this situation, oxidative destruction of polyunsaturated fatty acids in the membrane could be promoted, the permeability could be increased and endogenous phospholipase could be activated to break down membrane phospholipids.

According to the second hypothesis, vitamin E captures the free radicals that are formed as a result of the activity of a membrane-bound enzyme system involving electron transport. In biochemical experiments it was found that rat liver microsomes and mitochondria metabolize all vitamin E present in the membrane before peroxidizing the membrane polyunsaturated fatty acids upon incubation in vitro in the presence of inorganic iron and NADPH. If the same system functions in vivo, the reaction should proceed at a much lower rate since it was found that of a given dose in a period of three weeks a maximum of 30% and a minimum of 1% could be recovered as breakdown products in urine (17, 18).

The third hypothesis, the antioxidant theory, has for many years been predominant in vitamin E research. However the failure to demonstrate peroxides in vitamin E deficient tissues has brought many to reject this hypothesis. Yet in vitamin E deficient rat adipose tissue an increase in peroxides has been assessed (19, 20).

The above-mentioned hypotheses have been combined by Molenaar, Vos and Hommes (21) as follows:
Vitamin E, if present in a given membrane, is probably located
within it as a complex with the polyunsaturated fatty acids of the
phospholipids. This state is especially suited for one function of the
α-tocopherol molecule: inhibiting the peroxidation of membrane-
bound polyunsaturated fatty acids during electron transport functions
as stated above. Protection by vitamin E against peroxidation according to the antioxidant theory is only found in adipose tissue, where
fat is stored as large droplets in the vacuoles of fat cells. Whether
vitamin E has a function in chylomicrons remains to be seen and will
be discussed below.

EFFECTS OF VITAMIN E DEFICIENCY ON CELLULAR MEMBRANES

During the past five years, our group has studied intensively the effect
of vitamin E deficiency on the ultrastructure and chemical composition
of cellular membranes, especially of jejunal and liver epithelial cells.
A morphological investigation of a clinical vitamin E deficiency in two
children suffering from a-β-lipoproteinaemia and the effect of vitamin
E medication was followed by experiments in which ducklings were
made vitamin E deficient by means of a semi-synthetic diet. Thus far
these experiments have yielded the following evidence (21, 22, 23, 24,
25, 26, 27):

1) Cellular membranes of jejunal epithelial cells of patients with
   a-β-lipoproteinaemia and a resulting vitamin E deficiency and of
   ducklings with induced vitamin E deficiency could not be visualized
   in the usual fashion with the electron microscope (fig. 6). After
   fixation with osmium tetroxide, a decrease in positive membrane
   contrast could be observed in comparison with controls. The liver
   epithelial cells of vitamin E deficient ducklings showed the same
   phenomenon.
2) The vitamin E deficient patients needed a four months' treatment
   with vitamin E before a completely normal cellular ultrastructure
   could be observed (fig. 6).
3) Morphologically, those most affected were the mitochondrial
   membranes, endoplasmic reticular membranes and nuclear outer
   membranes in contrast with plasma membranes and the membranes
   of Golgi lamellae and vesicles. The loss of contrast appeared first

and was the greatest in the outer mitochondrial membrane (fig. 7).

4) The integrity of isolated mitochondrial membranes (especially outer membranes) decreased or changed under the influence of vitamin E deficiency, as can be inferred from electron micrographs of these membrane fractions (fig. 8). In this respect microsomal membranes did not differ from controls.

5) Biochemical analysis of isolated mitochondrial inner and outer membranes and microsomes of the liver of vitamin E deficient ducklings showed a specific loss of arachidonic acid. Especially the outer mitochondrial membrane showed a marked decrease in arachidonic content (67%) while the decreases for the inner mitochondrial and microsomal membranes were less (43% and 13%, respectively). An analogous decrease was observed in the linoleic acid content of outer mitochondrial membranes (44%), but not for inner mitochondrial and microsomal membranes (<10%) (table 1).

6) These relative decreases were found to be balanced by increases in palmitoleic and oleic acid in outer and inner mitochondrial

Table 1. *Fatty acid composition of inner and outer mitochondrial membranes and microsomes from vitamin E-deficient duckling livers (D) and controls (C).*

| | Content (wt % of total fatty acids) | | | | | |
| | Inner mitochondrial membrane[1] | | Outer mitochondrial membrane[2] | | Microsomes[3] | |
Fatty acid	C	D	C	D	C	D
C 16:0	20.4	24.1	29.6	27.2	25.6	23.9
C 16:1ω7	1.9	3.3	1.9	3.4	1.6	1.6
C 18:0	25.0	22.1	25.3	26.4	18.2	20.9
C 18:1ω9	20.9	25.3	21.9	25.2	21.6	20.5
C 18:2ω6	13.3	12.2	6.8	3.6	4.5	4.7
C 22:0	1.1	0.2	+	+	0.4	1.2
C 20:4ω6	13.3	7.6	9.4	3.3	16.9	14.7
C 24:0	+	+	0.7	+	1.6	2.2
C 22:6ω3	1.6	1.0	1.2	2.0	2.0	3.4
Unidentified	2.5	4.0	3.2	8.9	7.6	6.9
Total saturated	46.5	46.4	55.6	53.6	45.8	48.2
C 16:1ω7 + C 18:1ω9	22.8	28.8	23.8	28.6	23.2	22.1
C 18:2ω6 + C 20:4ω6	26.6	19.8	16.2	6.9	21.4	19.4

1. Average of 4 determinations, 10 control and 10 deficient animals.
2. Determination of 3 combined fractions, 8 control and 8 deficient animals.
3. Average of 3 determinations, 8 control and 9 deficient animals.

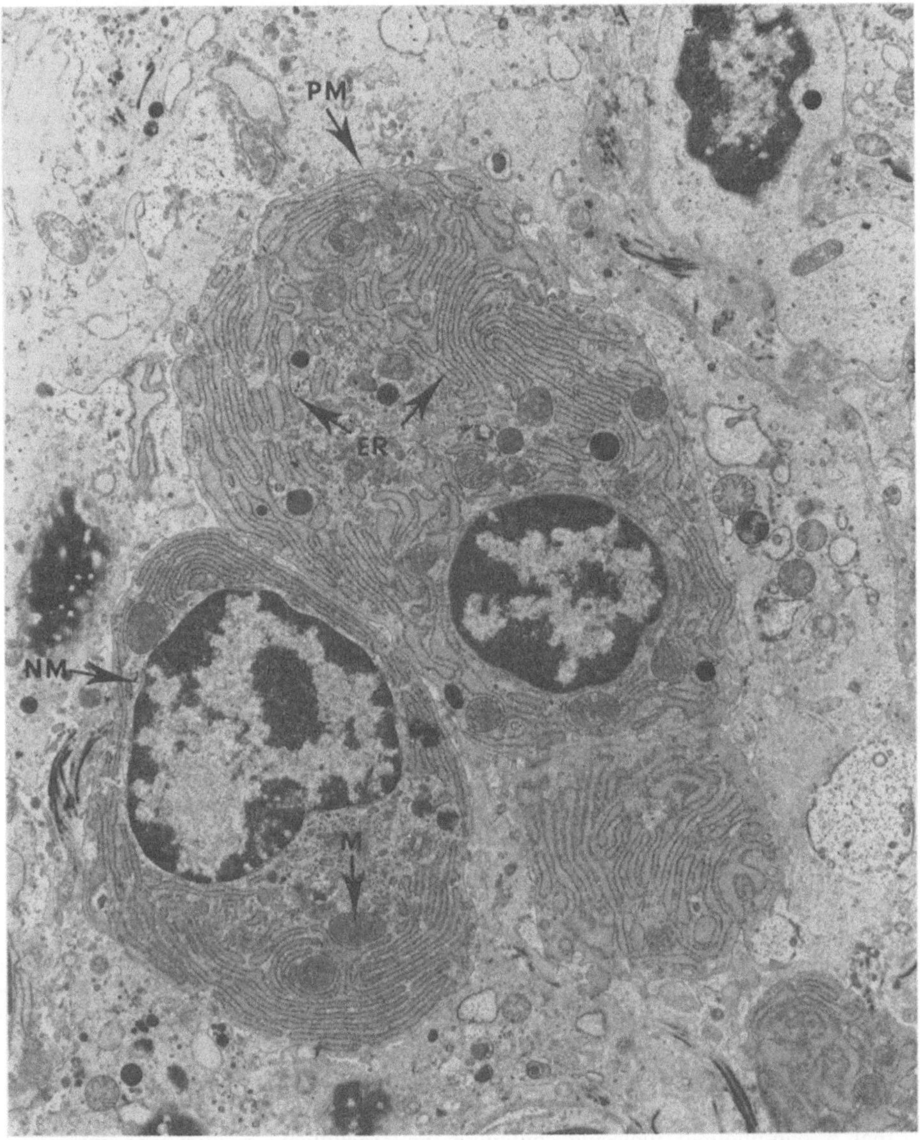

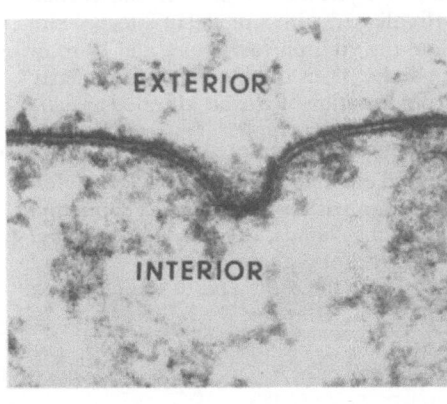

Fig. 2. Electron micrograph of two plasma cells. Note the extensive membrane systems in the cytoplasm. pm = plasma membrane, er = endoplasmic reticular membranes, m = mitochondrial membranes, nm = nuclear membrane. Glutaraldehyde fixation with postfixation in osmium tetroxide. Magnification x 9000.

Fig. 3. Electron micrograph of plasma membrane of an egg cell of Limnea stagnalis. Note two dark lines with a light zone in between. Compare with fig. 1. Osmium tetroxide fixation. Magnification x 120.000.

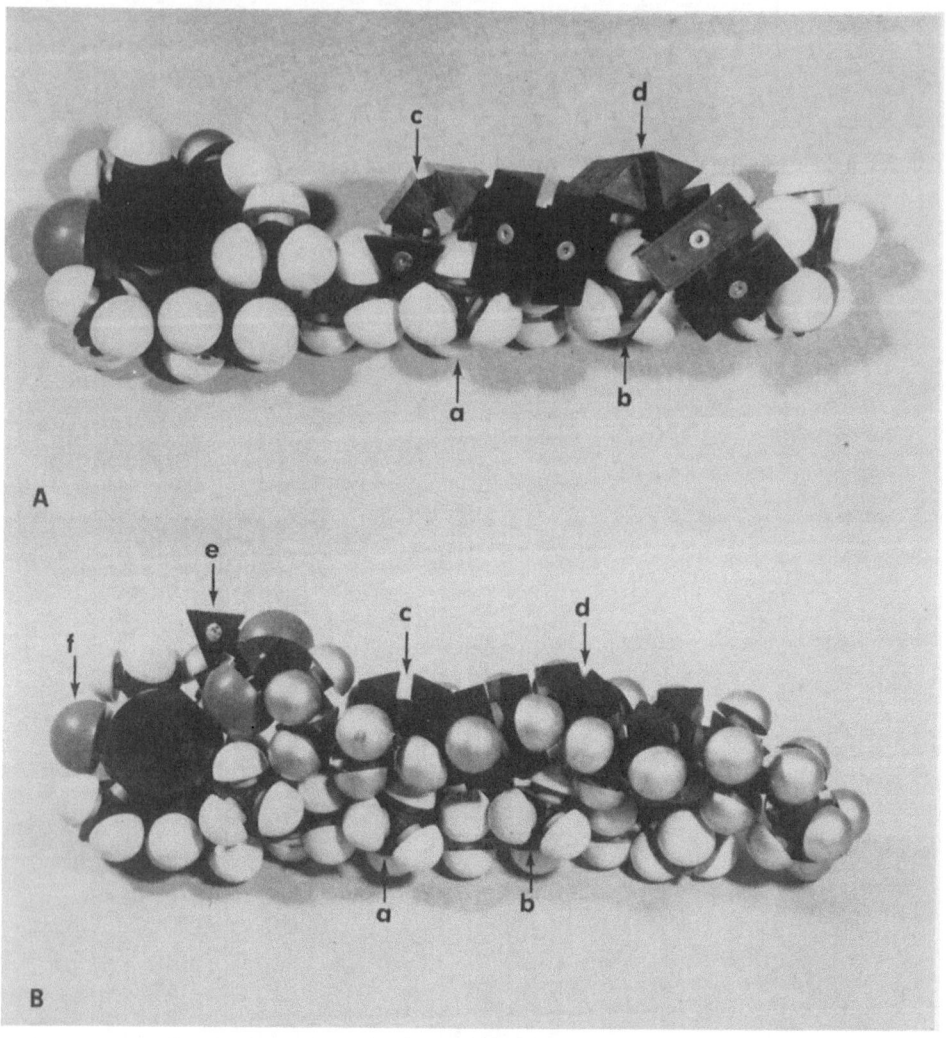

Fig. 5. Space-filling molecular models illustrating the way in which it is proposed that a phospholipid molecule containing an arachidonyl residue may interact with α-tocopherol in a biological membrane. (A) Model of part of the carbon skeleton of arachidonic acid (from C-4 to C-16) aligned with a model of α-tocopherol to allow the methyl groups at C-4, and C-8, of the vitamin (arrows: a and b) to fit into pockets created, respectively, by the $\triangle^5$ and $\triangle^{11}$ cis double bonds of the fatty acid (arrows: c and d). The quasi-helical conformation of the unsaturated arachidonyl chain that is required for the formation of the 'complex' between the two molecules is clearly apparent. (B) A similar model (reproduced at a slightly lower magnification) in which the complete unsaturated chain of an arachidonyl phospholipid, with its hydrogen atoms, is shown interacting with α-tocopherol. The methyl groups of α-tocopherol, and the arachidonyl double bonds, are labeled as before. The carbon skeleton of the glycerol moiety of the phospholipid (arrow: e), and the hydroxyl group of α-tocopherol (arrow: f) lie at the same end of the complex. (By courtesy of PROFESSOR J. A. LUCY and DR. A. T. DIPLOCK.)

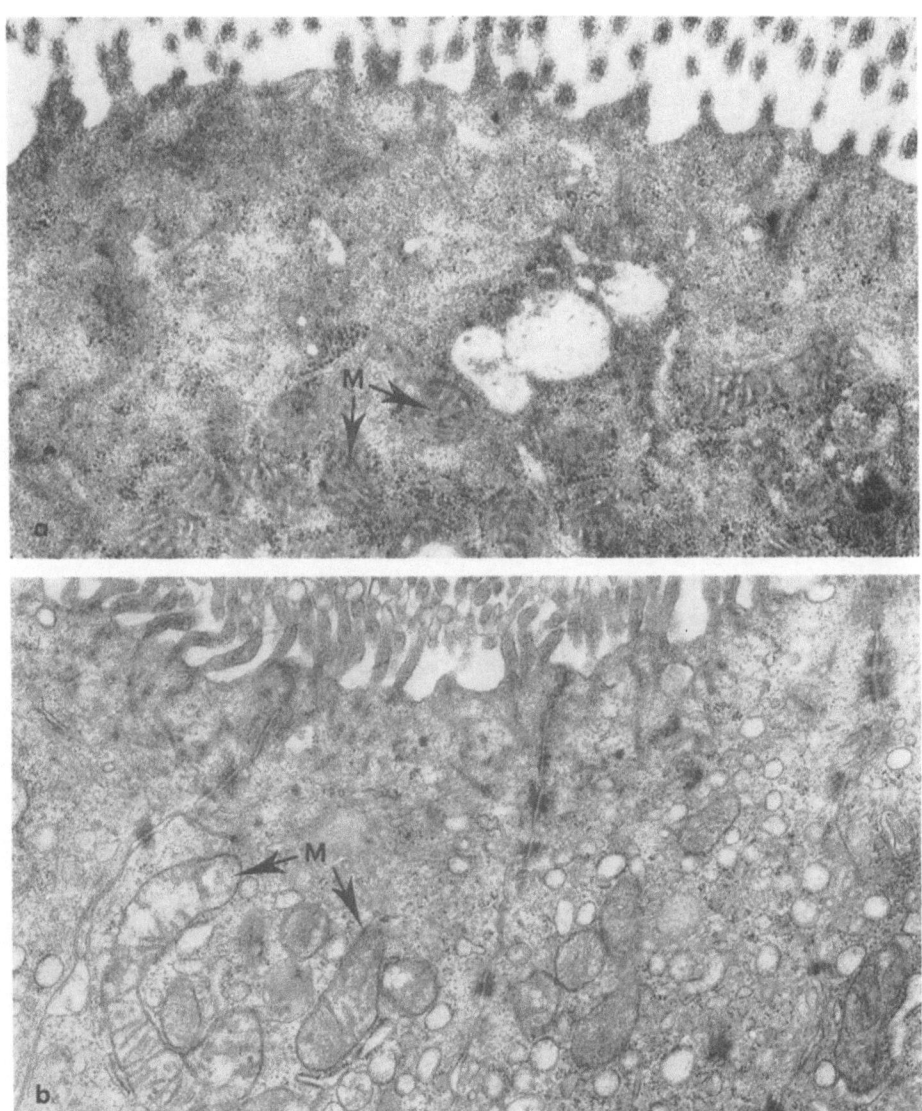

Fig. 6. Jejunal epithelial cells with parts of microvilli at the top from a patient with a-β-lipoproteinania resulting in hypovitaminosis E, before (a) and after (b) 4 months of treatment with vitamin E. a. Note the lack of membranes in general. Mitochondria (m) show their matrix, but lack positively contrasted membranes. Magnification x 25.000. b. The cells in general and the mitochondrial membranes in particular have a normal ultrastructural appearance. Membranes are visible in normal contrast. Magnification x 20.000.

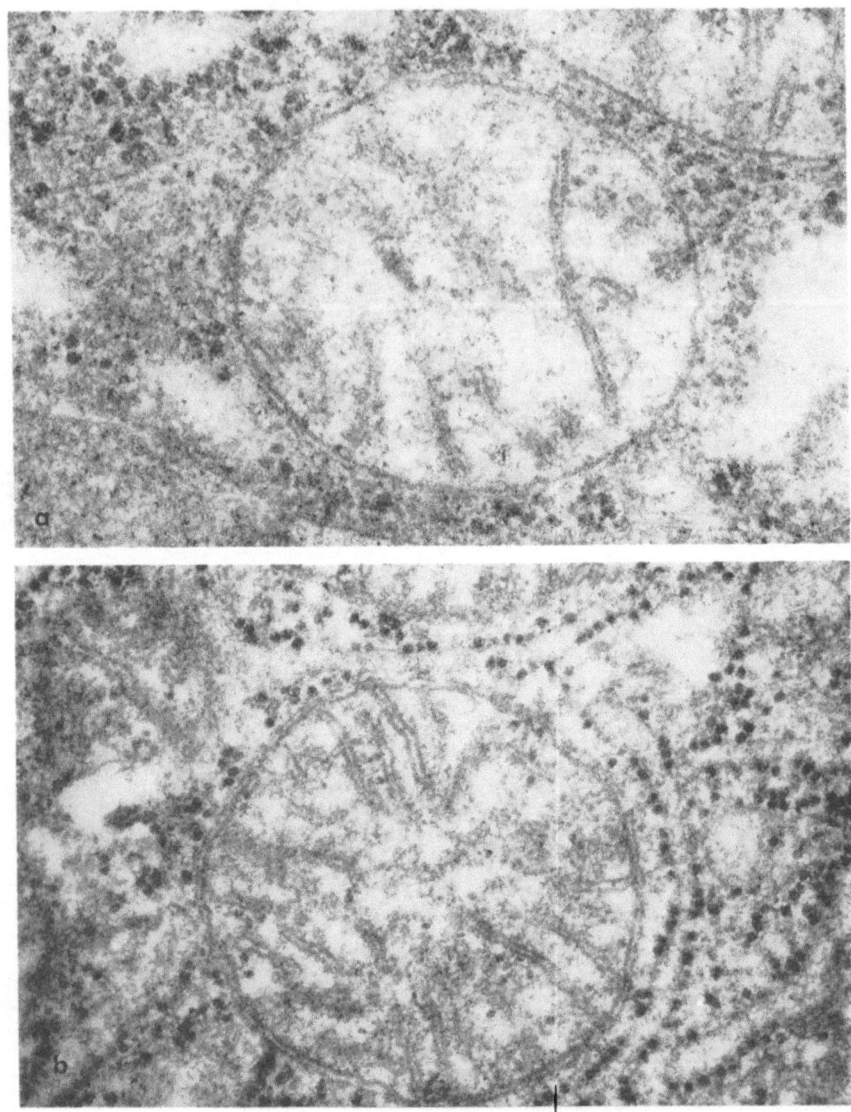

Fig. 7. (a). Vitamin E-deficient duckling; jejunal epithelial cell. Note the big difference in contrast between inner and outer mitochondrial membrane; compare with lower micrograph. Magnification x 80.000. From MOLENAAR, I., VOS, J., JAGER, F. C. and HOMMES, F. A. (1970). ref. (23). b. Non-vitamin E-deficient duckling; jejunal epithelial cell. The electron density of both mitochondrial membranes is almost the same. Compare with upper micrograph. Magnification 60.000 x. From MOLENAAR, I., VOS, J., JAGER, F. C. and HOMMES, F. A. (1970) ref. (23).

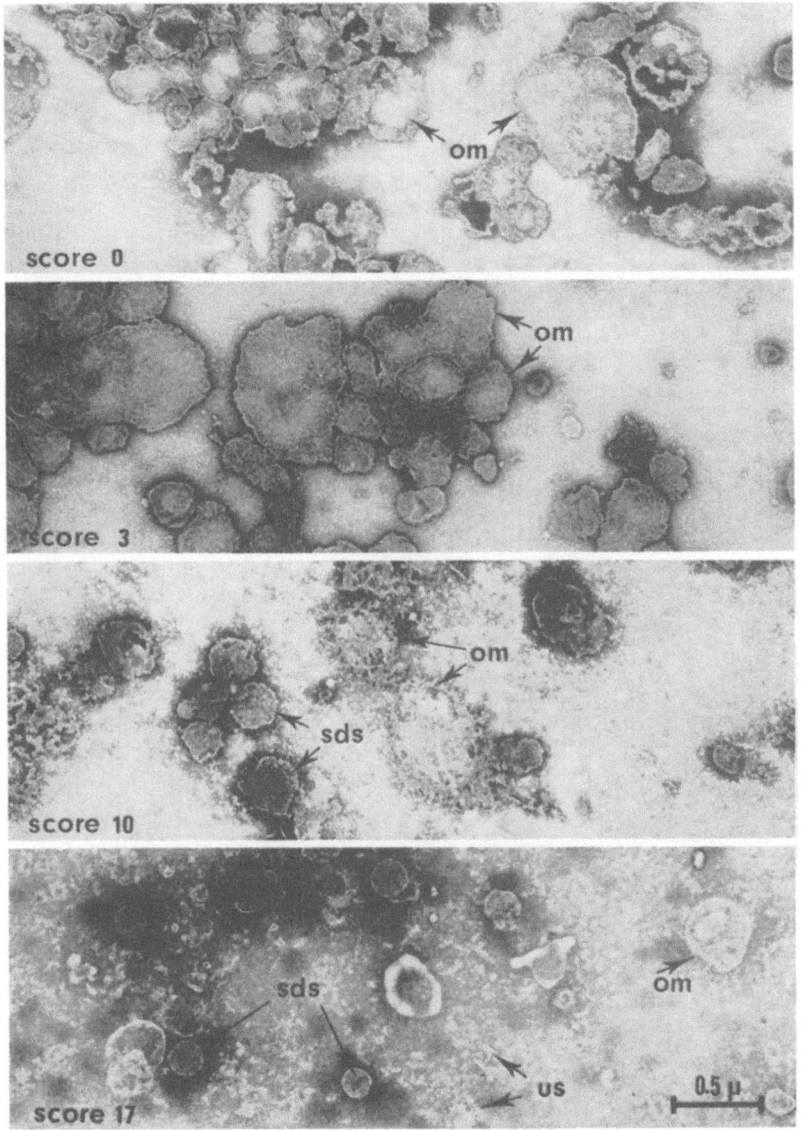

Fig. 8. Variation in ultrastructural aspect of outer mitochondrial membrane fraction from groups of ducklings with different degrees of vitamin E deficiency as judged by myopathy scores (0–17).

The preparations are 'negatively' stained with phosphotungstic acid. Note the gradual deterioration of outer membrane (om) integrity and the increase in the number of unidentified structures (us). Small dense sacs (sds) are not derived from outer membranes. Magnification x 26.000.

membranes and by an increase in the content of stearic acid in microsomal membranes (table 1).

7) The observed decrease in membrane-bound polyunsaturated fatty acids seems highly consistent with the decreased contrast of certain cellular membranes observed in vitamin E deficiency (sub 1, 2 and 3).

These results prompted us to investigate, in addition to membrane lipids, the membrane proteins and especially the membrane-bound enzymes. Histochemically as well as biochemically a stimulation of glucose-6-phosphatase, an enzyme of the endoplasmic reticular membrane, and 5′-nucleotidase, an enzyme of the plasma membrane of the bile capillary, has been found in vitamin E deficient duckling livers. Full results will be published elsewhere.

Summarizing, we state that in man and experimental animals vitamin E deficiency causes changes in membrane ultrastructure which can be correlated with a change in chemical composition and function.

UPTAKE AND ABSORPTION OF VITAMIN E

In the former paragraphs it was demonstrated that vitamin E is of vital importance for the proper functioning of the tissues and their cells. Furthermore it was shown that cellular membranes appeared here to be of paramount importance. The clinician who wants to prevent or cure a deficiency is confronted with two problems, to which this membrane-vitamin E concept could contribute a better approach:

1. How can the vitamin E status of the patient be assessed?
2. If proven necessary, how should vitamin E be 'brought' to its functional site by either oral or parenteral routes?

Before the first question is to be answered it should be pointed out that *severe* vitamin E deficiency in man is rare. Firstly because the basic requirement for vitamin E can easily be met by an appropriate composition of the food. Plants especially, being the organisms where the vitamin is synthesized (28), form a rich source of vitamin E. It has long been known that the intake of polyunsaturated fatty acids (PUFA) may increase the vitamin E requirement. However it must be noted that there is no consensus about the relevance of a fixed critical vitamin E/PUFA ratio (mg d-α-tocopherol/g PUFA) for a diet

(29, 30) in evaluating the vitamin E adequacy of this diet. Whatever the significance of such a ratio, it can be stated that in general vegetable oils with a high linoleic acid content contain by nature sufficient vitamin E to cover the basic requirement plus the extra requirement caused by a high PUFA intake (31). This fact is probably the reason why natural diets which differ in PUFA content contain sufficient vitamin E.

Secondly, severe deficiency is rare because the vitamin E reserve is very large, owing to the storage of vitamin E in the enormous total membrane surface as well as in the vacuoles of fat cells. Thirdly, the metabolic consumption of vitamin E is probably low, as can be judged from the radioactivity measured in urine after administration of radioactive vitamin E to rats and rabbits (32, 33).

These three factors make it understandable that severe deficiency in man seldom occurs. Yet it is this grade of deficiency which is commonly studied in experimental animals. In humans however, the subdeficiency seems to be especially interesting to trace and investigate, the more so because industrial and cooking processes tend to destroy tocopherols in many foods (34, 35, 36). JAGER (37) even concludes that a rather high percentage of human beings are in fact borderline cases of vitamin E deficiency. Therefore it is important to know whether a reliable assessment of the vitamin E status is possible.

For this assessment terms such as 'uptake' and 'absorption' have to be well defined. We define *uptake* as oral intake minus loss in faeces. *Absorption* is judged by the appearance of the administered compound in the plasma. A good uptake does not necessarily mean good absorption (38) and in turn, good absorption does not necessarily mean adequate vitamin E in the tissue. It is the mere localization of vitamin E in the membrane which one has to bear in mind in interpreting plasma tocopherol levels. Evidence has been obtained that the body has two pools of the vitamin at its disposal: first a labile one, which mobilizes rapidly (particularly in the blood), and secondly a fixed component (39), which we think most probably corresponds to the membrane-bound vitamin E. However, as we have seen, the vitamin does not function in the plasma but in the cellular membrane, which is a completely different phase as the above-mentioned membrane model of Singer clearly demonstrates. Thus 'absorption' being expressed as mg tocopherol/100 ml plasma could be a misleading parameter for the vitamin E status in the tissues at that very moment (38, 40). Therefore, a more refined approach for assessment of the vitamin E status should be developed, for instance an analysis of subcutaneous tissue or a skin biopsy.

The answer to the second question, namely how should vitamin E be brought to its functional site in the event of an established or suspected deficiency, depends on where the route of transport of the vitamin is hampered. Three possibilities exist:

1. *Insufficient vitamin E in the lumen in the case of vitamin E deficient food.* Therapy in this case is of course the use of a diet well supplemented with vitamin E (see above).
2. *Insufficient transport of the vitamin across the plasma membrane of the intestinal epithelial cell.* For the resorption of vitamin E, the formation of micelles is important (41, 42) which in turn demands sufficient bile secretion (43). Thus insufficient bile production, being caused by liver disturbances, can lead to a lower uptake of vitamin E by the intestinal epithelial cell (44, 45). A deficient pancreas function as found in cystic fibrosis can have the same consequences (46). As therapy, enzyme replacement is necessary; in addition the therapeutical measures mentioned under 3 could be of avail. Furthermore addition of free fatty acids and monoglycerids to the diet to improve vitamin E uptake has been described (47).
3. *Insufficient chylomicron synthesis or insufficient transport of chylomicrons to the bloodstream.* The chylomicrons are formed by the endoplasmic reticulum of the intestinal epithelial cells and transport about 75% of the vitamin taken up (48). Disturbances of the function of the endoplasmic reticulum which endanger chylomicron synthesis can thus result in a vitamin E deficiency. This is for instance the case in a-β-lipoproteinaemia (22); this disease can be imitated in experiments with puromycin in rats. The same effect can be achieved if the release of formed chylomicrons is impaired by unknown epithelial cell injury (49). Whether the same applies to sprue remains to be seen. Furthermore a vitamin E deficiency due to deficient chylomicron transport was found in a case of stasis of chyle in the intestinal lymphatics (50 and VAN TONGEREN, personal communication).

In the above-mentioned cases, where chylomicron synthesis or transport is impaired, use of medium chain fatty acids as a supply of fats should be considered. These molecules can be used by the intestinal epithelial cell for synthesis of very low density lipoproteins which could function as carriers for the vitamin. Apart from this the possibility exists that these free fatty acids as such could function as carriers. In these cases intravenous administration of vitamin E should also be taken into consideration, at least theoretically. In long-term complete intravenous nutrition, an adequate supplement of vitamin E in the emulsion should be considered (51).

So far it seems that there is no danger of an overdose of vitamin E. When high doses of 500 mg vitamin E/day were given to healthy subjects, it turned out that the erythrocyte membrane has a limited capacity for taking up more vitamin E than is normally present (52). A reticulocyte response was the only abnormal sign observed.

Summarizing, the question 'Why can't we live without vitamin E?' can be read as: 'Why can't our cellular membranes function properly without it?' Although much is already known, a lot of work has to be done in the field of cell biology in order to provide and extend the basis for medical vitaminology.

SUMMARY

The study of vitamin E is complicated by the polymorphous findings in different mammals and birds with experimental vitamin E deficiency and the often extremely diverse approaches to the problem, both leading to a bewildering variance in therapeutic aims, measures and successes.

Yet, it is this very situation which could provide a clue if one tries to tackle the problem from the viewpoint of cell biology. Cells can only organize their cytoplasmic space thanks to cellular membranes, which not only surround but also compartmentalize the cell. Membrane properties define to a large extent cellular and tissue properties. Changes in membrane properties introduce functional and morphological aberrations, depending in character upon the kind of membrane affected.

In this membrane concept, vitamin E plays an important role as a membrane stabilizer giving the vitamin its significance as a *nutrient*. The hydrophobic side chain of a tocopherol molecule is thought to form a complex with an arachidonic acid molecule, thus contributing significantly to the stability of the membrane. Evidence has been produced that vitamin E deficiency leads to a decrease in membrane-bound arachidonic acid and a loss of integrity of certain cellular membranes.

The mere localization of vitamin E in the membrane complicates concepts such as 'uptake' and 'absorption'. This is demonstrated most clearly in the case of *absorption* which is commonly assessed by measurement in the blood. However the vitamin does not function in the plasma but in the cellular membrane, which is a completely different phase. Thus the concept 'absorption' used in the common clinical sense could be a misleading parameter. The *uptake* must also be considered in close relation to the membrane localization of the vitamin. The intestinal epithelial cell where chylomicrons are formed, which transport about 75% of the vitamin, plays a central role in incorporating the vitamin into these globules via the membranes of the endoplasmic reticulum. In conclusion it can be stated that success in diagnostics and therapy in the field of vitamin E is only to be expected if, considering the membrane localization of vitamin E, a more refined approach for assessment of vitamin E deficiency can be developed and therapeutical measures are worked out on the basis of this parameter.

REFERENCES

1. EVANS, H. M. and BISHOP, K. S. (1922), On the existence of a hitherto unrecognized dietary factor essential for reproduction. *Science* 54, 650.
2. SCOTT, M. L. (1970), Studies on vitamin E and related factors in nutrition and metabolism. In: *The fat-soluble vitamins*, p. 355, H. F. DE LUCA and J. W. SUTTIE (eds.). University of Wisconsin Press, Madison.
3. GORDON, W. H. (1958), Studies of tocopherol deficiency in infants and children. *Pediatrics* 21, 673.
4. HORWITT, M. K. (1961), Vitamin E in human nutrition – An interpretative review. *Rev. Nutr. Res.* 22, 1.
5. DANIELLI, J. F. and DAVSON, H. (1935), A contribution to the theory of permeability of thin films. *J. cell. comp. Physiol.* 5, 495.
6. SJÖSTRAND, F. S. (1953), Electron microscopy of mitochondria and cytoplasmic double membranes. *Nature* 171, 30.
7. SINGER, S. J. and NICOLSON, G. L. (1972), The fluid mosaic model of the structure of cell membrane. *Science* 175, 720.
8. HENNING, R., KAULEN, H. D. and STOFFEL, W. (1970), Isolation and chemical composition of the lysosomal and the plasma membrane of the rat liver cell. Hoppe-Seyler Z. *Physiol. Chemie* 351, 1191.
9. OLIVEIRA, M. M., WEGLICKI, W. B., NASON, A. and NAIR, P. P. (1969), Distribution of alpha-tocopherol in beef heart mitochondria. *Biochim. biophys. Acta* 180, 98.
10. SILBER, R., WINTER, R. and KAYDEN, H. J. (1969), Tocopherol transport in the rat erythrocyte. *J. clin. Invest.* 48, 2089.

11. McCay, P. B., Poyer, J. L., Pfeifer, P. M., May, H. E. and Gillian, J. M. (1971), A function for alpha-tocopherol: Stabilization of the microsomal membrane from radical attack during TPNH-dependent oxidation. *Lipids* 6, 297.

12. McCay, P. B., Pfeifer, P. M. and Stipe, W. H. (1972), Vitamin E protection of membrane lipids during electron transport functions. *Ann. New York Acad. Sci.* 203, 62.

13. Lucy, J. A. (1972), Functional and structural aspects of biological membranes: a suggested structural role for vitamin E in the control of membrane permeability and stability. *Ann. New York Acad. Sci.* 203, 4.

14. Diplock, A. T. and Lucy, J. A. (1972), The biochemical modes of action of vitamin E and selenium: a hypothesis. *Febs Letters* 29, 205.

15. Tappel, A. L. (1962), Vitamin E as the biological lipid antioxidant. *Vitam. and Horm.* 20, 493.

16. Tappel, A. L. (1972), Vitamin E and free radical peroxidation of lipids. *Ann. New York Acad. Sci.* 203, 12.

17. Simon, E. J., Gross, Ch. S. and Milhorat, A. T. (1956), The metabolism of vitamin E. *J. biol. Chem.* 221, 797.

18. Krishnamurthy, S. and Bieri, J. G. (1963), The absorption, storage, and metabolism of alpha-tocopherol-C^{14} in the rat and chicken. *J. Lipid Res.* 4, 330.

19. Green, J. and Bunyan, J. (1969), Vitamin E and the biological antioxidant theory. *Nutr. Abstr. Rev.* 39, 321.

20. Glavind, J., Christensen, F. and Sylvén, C. (1971), Intestinal absorption and in vivo formation of lipoperoxides in vitamin E deficient rats. *Acta chem. Scand.* 25, 3220.

21. Molenaar, I., Vos, J. and Hommes, F. A. (1972), Effect of vitamin E deficiency on cellular membranes. *Vitam. and Horm.* 30, 45.

22. Molenaar, I., Hommes, F. A., Braams, W. G. and Polman, H. A. (1968), Effect of vitamin E on membranes of the intestinal cell. *Proc. nat. Acad. Sci.* 61, 982.

23. Molenaar, I., Vos, J., Jager, F. C. and Hommes, F. A. (1970), The influence of vitamin E deficiency on biological membranes. An ultrastructural study on the intestinal epithelial cells of ducklings. *Nutr. and Metabol.* 12, 358.

24. Molenaar, I., Vos, J., Jager, F. C. and Hommes, F. A. (1972), The effect of vitamin E deficiency on the ultrastructure of intestinal epithelial cells and their membranes in particular. In: *International Symposium on Vitamin E. Recent Advance in Physiology and Clinical Use.* Hakone, Japan, September 8th–9th, 1970, p. 76, N. Shimazono and Y. Takagi (eds.) Kyoritsu Shuppan Co. Ltd., Tokyo.

25. Vos, J., Molenaar, I., Searle-van Leeuwen, M. and Hommes, F. A. (1973), Cellular membranes in vitamin E deficiency: an ultrastructural and biochemical study of isolated outer and inner mitochondrial membranes. *Acta agricult. Scand.* Suppl. 19, 192.

26. Vos, J., Molenaar, I., Searle-van Leeuwen, M. and Hommes, F. A. (1972), Mitochondrial and microsomal membranes from livers of vitamin E-deficient ducklings. *Ann. New York Acad. Sci.* 203, 74.

27. Vos, J. (1972), *Cellulaire membranen bij vitamine E gebrek.* Thesis (with summary in English). University of Groningen, Groningen.

28. Green, J. (1958), Distribution of tocopherols during the life-cycle of some plants. *J. Sci. Food Agricult.* 9, 801.

29. Witting, L. A. (1972), Recommended dietary allowance for vitamin E. The *Amer. J. clin. Nutr.* 25, 257.

30. Jager, F. C. (1972), Effect of dietary linoleic acid and selenium on the requirement of vitamin E in ducklings. *Nutr. and Metabol.* 14, 210.

31. VLES, R. O. and JAGER, F. C. (1970), Etude expérimentale des besoin en vitamine E d'ingestion élevée d'acide linoléique. *Intern. Z. Vitaminforsch.* 40, 138.
32. KRISHNAMURTHY, S. and BIERI, J. G. (1963), The absorption, storage and metabolism of α-tocopherol-C^{14} in the rat and chicken. *J. Lipid Res.* 4, 330.
33. SIMON, E. J., GROSS, CH. S. and MILHORAT, A. T. (1956), The metabolism of vitamin E. I. The absorption and excretion of d-α-tocopheryl-5-methyl-C^{14}-succinate. *J. biol. Chem.* 221, 797.
34. MOORE, T., SHARMAN, I. M. and WARD, R. J. (1957), The destruction of vitamin E in flour by chlorine dioxide. *J. Sci. Food Agricult.* 2, 97.
35. LOSOWSKY, M. S. and KELLEHER, J. (1970), Vitamin E research in man in the U.K. *Brit. J. Nutr.* 24, 1033.
36. SMITH, C. L., KELLEHER, J., LOSOWSKY, M. S. and MORRISH, N. (1971), The content of vitamin E in British diets. *Brit. J. Nutr.* 26, 89.
37. JAGER, F. C. (1973), *Linoleic acid intake and vitamin E requirement*. Thesis. Agricultural University, Wageningen.
38. LOSOWSKY, M.S., KELLEHER, J., WALKER, B. E., DAVIS, T. and SMITH, C. L. (1972), Intake and absorption of tocopherol. *Ann. New York Acad. Sci.* 203, 212.
39. BIERI, J. G. (1972), Kinetics of tissue α-tocopherol depletion and repletion, *Ann. New York Acad. Sci.* 203, 181.
40. UNDERWOOD, B. A., DENNING, C. R. and NAVAB, M. (1972), Polyunsaturated fatty acids and tocopherol levels in patients with cystic fibrosis. *Ann. New York Acad. Sci.* 203, 237.
41. MACMAHON, M. T. and NEALE, G. (1970), The absorption of α-tocopherol in control subjects and in patients with intestinal malabsorption. *Clin. Sci.* 38, 197.
42. PEARSON, C. K. and LEGGE, A. M. (1972), Uptake of vitamin E by rat small intestinal slices. *Biochim. biophys. Acta* 288, 404.
43. GALLO-TORRES, H. E. (1970), Obligatory role of bile for the intestinal absorption of vitamin E. *Lipids* 5, 379.
44. KATER, R. M. H., UNTERECKER, W. J., KIM, C. Y. and DAVIDSON, C. S. (1970), Relationship of serum tocopherol to beta-lipoprotein concentrations in liver diseases. *Amer. J. clin. Nutr.* 23, 913.
45. GÖRANSSON, G., NORDÉN, Å. and ÅKESSON, B. (1973), Low plasma tocopherol levels in patients with gastrointestinal disorders. *Scand. J. Gastroenterol.* 8, 21.
46. DARBY, C. W., DAVIDSON, A. G. F. and DESAI, I. D. (1973), Muscular performance in cystic fibrosis patients and its relation to vitamin E. *Arch. Dis. Childh.* 48, 72.
47. THOMPSON, J. N. and SCOTT, M. L. (1970), Impaired lipid and vitamin E absorption related to atrophy of the pancreas in selenium-deficient chicks. *J. Nutr.* 100, 797.
48. BLOMSTRAND, R. and FORSGREN, L. (1968), Labelled tocopherols in man. *Intern. Z. Vitaminforsch.* 38, 328.
49. AMENT, M. E., SHIMODA, S. S., SAUNDERS, D. R. and RUBIN, C. E. (1972), Pathogenesis of steatorrhea in three cases of small intestinal stasis syndrome. *Gastroenterology* 63, 728.
50. STOELINGA, G. B. A., VAN MUNSTER, P. J. J. and SLOOFF, J. P. (1963), Chylous effusions into the intestine in a patient with protein-losing gastroenteropathy. *Pediatrics* 31, 1011.
51. WRETLIND, A. (1972), Complete intravenous nutrition. Theoretical and experimental background. *Nutr. and Metabol.* 14, 1.
52. HRUBÀ, F., VULTERINOVÀ, NOVÁKOVÁ, V. and PLACER, Z. (1971), Reflection of tocopherol saturation in the haemogram of healthy subjects. International *J. Vitam. Nutr. Res.* 41, 521.

THERAPEUTIC EFFECTS OF LINOLEIC ACID

A. J. VERGROESEN*

The physiological importance of fats as nutrients can be separated into an unspecific, although useful, role as a source of calories and as carriers of fat-soluble vitamins on the one hand and into a specific activity as essential fatty acids (EFA) on the other. In this review I shall restrict myself to a discussion of the latter aspect.

Except in cases of chronic fat malabsorption, or diets of extremely abnormal composition, the syndrome of EFA-deficiency in children as described by HANSEN (1, 2) is a rare phenomenon which can easily be cured by the addition of a few cal% of linoleic acid to the diet, if necessary by parenteral nutrition (3). Especially in infants with protein malnutrition who start to gain weight during treatment with high-protein diets, EFA-deficient diets given for only 5–10 days can cause perceptible depletion of the reserves of EFA. If these children are maintained for longer periods on such a diet, the ratio of 20:3 (n—9)/20:4 (n—6) in tissue and serum phospholipids will reach values up to 18, severe dermal lesions will develop and, what is probably even more important, an increased susceptibility to infection will occur (3).

Much more important is the role of cis-cis linoleic acid – the most common EFA in human nutrition – in the prevention of atherosclerosis. Although usually not diagnosed before the age of 40, the onset of this disease is in infancy and childhood. Recent papers (4, 5, 6) underline the necessity for reorientation in the prevention of cardiovascular diseases by giving priority to children instead of adults. As many as 13–33% of the school children (5) in the USA have serum cholesterol levels above 200 mg per 100 ml serum, which is thought generally to be too high. Mean blood cholesterol levels in Mexican and Wisconsin school children are 100 and 186 mg per 100 ml, respectively, without appreciable differences between the 5–9 and 10–14 year old children in either of the populations studied and without noticeable differences

* Unilever Research, Vlaardingen, The Netherlands

between the sexes (7). Apparently blood lipid composition patterns are already established early in life by social and nutritional habits; preventive measures should therefore be taken as early as possible. Neonatal familial Type II hyperlipoproteinaemia (FREDRICKSON's classification) has been diagnosed in circa 1% of 1800 consecutive unselected live births in a general hospital (8). Early recognition of this condition is important as the disease may be fatal even in childhood if left untreated, whereas the blood cholesterol levels can be normalized to a large extent by dietary measures (9).

In juvenile diabetes mellitus and in diabetic adults during periods of inadequate control, abnormal serum lipid compositions are also commonly observed (10); it is now recognized that this hyperlipidaemia is associated with atheromatous lesions which tend to appear at an early age and which progress rapidly. Thus prevention of hyperlipidaemia is an important consideration in the management of diabetes, particularly in children.

Consumption of a diet rich in EFA has been shown to reduce the levels of serum lipids in healthy volunteers, in diabetics and in patients with hypercholesterolaemia (see for a recent review, Ref. 11). However, considerable confusion still exists as to which dietary modification is most effective and yet still acceptable for consumption on a long-term basis. The availability of sufficient products rich in linoleic acid is essential for dietary control of hyperlipidaemia, as was demonstrated by the eventual failure of an initially successful treatment of juvenile diabetes patients with corn oil diets (12, 13).

With respect to the efficacy of blood-lipid-lowering diets, our data (14, 15) indicate that – contrary to the opinion of for instance GROEN (16) – substitution of saturated fat in the diet by monosaccharides or polysaccharides decreases serum cholesterol levels less than substitution by linoleic acid. It is claimed that for many dietary changes satisfactory prediction of the average change in the serum cholesterol level of man can be made using Keys' equation: $\triangle$ chol. (mg per 100 ml serum) $=1.35$ ($2 \triangle S - \triangle P$) $+ 1.5 \triangle Z$, where S and P are percentages of total calories provided by saturated and polyunsaturated fatty acids in the diet and $Z^2 =$ mg of dietary cholesterol per 1000 kcal (17). Although KEYS himself stated that this equation is of limited value and only applicable to the dietary compositions actually studied, the formula is generally interpreted in the sense that a reduction of saturated fatty acids is twice as effective as the same increase in polyunsaturated fatty acids. The real situation is however much more complex. The different saturated fatty acids have different quantitative effects on blood cholesterol levels – lauric, myristic and palmitic acid probably being the most effective and the saturated fatty acids with less than 12 carbon atoms being comparable to oleic acid (14, 17, 18, 19). Furthermore, we recently observed that elaidic acid (18:1 ω9-trans) in the presence – but not in the absence – of dietary cholesterol has a definite serum-cholesterol-increasing effect compared with oleic acid (18:1 ω9-cis). In fact, 18:1 ω9-trans was only slightly less active than a mixture of lauric and myristic acid consumed in equal amounts (15). Moreover, variations in poly-unsaturated fatty acids ($\triangle$P) cannot always be clearly related to blood lipid concentrations; increasing the linoleic acid concentration of a liquid formula diet containing 40 cal% fat (including 115 mg cholesterol/1000 kcal) from 10 to 34% at the expense of oleic acid decreased the effect of a 37% mixture of lauric and myristic fatty acid on the serum cholesterol concentration but not that of 34% elaidic acid or 36% oleic acid (15) (Fig. 1). It was further observed that even extremely large amounts of linoleic acid – up to 95% linoleic acid in a cholesterol-free liquid formula diet containing 50 cal% fat – do not improve the 20–25% reduction in blood cholesterol concentration obtainable with 35 cal% safflower oil containing 75% linoleic acid and 18% palmitic acid (14). In fact, the same 20–25% reduction in blood cholesterol was observed in a group of about 100 adolescents (12–18 years old, 80% of whom were boys) consuming a 'normal' Dutch diet (35–45 cal% fat and a daily intake of 200–500 mg cholesterol) in which margarine with 50–55% linoleic acid and about 25% saturated fatty acids, sunflower seed oil and a filled milk (3.5% safflower seed oil in skimmed milk) were substituted for butter, lard and normal milk (3.5% butterfat) (14). During the high linoleic acid period the children consumed 20–25 cal% linoleic acid, which is sufficient to fully com-pensate for the blood-lipid-increasing effects of saturated fatty acids (about 10 cal%) and cholesterol. This is in good agreement with the conclusions drawn by BROWN (11) from her own, KEYS' and HEG-STED's dietary studies predicting that under the above-mentioned conditions, the maximum effect of linoleic acid will manifest itself at 17 cal%. Quite interestingly, McGANDY et al. in a somewhat similar study, (20) in which the linoleic acid intake was increased by 10 cal% to a total of 13 cal%, induced a mean fall in blood cholesterol con-

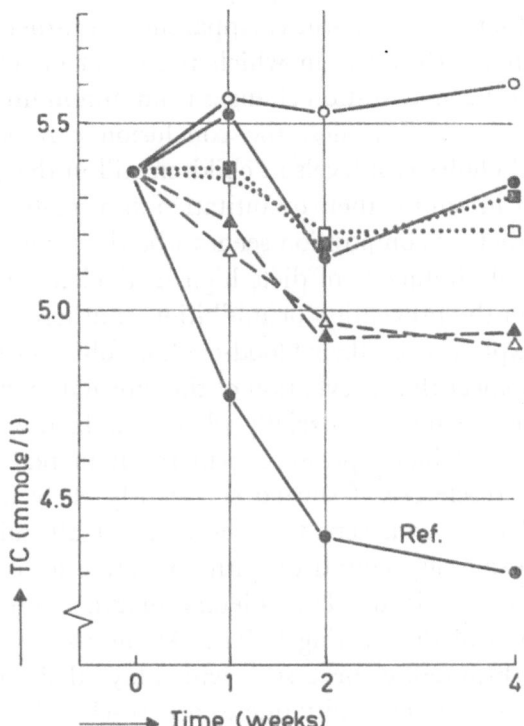

Fig. 1. Influence of a liquid formula diet (LFD), with 40 cal% fat, given for 4 weeks, on total fasting serum cholesterol concentrations (TC) in male and female volunteers. The percentage composition of the experimental fatty acid mixtures (prepared by mixing coconut oil or unhardened olive oil with safflower seed oil) was as follows:

							Reference
Experimental group	△	□	○	▲	■	◐	diet
Number of volunteers	12	12	12	11	12	12	17
Palmitic + stearic acid	13	14	12	12	13	11	10
Lauric + myristic acid	–	–	37	–	–	37	–
Elaidic acid	–	34	–	–	34	–	–
Oleic acid (extra)	36	–	–	36	–	–	–
Oleic acid		41			18		14
Linoleic acid		10			34		76

Dried egg yolk was added to these mixtures to obtain a LFD containing 115 mg cholesterol/1000 kcal (4.184 MJ) (average daily LFD consumption about 1900 kcal (7.949 MJ). A cholesterol–free LFD, with 40 cal% fat in safflower seed oil, was used as reference diet.

centration which although still highly significant was much less than the decrease observed in our study. Apparently, a rather narrow range exists (between 12–16 cal%) in which the effect of linoleic acid on serum cholesterol concentration changes from minimum to maximum. From these and other studies, the conclusion can be drawn that although blood cholesterol levels in children still in the growth period are lower than in adults, their quantitative and qualitative responses to changes in dietary composition seem to be the same.

The favourable influence of diets high in linoleic acid and low in saturated fat on the prevention or inhibition of atherosclerotic disease is commonly explained by their blood-cholesterol-lowering effect. It is reasonable to expect that prevention of the 'normal' increase in blood lipoprotein levels with age, especially when combined with prevention of a rise in arterial blood pressure, will result in real primary prevention of atherosclerosis if started sufficiently early in life. Nevertheless we still have to accept that most, if not all, adults living in developed (prosperous) countries with moderate-to-serious atherosclerosis will respond, if at all, to dietary modifications with only a partial regression of the existing lesions. At the sites of these lesions, intra-arterial thrombotic processes will play their primary and secondary roles in the morbidity due to atherosclerosis.

In this respect the studies of HORNSTRA (21, 22, 23) may be of great importance, as they can provide an additional explanation for the efficacy of high-linoleic-acid diets in primary and secondary prevention trials. In his experiments, HORNSTRA inserted a polyethylene cannula in the aorta of rats. At the tip of the cannula, platelet thrombi develop which after a variable time (the obturation time, OT) block the aorta completely. When the rats are fed diets containing increasing concentrations of linoleic acid, the OT appears to be dependent upon the dose and increases from 3.8 days (3 cal% linoleic acid) to 7.0 days (37 cal% linoleic acid) (21). Possibly this effect can be explained by a change in the fatty acid composition of the cellular membranes of endothelium and platelets, resulting in decreased thrombotic properties of these tissues. Furthermore, the high-linoleic-acid diets will change the fatty acid composition of adipose tissue and therefore the type of fatty acids released into the blood under, for instance, the influence of higher catecholamine concentrations. It has been demonstrated in vitro that albumin-bound linoleic acid has much less effect than, for instance, oleic and palmitic acid, which enhance platelet aggregation (24). Another explanation can be found in the possibility of an increased biosynthesis of prostaglandin E_1 (PGE_1), a very potent inhibitor of platelet adhesion and aggregation. In nearly all organs, PGE_1 is synthesized in response to a stimulation of the organ (nervous or hormonal) from dihomo-γ-linolenic acid (20:3 ω 6, 9, 12), an intermediate formed during the conversion of linoleic acid (18:2 ω 6, 9) into arachidonic acid (20:4 ω 6, 9, 12, 15). Both 20:3 ω 6, 9, 12 and 20:4 ω 6, 9, 12, 15 are present in the phospholipids of cell membranes and after release by phospholipase A can be converted locally by PG-synthetase into PGE_1 and PGE_2, respectively. PGE_2 does not inhibit platelet aggregation; in fact, it has a slight stimulating effect. Since the feeding of increasing amounts of linoleic acid does not result in increasing concentrations of arachidonic acid in cell membranes, it is possible that PGE_1 biosynthesis from 20:3 ω 6, 9, 12 is stimulated (25).

Apart from the inhibiting effect of PGE_1 on platelet aggregation and adhesion, PGE_1 (as well as PGE_2) has hypotensive effects, antagonizes the hypertensive properties of adrenaline and angiotensin, is a potent inhibitor of catecholamine-induced free fatty acid release from adipose tissue, increases natriuresis especially after its inhibition by vasopressin and finally decreases the influence of both sympathetic and parasympathetic nerve stimulation on myocardial tissue (26, 27). Thus the PGs can influence most of the recognized risk factors in atherosclerotic heart disease, suggesting a preventive or curative role of linoleic acid through increased PG synthesis. However mainly because of analytical problems, no quantitative relationship between the amounts of dietary linoleic acid and PG-biosynthesis in vivo has so far been measured. Nevertheless, the results of the following experiment might contribute to a better understanding of the role of high-linoleic acid diets in the reduction of cardiovascular diseases.

A newly developed method (23) for measuring platelet 'stickiness' directly in venous blood was used on a sample from the participants of a primary prevention trial performed in Finland (28). In this trial the use of a blood-cholesterol-lowering diet (linoleic acid concentration about 12 cal%) was associated with considerably and significantly reduced mortality from ischemic heart disease in comparison with the men consuming a 'normal' Finnish diet (linoleic acid concentration about 4 cal%). Venous blood was drawn from fasting men (73 controls, 63 from the high-linoleic acid group) through a microfilter, pore size: 20 μm, into a motor-driven syringe at a constant rate of 2.25 ml/minute. This filtration method is based on the use of a pore size which permits passage of red and white cells and platelets but is occluded by platelet aggregates. Heparin was infused into the siliconized system proximal to the filter at an anticoagulant concentration of 5 units/ml blood. Pressure was monitored proximal and distal to the filter, the rise in pressure difference reflecting occlusion of the filter by aggregated platelets. Macroscopic inspection and scanning electron microscopy of the filter confirmed the presence of aggregated platelets and the absence of blood clots. The aggregation time (AT) was taken to be the number of seconds required to reach the arbitrarily chosen pressure gradient of 5 mm Hg. The mean AT for the control group was 72 seconds compared with 114 seconds for the experimental group; this difference is highly significant statistically ($p_2 < 0.001$). It can therefore be concluded that the platelet function, as assessed by the filter method, was profoundly different in the control and experimental subjects. The prolonged aggregation time in the subjects receiving a diet low in saturated fat and high in linoleic acid implies decreased aggregatability of platelets, which is in good agreement with the decreased tendency toward arterial thrombus formation observed in rats receiving the same diet (21). It is therefore conceivable that the alteration in platelet function observed in this study contributed to the reduction in ischemic heart disease mortality in the Helsinki trial (28). Unpublished results from other clinical centers strongly suggest that patients with hyperlipaemia, diabetes or after a myocardial infarction normally display short ATs which gradually become longer after shifting to high-linoleic-acid diets. The implications of these results for the treatment of patients with cardiovascular diseases seem to be evident.

REFERENCES

1. HANSEN, A. E., HAGGARD, M. E., BOELSCHE, A. E., ADAM, D. J. D. and WIESE, H. F. (1958), Essential fatty acids in infant nutrition. III. Clinical Manifestation of linoleic acid deficiency. *J. Nutr.* 66, 565.
2. HANSEN, A. E., WIESE, H. F., BOELSCHE, A. N., HAGGARD, M. E., ADAM, D. J. D. and DAVIES, H. (1963), Role of linoleic acid in infant nutrition. Clinical and chemical study of 428 infants fed on milk mixtures varying in kind and amount of fat. *Pediatrics* 31 (Suppl. 1), 171.
3. PAULSRUD, J. R., PENSLER, L., WHITTEN, C. F., STEWART, S. and HOLMAN, R. T. (1972), Essential fatty acid deficiency in infants induced by fat-free intravenous feeding. *Amer. J. clin. Nutr.* 25, 897.

4. KANNEL, W. B., DAWBER, T. R. (1972), Atherosclerosis as a pediatric problem. *J. Pediatr.* 80, 544.
5. HAAS, J. H. DE (1973), Primary prevention of coronary heart disease, a socio-pediatric problem. *Hart Bull.* 4, 3.
6. FREDRICKSON, D. S. (1972), Introduction to symposium: Factors in childhood that influence the development of atherosclerosis and hypertension. *Amer. J. clin. Nutr.* 25, 221.
7. GOLUBJATNIKOV, R., PASKEY, T. and INHORN, S. L. (1972), Serum cholesterol levels of Mexican and Wisconsin school children. *Amer. J. Epidemiol.* 96, 36.
8. GLUECK, C. J. and TSANG, R. C. (1972), Pediatric familial type. II. hyperlipoproteinemia: effects of diet on plasma cholesterol in the first year of life. *Amer. J. clin. Nutr.* 25, 224.
9. KWITEROVICH, P. O., LEVY, R. I. and FREDRICKSON, D. S. (1970), Early detection and treatment of familial type. II. hyperlipoproteinemia. *Circulation* (Suppl. III) 62, 37.
10. CHANCE, G. W., ALBUTT, E. C. and EDKINS, S. M. (1969), Serum lipids and lipoproteins in untreated diabetic children. *Lancet* i, 1126.
11. BROWN, H. B. (1971), Food patterns that lower blood lipids in man. *J. Amer. diet. Ass.* 58, 303.
12. LLOYD, J. K. (1966), Control of dietary fat in relation to diabetic complications in children. *Proc. Nutr. Soc.* 25, 74.
13. CHANCE, G. W., ALBUTT, E. C. and EDKINS, S. M. (1969), Control of hyperlipidaemia in Juvenile Diabetes. Standard and corn oil diets compared over a period of 10 years. *Brit. med. J.* 3, 616.
14. VERGROESEN, A. J. and DE BOER, J. (1971), Effecten van meervoudig onverzadigde en andere vetzuren in de voeding. *Voeding* 32, 278.
15. VERGROESEN, A. J. (1972), Dietary fat and cardiovascular disease: possible modes of action of linoleic acid. *Proc. Nutr. Soc.* 31, 323.
16. GROEN, J. J. (1967), Effect of bread in the diet on serum cholesterol. *Amer. J. clin. Nutr.* 20, 191.
17. KEYS, A., ANDERSON, J. T. and GRANDE, F. (1965), Serum cholesterol response to changes in the diet. IV Particular saturated fatty acids in the diet. *Metabolism* 14, 776.
18. HEGSTED, D. M., McGANDY, R. B., MYERS, M. L. and STARE, F. J. (1965), Quantitative effects of dietary fat on serum cholesterol in man. *Amer. J. clin. Nutr.* 17, 281.
19. HEGSTED, D. M., McGANDY, R. B., MYERS, M. L. and STARE, F. J. (1968), Effects of Specific Fatty Acids on Serum Cholesterol in Man: Studies with Semi-synthetic Materials. In: *Symposium Dairy Lipids and Lipid Metabolism. Chicago, 1967*, M. F. Brink and D. Kritchevsky (eds.). The Air Publishing Company, Westport, Connecticut, 161.
20. McGANDY, R. B., HALL, B., FORD, C. and STARE, F. J. (1972), Dietary regulation of blood cholesterol in adolescent males: A pilot study. *Amer. J. clin. Nutr.* 25, 61.
21. HORNSTRA, G. (1971), The influence of dietary sunflowerseed oil and hardened coconut oil on intra-arterial occlusive thrombosis in rats. *Nutr. and Metabol.* 13, 140.
22. HORNSTRA, G. and VENDELMANS, A. (1973), Induction of experimental arterial occlusive thrombi in rats. *Atherosclerosis* 17, 369.
23. HORNSTRA, G., LEWIS, B., CHAIT, A., TURPEINEN, O., KARVONEN, M. J. and VERGROESEN, A. J. (1973), Influence of dietary fat on platelet function in men. *Lancet* i, 1155.

24. HOAK, J. C., SPECTOR, A. A., FRY, G. L. and WARNER, E. D. (1970), Effect of free fatty acids on ADP-induced platelet aggregation. *Nature* 228, 1330.
25. THOMASSON, H. J. (1969), Prostaglandins and cardiovascular disease. *Nutr. et Dieta (Basel)* 11, 228.
26. RAMWELL, P. (ed.) (1973), *The prostaglandins*. Plenum Press, New York, London.
27. HORTON, E. W. (1972), *Prostaglandins*. Springer Verlag, Berlin, Heidelberg, New York.
28. MIETTINEN, M., TURPEINEN, O., KARVONEN, M. J., ELOSUO, R. and PAAVILAINEN, E. (1972), Effect of cholesterol-lowering diet on mortality from coronary heart disease and other causes. A twelve-year Clinical Trial in Men and Women. *Lancet* ii, 835.

PROTEIN AND AMINO ACIDS

D. M. HEGSTED*

The Joint FAO/WHO Expert Committee on Energy and Protein Requirements has recently considered protein and amino acid requirements and the report of this Committee is expected to be published shortly. My approach today will be to briefly consider the findings of this Committee and then comment on some of the inadequacies, uncertainties and disagreements in this field. Some of the concepts of protein and amino acid metabolism which have been generally accepted for many years are now being recognized as less than adequate. The field is in transition and it is a difficult time to develop a concensus.

For the past 15 to 20 years protein requirements at different ages have been estimated by the so-called 'factorial method' (1–4). This can be briefly described as follows.

First, the minimal obligatory nitrogen excretion which develops a few days to a week after a protein-free or very low protein diet is fed is estimated. The urinary nitrogen falls rather rapidly under such conditions and is the major nitrogen loss. In the past the minimal urinary nitrogen excretion has been assumed to be approximated by 2 mg nitrogen/basal calorie/day. To this obligatory nitrogen loss are added estimates of minimal fecal loss, excretion through the skin, etc. to arrive at a total minimal obligatory nitrogen loss.

Second, for infants and children and during pregnancy and lactation an addition is made for the minimal nitrogen needs required for the formation of new tissues or for milk. The amount of nitrogen involved is estimated from the rates of tissue growth or the amount of milk produced.

Third, it is assumed that these minimal nitrogen needs can be directly translated into minimal protein needs. That is, it has been

* Department of Nutrition, Harvard School of Public Health, Boston, Massachusetts.

assumed that certain proteins are 100% efficient in fulfilling these obligatory nitrogen needs.

Fourth, since most diets contain proteins which are not 100% utilized, a correction is made to convert the minimal protein needs into the needs for proteins which are less efficiently utilized. Measurements of biological value (BV) as defined by MITCHELL (5) or of net protein utilization (NPU) (6) have been assumed to be adequate measures of protein quality. Thus, if the BV of the protein in a diet were 50%, i.e., only 50% as efficient as the best quality protein, the minimal requirement would be doubled.

Finally, since these kinds of estimates are based upon average values and it is recognized that individuals do vary, some correction is added to cover individual differences, an allowance for safety, a fudge factor to cover ignorance, etc. Since information is minimal this kind of correction has been based almost entirely upon the judgment of the group making the recommendation.

The findings of the most recent FAO/WHO Committee differ in several respects from the prior reports. In the first place there are convincing data available to show that the minimal urinary nitrogen is less than 2 mg nitrogen/basal calorie/day and on the average is nearer to 1.4 mg nitrogen/basal calorie/day (7–9). This finding would normally lower the requirement by about 30%. However, the same papers also demonstrate that highest quality proteins, such as egg protein, are not as efficiently utilized in adult man or adult rats as was formerly thought. Rather, they appear to be only about 60 to 70% efficient in replacing the obligatory nitrogen losses. Thus, although the Committee found that the obligatory nitrogen losses were less than previous estimates, they found it necessary to raise the amount of protein required to replace these losses. The difference in net protein required was small and not very significant.

In fig. 1 I have indicated several of the published recommendations for different ages starting with the report of HEGSTED in 1957 (1). That report did not include any allowance for safety or for individual variation and is therefore considerably below subsequent recommendations. If an additional 30% or so were added to these values, they would approach several of the other estimates.

It is clear that not much change has been made in the estimated requirements of infants. These values are influenced greatly by the protein content of breast milk. Nevertheless, it is of interest that the theoretical approach which I have outlined above does, in fact, yield estimates very close to the protein consumed by breast fed infants, assuming that protein in breast milk is 100% utilizable for maintenance and for growth. Since it is assumed that such young infants will ordinarily consume diets of very high quality, no correction for protein quality is applied until 6 months or so of age.

Since infants have the highest relative growth rate of any group, their protein needs per unit weight are much higher than for any other group. It is of interest, therefore, that the protein content of breast milk and many of the commercial formulae are quite low-6 to 7% of the total calories being supplied as protein. Few staple foods except for rice, cassava, etc., have a protein content this low and this has undoubtedly influenced thinking about protein needs of other age groups.

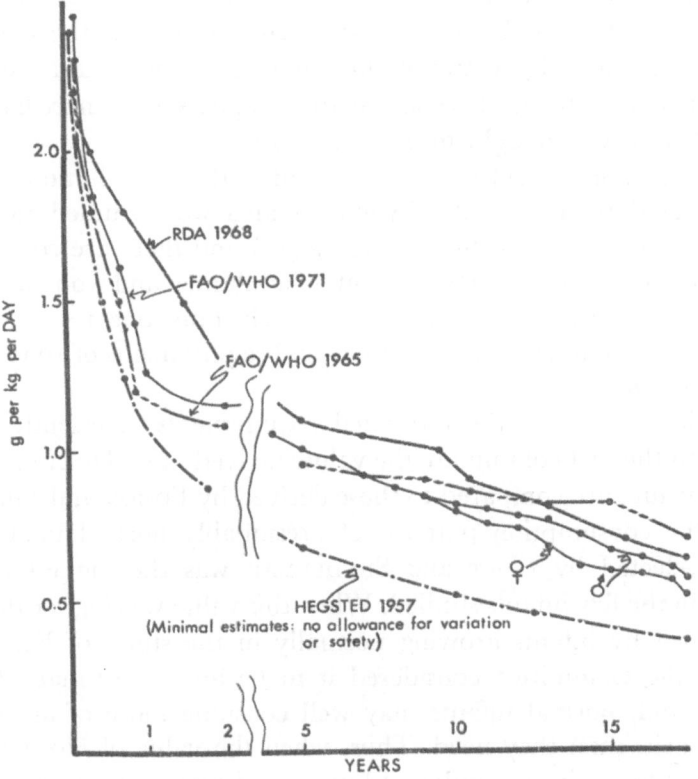

Fig. 1. Recommended intakes from various groups compared to minimal estimates made in 1957.

It is not possible to discuss the reasons for the differences in the curves shown in fig. 1. Most of the difference with age is related or justified by changes in rate of growth. Other differences represent compromises arrived at by the Committees and often the reasons for these are not clearly discernible. Some differences in the published values represent differences in the assumed quality of the protein in the usual diet.

It should be clear to everyone that these curves are derived largely by extrapolation from limited data obtained at a few ages. The data on protein needs of young infants seem reasonably secure in that feeding practice and theory apparently agree. There are also a considerable amount of data obtained with adult subjects. An inspection of these data in the literature reveals numerous discrepancies and inconsistencies, probably due to differences in the design of the studies, differences in the degree of control, etc. However, the major point to be made is that in between infancy and adulthood the curves are influenced more by extrapolation than by actual data. As I will indicate in a moment, this extrapolation appears to be more hazardous now than it was thought to be in the past.

Data on amino acid requirements suffer the same limitations. The amino acid requirements of young infants were studied rather extensively by HOLT and his colleagues (10) and there are considerable data on the amino acid requirements of adult men and women (11, 12). In between these extremes there is really only one report, that of NAKAGAWA et al. (13) on the amino acid requirements of 10 to 12 year old children.

Table 1 indicates the estimated requirements of essential amino acids. In the first column are the values arrived at by HOLT et al. (10). These values are compared to those derived by FOMON and FILER (14) from the consumption patterns of presumably normal infants. The value selected by HOLT and SNYDERMAN was the highest estimate found in the few infants studied. When this value was higher than that consumed by infants growing normally in the study of FOMON and FILER, the Committee considered it to be an overestimate. On the other hand, normal infants may well consume more of an essential amino acid than they need. Thus, when the value of HOLT was less than that found in the studies of FOMON and FILER, the value given by HOLT was selected as the best estimate of requirement. In the last column are given the amounts of each amino acid which would be

Table 1. *Estimated amino acid requirements of infants*

Amino Acids	Estimated Requirements		Composite of Lower Values	Suggested Pattern[3]
	Holt & Sniperman[1]	Fomon & Filer[2]		
	mg/kg/day	mg/kg/day	mg/kg/day	mg/g protein
Histidine	34	28	28	14
Isoleucine	119	70	70	35
Leucine	229	161	161	80
Lysine	103	161	103	52
Methionine + cystine	45 + Cys	58[4]	58	29
Phenylalanine + tyrosine	90 + Tyr	125[4]	125	63
Threonine	87	116	87	44
Tryptophan	22	17	17	8.5
Valine	105	93	93	47

Taken from FAO/WHO report (4).

1. Requirements estimated when amino acids were fed or incorporated in basal formulas. The values represent estimates of maximal individual requirements to achieve normal growth (10).
2. Calculated intakes of amino acids when formulas were fed in amounts sufficient to maintain good growth in all the infants studied – the amino acids were not varied independently (14).
3. Based on a safe level of intake of 2 g protein/kg/day, the average of suggested levels for the period 0–6 months.
4. The values for cystine and tyrosine were estimated on the basis of the methionine:cystine and phenylalanine:tyrosine ratios in human milk.

Table 2. *Estimated amino acid requirements of adults.*

Amino Acids	Some Reported Amino Acid Requirements			Combined Adult Value[4]	Suggested Pattern[5]
	Men[1]	Women			
		Observed[2]	Recalculated[3]		
	mg/day	mg/day	mg/day	mg/kg/day	mg/g protein
Histidine	0	0	0	0	0
Isoleucine	700	450	550	10	18
Leucine	1100	710	730	14	25
Lysine	800	700	545	12	22
Methionine + cystine	1100	550	700	13	24
Phenylalanine + tyrosine	1100	700	—	14	25
Threonine	500	310	375	7	13
Tryptophan	250	160	168	3.5	6.5
Valine	800	650	622	10	18

Taken from FAO/WHO report (4).

1. Taken from ROSE (11). The values represent the highest estimate of individual requirement to achieve positive nitrogen balance.
2. Taken from LEVERTON and co-workers (references summarized by IRWIN & HEGSTED, *J. Nutr.* 101, 539, 1971). The values represent the highest estimate of individual requirement to achieve the zone of nitrogen equilibrium (balance of 0 ± 5% of intake).
3. Data of some of the above authors recalculated by HEGSTED (12) using regression analysis to estimate the average requirement to achieve nitrogen equilibrium.
4. Derived estimate emphasizing the upper range of individual requirements.
5. Assuming a safe level of protein intake of 0.55 g/kg/day (averaged value for men and women).

required in the dietary protein, assuming that the infant required 2 g of protein/kg/day.

Table 2 indicates the origin of the estimated requirements of amino acids for adults. These values are largely those derived by ROSE in his classic studies (11) and those on adult women (12). Again, in the last column is the mg of amino acid required per gm of protein assuming that the minimal protein need of the adult was 0.55 g/kg/day.

Table 3. *Essential amino acid requirements per unit protein**

Age	Protein requirements	Total amino acid requirements	
	g/kg	mg/kg	mg/g protein
Infants	2.0	742	373
10–12 years	0.8	262	326
Adult	0.55	84	152

* Taken from WHO/FAO Report (4).

Table 3 indicates the problem that has to be dealt with. In the first column are the estimates of the total protein need. These fall from 2 g/kg in infancy to 0.55 in adulthood. The adult is assumed to need only about 25% as much protein as the infant. Yet as shown in the next column the estimated need for essential amino acids is only about 11% that of the infant. The essential amino acid needs appear to fall much lower than the nitrogen need. Thus, when the essential amino acid need is expressed per unit protein (last column), the Committee concludes that a protein which contained only 152 mg of essential amino acid/g or 15% of essential amino acids would supply all of the essential amino acids in adequate amounts even though fed at a minimal level. In contrast, the protein required by infants would have to contain 373 mg/g or 37% in order to be adequate at the minimal level.

High quality proteins like egg and milk contain nearly 50% of their total amino acids as essential amino acids. There are no proteins which have as little as 15% of their total amino acids as essential amino acids. The net conclusion is that protein quality is of little importance in adults whereas it may be very important in infants or young children. This implies that protein quality is not only a function of the protein but also a function of the individual who eats it. Thus, the problem of calculating the protein needs of a population becomes extremely complicated.

A further complication is provided by the data on the 10 to 12 year olds studied by NAKAGAWA et al. These estimates are relatively high compared to the rate of growth of these children. If growth rate is not the factor which influences the amino acid requirements, then we are left with no indication of what factors do influence these needs. Extrapolation thus becomes very difficult. It is possible or likely that the estimate derived by NAKAGAWA et al. is simply more generous than that developed for adults but since few individuals were studied there is no satisfactory way to explain the differences.

Now, I should like to turn to some other studies which bear on these problems and indicate the nature of some of the disagreements and uncertainties which need solution. There is abundant evidence that the young rat is a very efficient utilizer of protein. Figure 2, for example,

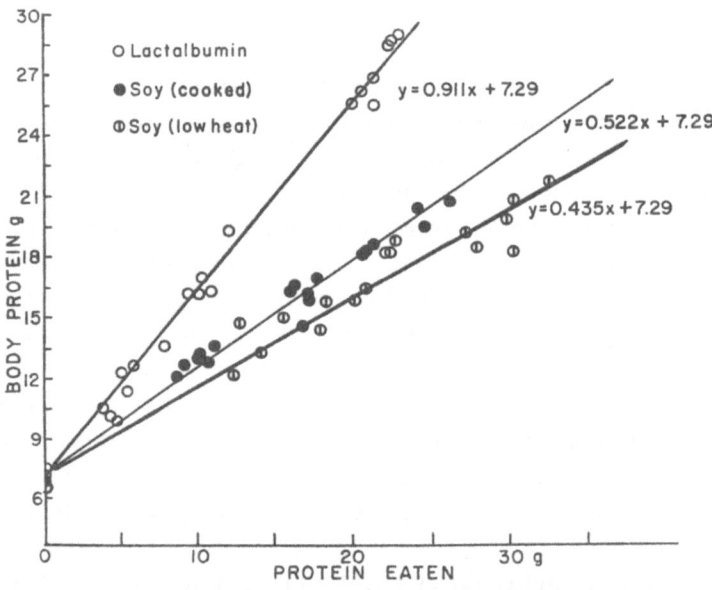

Fig. 2. Change in body protein of young rats fed diets with different protein contents for three weeks.

shows the change in body protein of young rats fed diets containing different amounts of a high quality protein, such as lactalbumin. This line has a slope of 0.91 indicating that 91% of the lactalbumin consumed can be accounted for in new body protein, i.e., for each gram of lactalbumin protein consumed the body protein increased by 0.91 g.

This is not a maximum value and many values have been reported for egg protein which approach 95–100%.

As I will indicate later, the slope of such a line is the best estimate of the relative protein quality of a protein for the young rat.

We have studied the protein needs of infant cebus monkeys (15) and the data from one of the proteins are shown in fig. 3. The technique was simply to feed infant monkeys a liquid formula which varied in protein content, to measure the food consumed accurately, and to measure the growth rate over a three week test period. The protein content of the diet was then changed and another three week test period followed. The monkeys ranged in age from 8 weeks to about one year.

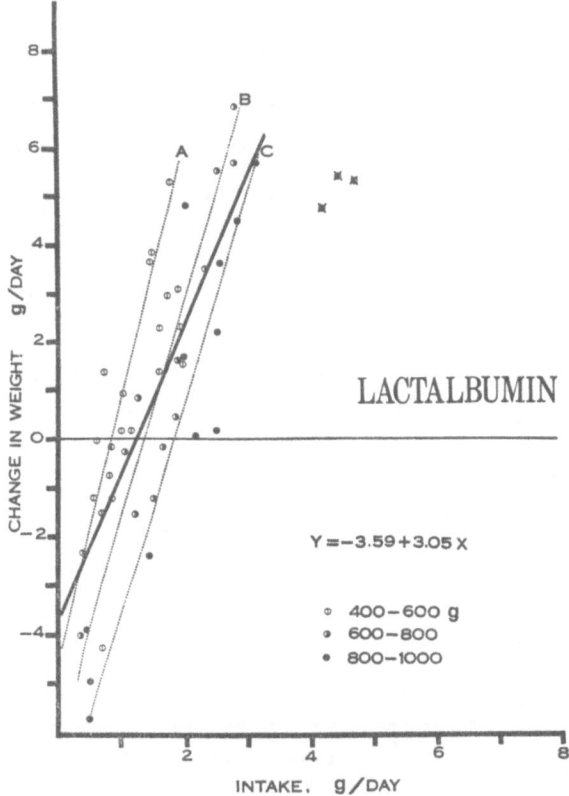

Fig. 3. Change in body weight of infant cebus monkeys fed different quantities of lactalbumin. Taken from Samonds and Hegsted (15).

As shown in fig. 3 and as would be expected, larger animals consumed more food and the data were arbitrarily divided into three
weight groups – those between 400 and 600 g, 600–800 g, and 800–
1000 g. Three distinct regression lines could be calculated which have a
similar slope. The usual procedure to correct for differences in weight
is to report the intake per unit weight. When this is done (fig. 4) it is of
interest that the maintenance requirement, the amount required to just
maintain weight, is essentially constant at approximately 2 g/kg.
However, a family of lines with different slopes are generated, the
smaller animals having a much lower slope than the larger animals.
This seems readily explicable even though we did not expect it. An
animal of 500 g which received 1 g/kg in excess of his maintenance

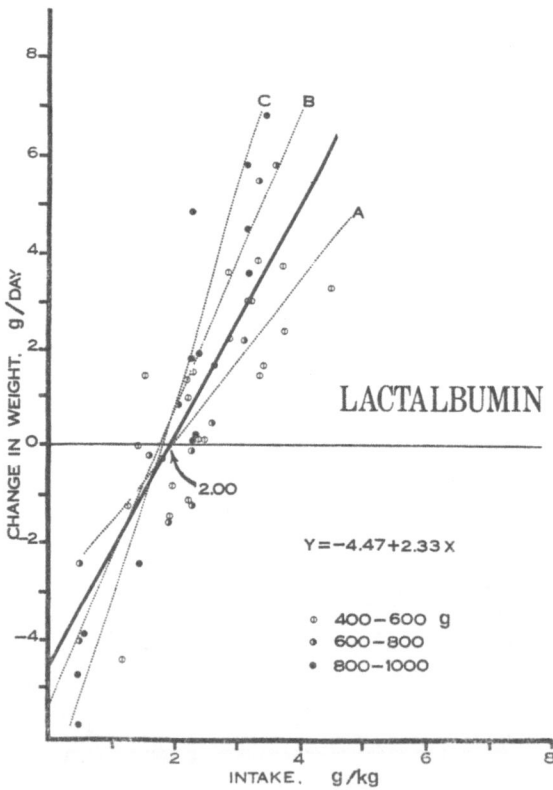

Fig. 4. Change in weight of infant cebus monkeys fed different quantities of lactalbumin (intake expressed per unit body weight; same data as in Fig. 3). Taken from
SAMONDS and HEGSTED (15).

requirement (3 g/kg) will receive 0.5 g of protein which can be utilized for growth whereas a 1000 gm animal fed 3 g/kg will receive 1.0 g of protein which can be utilized for growth. Thus, the larger animal has twice as much protein available for growth as the smaller animal even though the intake per unit weight is the same and consequently the larger animals grow at nearly twice the rate. This may have implications in defining protein needs for infants since it would seem certain that the same principles apply and may explain some of the difficulties or inconsistencies found in the various estimates of protein needs of infants and young children.

We have also tried to estimate the efficiency with which the young monkey converts protein into new tissue. Although we do not have extensive data on the body composition of the young monkeys as yet, such data as we do have indicate a body composition of approximately 20% protein. Using this value, the data show that the infant monkey is only about 70% efficient in converting lactalbumin into new tissue whereas the rat is 90 to 95% efficient. The value for monkeys is much nearer to the value in man found by CALLOWAY and MARGEN (8).

It seems likely that this lower value is due to the fact that the maintenance of body tissue protein is a less efficient process that the conversion of protein into new tissue. Relatively low efficiencies have been reported for adult man, adult rats, and young monkeys whereas young rats and very young human infants appear to have high efficiencies. However, as I have already indicated we do not have enough data to be sure that growth rate is the factor and this makes extrapolation to other age groups suspect.

Now, I wish to discuss briefly some of the problems related to the estimation of protein quality. The estimation of biological value (BV), generally thought to be the best estimate of protein quality, has been based upon the change in nitrogen retention with change in intake as shown in fig. 5. That is, at low levels of intake, it has been assumed that the nitrogen retention will be linearly related to intake. Thus, the practice has been simply to measure nitrogen balance at two points at a very low or zero intake and at some arbitrarily selected intake. Net protein utilization (NPU) is based upon the same assumptions except that the abscissa is total nitrogen consumed rather than nitrogen absorbed. However, the point that I want to emphasize is that both of these measures are slopes, $\frac{y}{x}$.

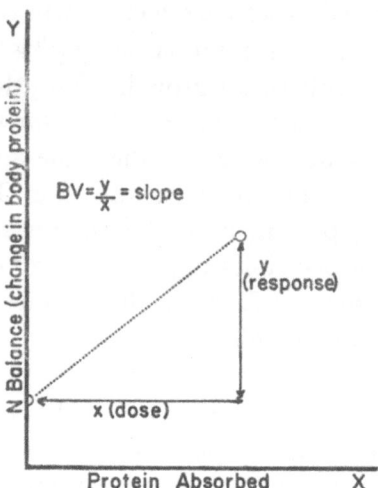

Fig. 5. Biological value by definition is the slope of an assumed linear line relating nitrogen balance to absorbed protein.

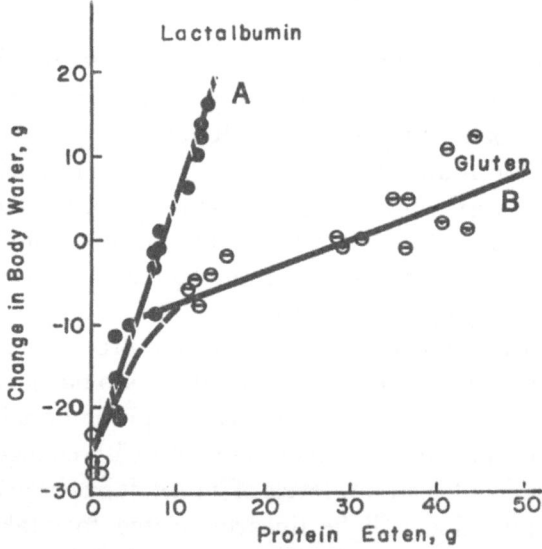

Fig. 6. Actual change in body water in adult rats fed different quantities of lactalbumin or wheat gluten. Taken from SAID and HEGSTED (16).

It is now becoming entirely clear that the assumption that the slope could be calculated from any two points is not true for many proteins. As shown in fig. 6 from the paper of SAID and HEGSTED (16), the slope is approximately linear for some proteins, such as lactalbumin in this

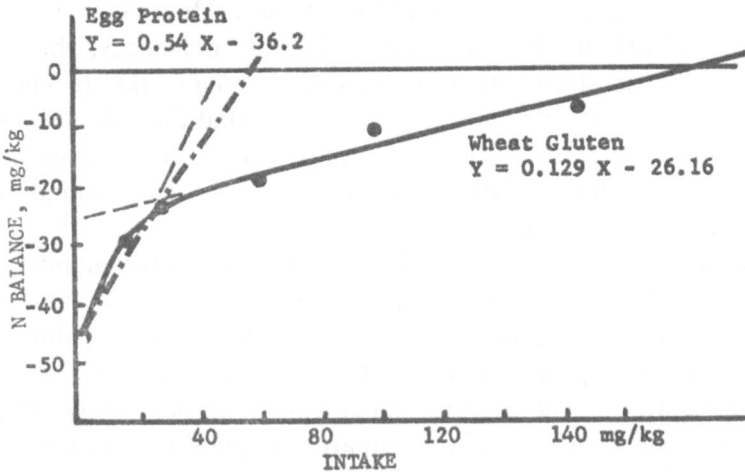

Fig. 7. Change in nitrogen balance in adult men fed different quantities of egg protein or wheat gluten. Taken from INOUE et al. (17).

instance, but not for many, perhaps most, as demonstrated by wheat gluten. Comparable data on man have been presented by INOUE et al. (17). Figure 7 shows the nitrogen balance data of INOUE et al. obtained with adult human subjects. It is clear from these slides that the biological values of wheat gluten and lactalbumin or egg are the same at low levels of intake whereas they are markedly different at higher intakes. Thus, the BV or NPU which one obtains for wheat gluten depends almost entirely upon the level of gluten which happens to be selected, certainly an unsatisfactory situation.

The reason for this also now is becoming clear. The general assumption made in the calculation of BV, NPU or amino acid score is that all essential amino acids must be present at the site of protein synthesis and therefore any deficiency of any essential amino acid will affect protein utilization to the same degree. This theory fails to account for the fact that the body has great but varying ability to conserve certain amino acids when they are in short supply. For example, fig. 8 shows the changes in weight of adult rats fed diets which were lacking in either lysine, methionine, threonine or total protein (18). The theory would say that a protein completely lacking in any essential amino acid should not be utilizable; it should be the nutritional equivalent of no protein at all. It is apparent that a threonine-free diet approximately fulfills this expectation. These animals lose weight and tissue at rates which approximate the protein-free group. However, with most amino acid deficiencies and especially lysine deficiency, the loss of tissue is much slower than expected. Although the biochemical mechanisms are not yet known, it seems clear that the animals must be able to conserve amino acids and reutilize them. Thus, a lysine-free diet will yield a BV or NPU as high as 40 to 50% even though such a diet will not allow survival in the long run.

Since most proteins are either limiting in lysine or methionine, most of the published values for BV or NPU are gross overestimates of the true nutritive value. The best estimate of the nutritive value is the slope of the linear part of the curve. For example, in fig. 7 INOUE et al.'s data indicate an efficiency of wheat gluten of only about 13% in fulfilling protein needs. This compares to published values in the literature of 40%.

This is a very important problem which is not yet sufficiently appreciated and is ignored in the FAO/WHO report (4). For example, if the protein requirement of an individual for egg protein is assumed to be 0.6 g/kg/day the requirement for gluten, assuming a BV of 40%, would be estimated as 1.5 mg/kg/day. On the other hand, if the quality is as low as 15%, the requirement would be calculated as 4 g/kg/day. This is nearly a three-fold difference.

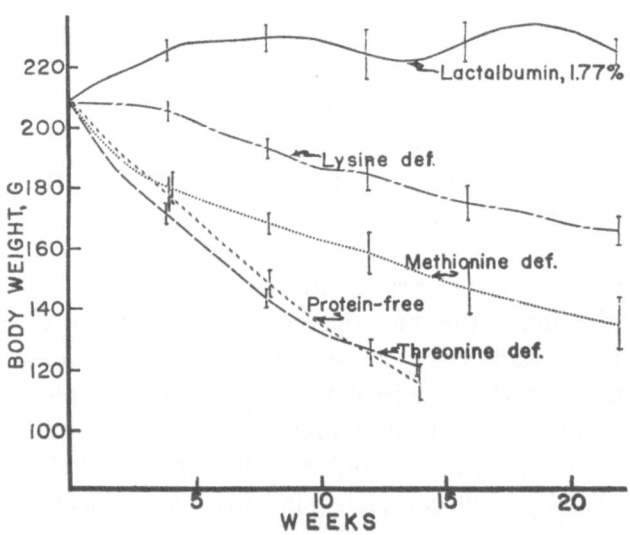

Fig. 8. Change in weight of adult rats fed diets completely free of lysine, methionine, threonine or total protein.

The major point to be made is that underestimating protein needs is a more serious error than overestimation since this will lead to recommendations of diets which do not meet requirements. And that the current values used to calculate protein needs of diets with poor protein quality will lead to underestimates of the true protein needs. This whole area requires much more consideration than it has received to date.

SUMMARY

The major conclusions I would draw are that estimates of total protein needs when high quality proteins are in the diet are relatively low. They are only reasonably secure for very young infants and adults. Other values are derived by extrapolation but there are reasons to be suspicious of the basis of this extrapolation.

Estimates of amino acid needs have similar limitations. Indeed, these estimates are so low that very few diets will be found which do not meet the amino acid requirements of adults if the estimates are correct. No rational explanation is yet available to explain the variable estimates for amino acid needs at different ages.

Finally, the current methods of estimating protein quality are clearly inadequate and thus the values in the literature which have been used to calculate protein needs when poor quality proteins are eaten are suspect. Better methods, however, are now available and it can be expected that this whole area will be revised in the very near future.

REFERENCES

1. HEGSTED, D. M. (1957), Theoretical estimates of the protein requirements of children. *J. Amer. diet. Ass.* 33, 225.
2. World Health Organization (1965), *Protein Requirements*. WHO Technical Report Series no. 301, Geneva, Switzerland.
3. Food and Nutrition Board (1968), *Recommended Dietary Allowances*, 7th ed. National Academy of Sciences – National Research Council Publ. 1694, Washington, D.C.
4. World Health Organization (1973), *Energy and Protein Requirements*. Report of a Joint FAO/WHO *ad hoc* Expert Committee. WHO Technical Report Series no. 522, Geneva, Switzerland.
5. MITCHEL, H. H. (1924), A method for determining the biological value of protein. *J. biol. Chem.* 58, 873.
6. MILLER, D. S. and BENDER, A. E. (1955), The determination of the net utilization of proteins by a shortened method. *Brit. J. Nutr.* 9, 382.

7. YOUNG, V. R. and SCRIMSHAW, N. S. (1968), Endogenous nitrogen metabolism and plasma free amino acids in young adults given a 'proteinfree' diet. *Brit. J. Nutr.* 22, 9.

8. CALLOWAY, D. H. and MARGEN, S. (1971), Variation in endogenous nitrogen excretion and dietary nitrogen utilization as determinants of human protein requirements. *J. Nutr.* 101, 205.

9. FOMAN, S. J., DeMAEYER, E. M. and OWEN, G. E. (1965), Urinary and fecal excretion of endogenous nitrogen by infants and children. *J. Nutr.* 85, 235.

10. HOLT, L. E. and SNYDERMAN, S. E. (1967), The amino acid requirements of children. In: *Amino acid metabolism and genetic variation,* p. 381, W. L. Nyan (ed.). McGraw Hill, New York.

11. ROSE, W. C. (1957), The amino acid requirements of adult man. *Nutr. Abstr. Rev.* 27, 631.

12. HEGSTED, D. M. (1963), Variation in requirements of nutrients–amino acids. *Fed. Proc.* 22, 1424.

13. NAKAGAWA, I., TAKAHASHI, T., SUZUKI, T. and KOBAYASHI, K. (1963), Amino acid requirements of children: Minimal needs of tryptophan, arginine and histidine based on nitrogen balance method. *J. Nutr.* 80, 305.

14. FOMON, S. J. and FILER, L. J. (1967), Amino acid requirements of normal growth. In: *Amino acid metabolism and genetic variation,* p. 391, W. L. Nyan (ed.). McGraw Hill, New York.

15. SAMONDS, K. W. and HEGSTED, D. M. (1973), Protein requirements of young cebus monkeys *(Cebus albifrons and apella). Amer. J. clin. Nutr.* 26, 30.

16. SAID, A. K. and HEGSTED, D. M. (1969), Evaluation of dietary protein quality in adult rats. *J. Nutr.* 99, 474.

17. INOUE, G., FUJITA, Y., KISHI, K. and NIIYAMA, Y., Nutritive values of egg protein and wheat gluten in young men. *Proceedings of the 9th International Congress of Nutrition,* in press.

18. SAID, A. K., HEGSTED, D. M. and HAYES, K. C., Response of adult rats to deficiencies of different essential amino acids. Brit. J. Nutr., in press.

CARBOHYDRATES AS NUTRIENTS

I. MACDONALD*

Carbohydrate in the diet has been accepted over the centuries as a pleasant and cheap source of energy for the body and neither excess nor deficiency states appear to have resulted from dietary carbohydrates per se. Consequently more attention has, perhaps rightly, been drawn to the proteins and fats in the diet. However, there has recently been a tendency to question the long held views that dietary carbohydrates have no specific role either for good or for evil and are merely cheap and satisfying sources of energy. I should therefore like to consider those aspects of nutrition in which dietary carbohydrates seem to play a special role.

A. PARTICULAR ROLE OF DIETARY CARBOHYDRATES IN PHYSIOLOGY

The ultimate fate of dietary carbohydrate is of course, its breakdown to carbon dioxide and water with the liberation of energy. This can be done directly or the carbohydrate can first be converted to glycogen or fat and stored as such before its breakdown to release energy. The energy aspect of dietary carbohydrates can theoretically be taken over by the proteins and fats, though a diet without carbohydrate would not be to everyone's taste. In fact, it has long been known that a high fat: low carbohydrate diet leads to an incomplete breakdown of fat with the formation of ketone bodies.

1. *Protein sparing*

Dietary carbohydrate has been called a 'protein sparer' meaning that the addition of carbohydrate to a diet allows more of the protein to be used for those purposes specific to proteins rather than as an energy

* Department of Physiology Guy's Hospital Medical School, London, U.K.

source. This is another way of recognising the fact that in nutritional terms, the body gives a higher priority to energy production than it does to protein metabolism. The circumstances in which dietary carbohydrate acts as a 'protein sparer' can only operate in states of inadequate energy intake and it is theoretically possible that the addition of fat to such a diet would also make it a 'protein sparer'.

2. *Glucose in metabolism*

Glucose is the common currency of metabolic energy and there are tissues in the body such as the brain that can only utilize glucose in normal circumstances. This fact does not, however, mean that dietary carbohydrates are essential because protein, though not fat, can be converted in the body to glucose. It is apparent, however, that under conditions of starvation there is not enough glucose produced either from protein breakdown, or from the glycerol moiety of triglyceride breakdown, to provide the brain with sufficient glucose and the continued normal function of the brain in starvation is due to its ability to adapt and obtain its energy from ketone bodies (1).

3. *Lactose and calcium metabolism*

It is not easy to speculate on the advantages of lactose, as opposed to the more easily produced disaccharide maltose, in breast milk except possibly in calcium metabolism. It has been found that lactose in the diet increases retention of dietary calcium by, apparently, improving the utilisation of calcium already absorbed. Lactose also increases the mineral content of bones and prevents loss of minerals from the skeleton of lactating rats (2). If these findings were confirmed then it is possible they might have some clinical significance in man, but it is also possible that this interrelation of lactose and calcium is of more consequence to the rapidly growing long-legged animal whose fleet movement in early life is essential for survival.

4. *Carbohydrates and blood glucose levels in infancy*

There is a relative deficiency of pancreatic amylase during the first few weeks of life (3) so that the blood glucose after cooked starch shows only a slight rise compared with an equal amount of glucose (4).

It should be possible to prevent the reactive hypoglycaemia following glucose ingestion by giving to infants starch that is only partially hydrolysed, such as 'glucose syrup' – a water soluble carbohydrate mixture resulting from partial hydrolysis of starch.

B. PARTICULAR ROLE OF DIETARY CARBOHYDRATES IN PATHOLOGY

It is only in the past 30 years or so that the carbohydrates in the diet have been considered to have any effect in the initiation of pathology in man. It has obviously been accepted for a long time that dietary carbohydrate can be converted by the body into fat and stored as such, but this transference of energy from one chemical compound to another is not a special feature of carbohydrates. There is now a general awareness that dietary carbohydrates can have effects on metabolism which are specific not only for carbohydrates as a group but are also specific for individual carbohydrates in the diet.

1. *Kwashiorkor*

An example of a disorder which relies on dietary carbohydrate for its clinical appearance is kwashiorkor. This malnutritional state in children in tropical regions has at least two important aetiological factors, one of these is an inadequate protein intake and the other is an energy intake that is in relative excess compared to the dietary protein. In the circumstances in which this condition is found the relative (but not absolute) excess intake of energy comes from carbohydrate. It is possible, that an excess of energy from fat instead of carbohydrate could produce the same clinical picture but in the condition as seen clinically the energy is derived mainly from carbohydrate.

The features of kwashiorkor that are the responsibility of the carbohydrate intake are the large quantities of liver fat and the presence of depot fat. In marasmus both these features are absent.

In kwashiorkor the serum protein pattern is characterised by a low concentration of albumin and a raised level of gamma globulin. There is evidence to suggest that these features also are a consequence of the dietary carbohydrate. In healthy adult men a diet adequate in protein but high in carbohydrate produces, within a few days, a fall in the serum albumin level with a rise in the gamma globulin concentration (5). Experiments in animals on low protein, high carbo-hydrate intakes show a similar trend in serum protein pattern (6).

2. Obesity

Dietary carbohydrates are implicated in the aetiology of obesity as indeed is any source of energy. The special place apparently reserved for carbohydrates in the production of over-weight is not due to any physiological phenomenon but to the psychology of dietary carbo-hydrates. Carbohydrates can gratify hunger (for short periods) are pleasant to taste, cheap to buy, have a high convenience value, and are often consumed to satisfy appetite rather than hunger (eg sweets). For these reasons and in the knowledge that refined carbohydrates contain little else of nutritional value, the dietary advice in obesity is to restrict the carbohydrate intake, though at any given weight fat contains more than twice as much energy as carbohydrate.

The role of dietary carbohydrate in relation to body weight may not be as simple as first appears. There is evidence that a high carbohydrate diet is associated with water retention (7) and also that not all dietary carbohydrates appear to be equal in the degree of body weight and body fat increase they produce in experimental animals. Sucrose seems to result in a greater increase in body fat than glucose or its polymers (8, 9).

3. Diabetes

There is no evidence that an excessive consumption of carbohydrate can lead to the development of diabetes mellitus, in fact quite the reverse, as witnessed by the low incidence of diabetes in those popula-tions whose diet contains large proportions of carbohydrate. There is a suggestion, however, that switching from starchy foods to more refined carbohydrates, and sucrose in particular, may be associated with an increase in the incidence of diabetes (10, 11). Some evidence to support this hypothesis comes from recent experimental work in rats in which it was shown that there is an interaction between genetic factor(s) and the amount of sucrose in the diet in the development of diabetes (12). The close association in man between carbohydrate-induced hypertriglyceridaemia and a poor glucose tolerance test would be compatible with the findings described in rats.

4. Dental caries

It is widely known that dietary carbohydrate is necessary for dental caries to develop and there are many reports both in the clinical and experimental situation, confirming this. The greater propensity of dietary sucrose, compared with other carbohydrates, to lead to caries is also well documented. Studies using glucose syrup (a partial hydrolysate of starch) in place of sucrose have demonstrated that dental disease is reduced by this replacement (13, 14) yet a commercial attempt to market for pre-school children a vitamin C rich fruit drink in which glucose syrup replaced the sucrose, failed (15). The dental ravages of the slow persistent drip of fruit juice concentrates containing sucrose has been shown (16).

5. Hyperlipidaemia

The group of disorders that have, in recent times, highlighted the importance of diet in clinical therapy, are those disorders of lipid metabolism that manifest themselves as raised lipid levels in the blood. The increase in serum lipid concentration is in itself of little consequence, but the elevated level does have a very significant correlation with vascular disease (17). The lipid fraction of plasma that has a special relationship with dietary carbohydrate is the triglyceride moiety, and because of this it is possible that dietary carbohydrate can, in some persons, be associated with vascular disease.

About 13% of males in the apparently healthy adult population of developed countries are 'sensitive' to dietary carbohydrate (18) and this meant that their level of triglyceride in fasting serum is markedly increased with an increase in carbohydrate consumption. The incidence of this disorder (FREDRICKSON's Type IV) in children is not known but the high incidence of atheroma in young soldiers (19) and airmen (20) suggests that its frequency may not be zero, especially when it is considered that this condition may be genetically determined (21).

There is some evidence to suggest that the type of carbohydrate may influence the production of endogenous triglyceride, and that fructose is more triglycerogenic than is glucose (22). Certainly in experiments in man and animals the substitution of fructose for glucose results in raised fasting serum triglyceride levels (23) and it is possible that in hypertriglyceridaemia a comparable difference in response occurs (24, 25, 26), though in diabetic children given fructose no elevation in serum triglyceride level occurred (27).

6. *Skin*

The older textbooks of medicine and dermatology referred to dietary carbohydrate in the therapy of pustular acne and seborrhoeic states and advised mothers of children with such conditions to reduce the carbohydrate intake and especially 'sweets'. Subsequently it has been found that the amount of triglyceride on the surface of the skin can be reduced if the sucrose in the diet is replaced by starch (28) and the fatty acid composition of skin surface lipid depends on the type of dietary carbohydrate eaten (29). Thus it seems that the clinical observations may be substantiated by scientific findings.

C. 'NEW' CARBOHYDRATES

Modern techniques in food technology have led to the economical production of types of carbohydrate that were previously too expensive for widespread use. A consequence of this is the search for outlets for these now readily available compounds and in any situation where a demand has to be created, there are dangers in over zealous application. The food manufacturer having been criticised, in the past, for the impurity of his product now finds himself assailed for making compounds too refined (30, 31).

The changing habits of large groups of the population may also lead to dietary components which were previously innocuous, now becoming 'risk factors' in the aetiology of disease. As an example the oral contraceptive raises the serum triglyceride level and decreases the glucose tolerance (32) and the changes in these parameters are more exaggerated when the diet contains a high proportion of carbohydrate and especially sucrose (33).

1. *Fructose*

This monosaccharide is now available in pure form comparatively cheaply and because it does not stimulate insulin release it has been advocated for diabetes. To a degree, it is replacing sorbitol as a sweetner in diabetic 'foods.' Fructose is converted to some extent, to glucose and this offsets its non-insulinogenic virtue. As it is not actively absorbed, like glucose, it can give rise to osmotic diarrhoea. Fructose has been used extensively by surgeons in intravenous feeding mainly because, unlike glucose, it does not give rise to local problems at the site of injection. However, there are dangers in giving fructose intravenously, dangers that are not shared by glucose, the most serious of which is lactic acidosis, especially when the liver is damaged (34).

Publication of a recent symposium on the clinical and metabolic aspects of fructose reveals that its effects are more distinctive than was at one time thought (35).

2. Maltose and its polymers

The partial hydrolysis of starch produces a mixture of carbohydrates whose composition can vary depending on the degree of hydrolysis. Complete hydrolysis will, of course, lead to glucose, but cessation of the process before this stage is reached leads to a mixture containing maltose, maltotriose, maltotose and higher polysaccharides, all of which are water soluble. The misleading name 'glucose syrup' is given to this concoction.

The features of glucose syrup that distinguish it from common carbohydrates are that it has a low osmotic pressure per gram carbohydrate and that the end product of hydrolysis in the gut, which is rapid, is glucose.

The food manufacturer is using increasing quantities of glucose syrup because it possesses many of the physical properties he requires (36). After absorption its effects are very similar to those of glucose.

An unexpected finding is that it seems likely thatmaltose c an be metabolised by the body without prior conversion to glucose (37) and this makes the advantageous use of maltose for intravenous feeding a distinct possibility.

A short review of the effects on metabolism of maltose and higher saccharides has recently been published (38).

3. Xylitol

This sugar alcohol found in the pentose pathway can also be produced cheaply and has been extensively investigated. Its advantages are that its transport into muscle is not dependent on insulin and it is well metabolised by diabetics (39) and is useful in uraemia (40). Large amounts by mouth give rise to diarrhoea and its use as an intravenous source of energy has met with difficulties (41, 19).

4. *Sucrose*

Though not in any sense a 'new' carbohydrate, there has been considerable speculation as to its role in the cause of disease in recent years. There is no conclusive evidence that this very common article of the Western diet is implicated in the aetiology of these ills found in developed countries, though there is some evidence to support such a hypothesis. Many of the metabolic effects of sucrose that differentiate it from starch and its derivatives are due to the fructose contained within its molecule. Perhaps the most unfortunate property possessed by sucrose is its very acceptable sweetness as this tends to result in over-indulgence with its consequent increase in depot fat.

D. INTERRELATIONSHIPS OF CARBOHYDRATES AND OTHER VARIABLES

There is a tendency to consider each component of the diet in isolation and to over-look the fact that food is a mixture of such components. There have been few investigations in this difficult area but such as there has been would point to relationships that could have clinical significance. For example in healthy men the addition of a poly-unsaturated fat to the diet offsets the rise in fasting serum triglyceride level produced by dietary sucrose or fructose whereas a saturated fat has no such effect (42). It has also been shown that the substitution of dietary protein by an amino acid mixture in experiments using large quantities of sucrose leads to a marked rise in fasting serum triglyceride level – such a rise does not occur when the sucrose is replaced by glucose syrup (43).

The metabolism of carbohydrate is affected by the sex of the consumer in as much as pre-menopausal women do not have the propensity to form triglyceride from fructose, such as is found in men and post-menopausal women (44), an effect that may be reversed in those taking mixed steroid oral contraceptives (33).

There also appears to be a relationship between the carbohydrate in the diet and the frequency of eating. There are several reports on the different effects on the metabolism of children and adults eating the same food but at different intervals of time (45) and under experimental conditions the frequency of consuming sucrose affects both the triglyceride and phospholipid response in the fasting serum (46).

There is a considerable knowledge on the absorption and uptake of various dietary carbohydrates in children which have been considered in detail in this series on previous occasions and it would therefore be churlish to consider this aspect of carbohydrates now. Apart from absorption studies much of the knowledge about dietary carbohydrates as nutrients comes from studies in adults. Reasons for this include the lack of evidence that carbohydrates can be specifically harmful to children and consequent upon this, the reluctance to carry out experiments on this age group. With nutrition, the stimulus and the pathological response may be separated by years, so it is theoretically possible that certain dietary carbohydrates in childhood may be initiating a process whose clinical appearance occurs in adulthood. In the absence of any evidence this remains only a suggestion.

REFERENCES

1. OWEN, O. E., MORGAN, A. P., KEMP, H. G., SULLIVAN, J. M., HERRERA, M. G. and CAHILL, G. F. (1967) Brain metabolism during fasting. *Journal of Clinical Investigation* 46, 1589.
2. DUNCAN, D. L. (1955) The physiological effects of lactose. *Nutrition Abstracts and Reviews* 26, 309.
3. HADORN, B., ZOPPI, G., SHMERLING, D. H., PRADER, A., McINTYRE, I. and ANDERSON, C. M., (1968) Quantitative assessment of exocrine pancreatic functions in infants and children. *Journal of Paediatrics* 73, 39.
4. HUSBAND, J., HUSBAND, P. and MALLINSON, C.N., (1970) Gastric emptying of starch meals in the new-born. *Lancet* ii, 290.
5. COLES, B. L., (1969) The influence on serum protein concentration of the protein intake in high carbohydrate diets. *British Journal of Nutrition* 23, 401.
6. COLES, B. L. and MACDONALD, I., (1963) The influence of dietary carbohydrate intake on serum protein levels. *Journal of Physiology (London)* 165, 327.
7. BENEDICT, F. G. and MILNER, R. D., (1907) Experiments on the metabolism of matter and energy in the human body. *Bulletin of the U.S. Department of Agriculture* 175, 33.
8. ALLEN, R. J. L. and LEAHY, J. S., (1966) Some effects of dietary dextrose, fructose, liquid glucose and sucrose in the adult male rat. *British Journal of Nutrition* 20, 339.
9. BROOK, M. and NOEL, P., (1969) Influence of dietary liquid glucose, sucrose and fructose on body fat formation. *Nature* 222, 562.
10. COHEN, A. M., BAVLY, S. and POZNANSKI, R., (1961) Change of diet of Yemenite Jews in relation to diabetes and ischaemic heart disease. *Lancet* i, 1399.

11. CAMPBELL, G. D., (1963) Diabetes in Asians and Africans in and around Durban. *South African Medical Journal* 37, 1195.

12. COHEN, A. M., TEITELBAUM, A. and SALITERNIK, R., (1972) Genetics and diet as factors in development of diabetes mellitus. *Metabolism* 21, 235.

13. GRENBY, T. H., (1972) The effect of glucose syrup on dental caries in the rat. *Caries Research* 6, 52.

14. BULL, J. and GRENBY, T. H., (1973) Changes in the dental plaque after eating sweets containing starch hydrolysates instead of sucrose. *Proceedings of the Nutrition Society*. In press.

15. ALLEN, R. J. L., (1973) Personal communication.

16. WINTER, G. B., HAMILTON, M. C. and JAMES, P. M. C., (1966) Role of the comforter as an aetiological factor in rampant caries of the deciduous teeth. *Archives of Disease in Childhood* 41, 207.

17. CARLSON, L. A. and BOTTIGER, L. E., (1972) Ischaemic heartdisease in relation to fasting values of plasma triglyceride and cholesterol. *Lancet* i, 865.

18. WOOD, P. D. S., STERN, M. P., SILVERS, A., REAVEN, G. M. and GROEBEN, J., (1972) Prebalance of plasma lipoprotein abnormalities in a free-living population of the Central Valley, California. *Circulation* 45, 114.

19. ENOS, W. F., BEYER, J. C. and HOLMES, R., (1955) Pathogenesis of coronary disease in American soldiers killed in Korea. *Journal of the American Medical Association* 158, 912.

20. GLANTZ, W. M. and STEMBRIDGE, V. A., (1959) Coronary artery atherosclerosis as a factor in aircraft accident fatalities. *Journal of Aviation Medicine* 30, 75.

21. FREDRICKSON, D. S., LEVY, R. I. and LEES, R.S., (1967) Fat transport in lipoproteins – an integrated approach to mechanisms and disorders. *New England Journal of Medicine* 276, 32–44, 94–103, 148–156, 215–226, 273–281.

22. ZAKIM, D., (1972) The effect of fructose on hepatic synthesis of fatty acids. *Acta medica scandinavica Supplement* 542, 205.

23. MACDONALD, I., (1972) Dietary carbohydrate:triglyceride interrelationships in man. In: A. Albanese (ed), *Newer methods of nutritional biochemistry*, Academic Press, New York 5, 125.

24. KUO, P. T. and BASSETT, D. R., (1965) Dietary sugar in the production of hyperglyceridemia. *Annals of internal medicine* 62, 1199.

25. KAUFMANN, N. A., POZNANSKI, R., BLONDHEIM, S. A. and STEIN, Y., (1966) Changes in serum lipid levels of hyperlipidemic patients following the feeding of starches, sucrose and glucose. *American Journal of Clinical Nutrition* 18, 261.

26. ROBERTS, A. M., (1971) Some effects of a sucrose-free diet on fasting serum lipid levels. *Proceedings of the Nutrition Society* 30, 71A.

27. AKERBLOM, H. K., SILTANEN, I. and KALLIO, A. K., (1972) Does dietary fructose affect the control of diabetes in children? *Acta medica scandinavica Supplement* 542, 195.

28. LLEWELLYN, A. F., (1966) Variations of the skin surface lipid associated with dietary carbohydrates. *Proceedings of the Nutrition Society* 26, ii.

29. MACDONALD, I., (1964) Changes in the fatty acid composition of sebum associated with high carbohydrate diets. *Nature* 203, 1067.

30. CLEAVE, T. L. and CAMPBELL, G. D., (1969) *Diabetes, coronary thrombosis and the saccharide disease*. John Wright and Sons, Bristol.

31. BURKITT, D. P., (1972) Varicose veins, deep vein thrombosis and haemorrhoids: epidemiology and suggested aetiology. *British Medical Journal* 2, 556.

32. WYNN, V. and DOAR, J. W. H., (1969) Some effects of oral contraceptives on carbohydrate metabolism. *Lancet* ii, 761.

33. STOVIN, V. and MACDONALD, I., (1973) Some effects of diet with oral contra-

ceptive on carbohydrate:lipid metabolism in the baboon. *Proceedings of the Nutrition Society* (In press).

34. Woods, H. F. and Alberti, K. G. M. M., (1972) Dangers of intravenous fructose. *Lancet* ii, 1354.

35. Nikkila, E. A. and Huttunen, J. K. (eds.), (1972) Clinical and metabolic aspects of fructose. *Acta medica scandinivica, Supplement* 542.

36. Wood, F., (1964) Glucose syrups in food manufacture. *International Food Industry Congress* 153.

37. Young, J. M. and Weser, E., (1971) The metabolism of circulating maltose in man. *Journal of clinical investigation* 50, 986.

38. Macdonald, I., (1973) *The effects on metabolism of maltose and higher saccharides.* In press.

39. Yamagata, S., Goto, Y., Ohneda, A., Anzai, M., Kawashima, S., Chiba, M., Maruhama, Y. and Yamauchi, Y., (1965) Clinical effects of xylitol on carbohydrate and lipid metabolism in diabetes. *Lancet* ii, 918.

40. Spitz, I. M., Rubenstein, A. H., Bersohn, I. and Bassler, K. H., (1970) Metabolism of xylitol in healthy subjects and patients with renal disease. *Metabolism* 19, 24.

41. Thomas, D. W., Edwards, J. B., and Gilligan, J. G., (1972) Complications following intravenous administration of solutions containing xylitol. *Medical Journal of Australia* 1, 1238.

42. Macdonald, I., (1972) Relationship between dietary carbohydrates and fats in their influence on serum lipid concentrations. *Clinical Science* 43, 265.

43. Coles, B. L. and Macdonald, I., (1972) The influence of dietary protein on dietary carbohydrate:lipid interrelationships. *Nutrition and Metabolism* 14, 238.

44. Macdonald, I., (1966) Influence of fructose and glucose on serum lipid levels in men and pre- and post-menopausal women. *American Journal of Clinical Nutrition* 18, 369.

45. Fabry, P., (1967) *Feeding patterns and nutrition adaptation.* Butterworth, London.

46. Macdonald, I., Coles, B. L., Brice, J. and Jourdan, M. H., (1970) The influence of frequency of sucrose intake on serum lipid, protein and carbohydrate levels. *British Journal of Nutrition* 24, 413.

THE REQUIREMENTS FOR WATER AND SALT

R. A. MCCANCE[*]

Water and salt are among the most fundamental needs of man and indeed of all animals, but the requirements for them are not often seriously considered and were not accorded much prominence by the National Academy of Sciences (1) or by the panel set up in Britain (2).

It is now well known that for some days or weeks after birth the kidney of the newborn animal is not able to excrete either water or sodium salts with the facility it will later possess, and these facts must be taken into account in considering what the desirable or the limiting intakes of a healthy infant should be. These intakes, moreover, cannot be considered apart from the intakes of other nutrients required for growth and health.

DESIRABLE INTAKES

With due deference to the sponsors of this colloquium, let us agree for the moment that full term babies, and premature ones above a certain size, can make very satisfactory growth – for a few months at any rate – on human breast milk. This at once gives us intakes of our two nutrients which we can regard as satisfactory and table 1, which has been

Table 1. *Volumes of milk and quantities of Na, Cl and K taken by a baby on breast milk.*

Age	Milk ml/kg/day (50th centile)	Water ml/kg/day	Na	Cl	K
				m.eq./kg/day	
8 days[1]	145	126	2.9	3.4	2.6
3 weeks[2]	200	174	1.4	3.6	2.6
6 weeks[2]	190	165	1.35	3.4	2.5
11 weeks[2]	175	152	1.2	3.2	2.3
15 weeks[2]	160	139	1.1	2.9	2.1
19 weeks[2]	150	130	1.0	2.7	2.0

[1] Transitional milk   [2] Mature milk

[*] Sidney Sussex College, Cambridge, U.K.

compiled from FOMON (3), and The Composition of Foods (4), shows what these are likely to be, assuming that breast milk contains 13% of solids. The energy value of the diets may be calculated on the assumption that the protein, fat and carbohydrate in 100 g breast milk will provide about 75 kcal.

Let us assume that a healthy baby 3–4 weeks old will be getting 174 ml H_2O/kg/day from its milk and 150 kcal/kg/day. This water, reinforced by some water of oxidation will be excreted partly by the lungs and skin and to a limited extent by the bowel. At this age some of it will be incorporated into growing tissues, and the excess, which we may reckon (see later) to be between 120 and 145 ml/kg/day, will be excreted by the kidney. Experience shows that this volume of water will not tax the kidney and will normally be quite sufficient to excrete the necessary solutes. Much larger intakes may be dangerous, for some of the water is likely to be retained, the fluids of the body will become diluted and the result may be fatal.

According to DROESE et al. (5) a growing child should retain some 1.5 m eq of Na/day over the first six months of its life, during which its average weight may be assumed to be about 4 kg if it was a bit small at birth, and hence its daily retention some 0.4 m eq/kg/day. This is considerably less than it will have been receiving from breast milk (see Table 1) and, in fact, DROESE et al. (5) calculated that 70 to 80% of the intake of Na should normally be excreted, mostly by the kidney. The findings of SLATER (6) would support this estimate. The kidney of the neonatal baby, however, is only capable of maintaining a very low sodium clearance and fails to excrete all the sodium salts if the intakes become too large. Some water is necessarily retained as well and hypertonic expansion of the extracellular fluids follows. This is something very much to be avoided (5, 7).

So far so good, but if we are here to consider diets for children with renal and gastro-intestinal handicaps, synthetic diets of various kinds and, above all, diets for intravenous administration, it is a valuable exercise to consider what may be termed the minimal intakes or minimal requirements which must be maintained at all costs.

MINIMAL REQUIREMENTS

a. *Water*

Table 2 shows that infants obtain water in two ways and lose it in three, some of which can be subdivided. In a growing infant the left hand side should be greater than the right, but if the infant is not growing the two sides are better to be equal. Let us now consider the magnitude of these quantities and the extent to which they can be significantly or safely manipulated to the infants advantage.

Table 2. *The sources of water and channels of loss in infancy.*

Sources	Channels of Loss
1. Administration by mouth or vein.	3. Evaporation (lungs and skin).
2. Oxidation of the hydrogen in organic molecules.	4. The bowel (either end).
	5. The urine.

We have gathered from table 1 the volumes of milk obtainable at various ages from the breast and which we may regard as the desirable ones, however they are administered, and it is to be noted that these amounts of milk will carry enough nutrients for all the metabolic processes and growth. The only other source of water at any age comes from the water produced by metabolism. The resting metabolism of a healthy infant in its zone of thermo-neutrality amount to between 28 and 40 kcal/kg/24 h in the first hours after birth depending upon its maturity, and rises to near 48 kcal by the end of the first week or ten days. Forty eight kcal/kg/day will require the combustion of 10 l of oxygen per kg/day or 7 ml O_2/kg/min (8, 9, 10, 11, 12, 13, 14, 15). If this heat were derived entirely from the combustion of the protein, fat and carbohydrate in breast milk the water produced would be between 5 and 7 ml/kg/day (16, 17, 18).

If we turn now to the channels of loss it appears that at 34 °C some 23% of the heat of metabolism is lost by the dissipation of water (when the relative humidity of the environment is 45%). This relationship is present from birth and is independent of weight or surface area. Our hypothetical infant, therefore, with a resting metabolic rate of 48 kcal/kg/day at 34 °C will lose 48 × 23/100 = 11 kcal/kg/day in this way and from the latent heat of evaporation of water at 34 °C this will involve the dissipation of 19 g of water (19, 20). These estimates of losses from the

lungs and skin, derived from fundamental physiology, agree satisfactorily with those obtained by direct measurement (20). ZWEY-
MULLER and PREINING (21) found the losses from the lungs and skin in
infants less than 12 hours old to be 10 to 16 g/kg/day according to the
infants activity. FARANOFF et al. (22) recorded losses in growing infants
over 10 days old to be about 34 g/kg/day, but the environment was not
critically defined. JONXIS et al. (14) arrived at figures from 22 to
36 ml/kg/day according to the humidity (see also HEY and KATZ (20)),
and LITTLE, BRODSKY and GREATHOUSE (23) in the first few days of
life from 17 to 34 g/kg/day according to the infants maturity. Dr.
Oliver BROOKE (24), in work which has not yet been published, arrived
at a mean figure of 50 g/kg/day for malnourished children in the first
few days of treatment, 4–17 months of age with a mean weight of
4.4 kg.

The insensible loss of water is always accompanied by a loss of
carbon dioxide, and the insensible loss of weight has been used as a
guide to the insensible loss of water and the metabolic rate. Professor
JONXIS (14) discussed this briefly at the Nutricia Colloquium in 1967
and other references are given by HEY and KATZ (20). Since the
production of 48 kcal/kg/day involves the uptake of 10 l of oxygen,
given a R.Q. of 0.8, this will involve the liberation of 8 l of CO_2
which will weigh $44 \times 8/22.4 = 1.6$ g CO_2 so that in an infant with such
a metabolic rate $1.6 \times 100/1.6 + 19 = 8\%$ of the insensible loss of weight
will be carbon-dioxide and the rest water.

As already stated the losses of water by the skin and lungs depend
upon the metabolic rate, but even at rest this itself is affected by the
environmental temperature and particularly the gradient from the
skin to the environment, for the metabolic rate and therefore the
consumption of oxygen, and the internal turnover of water, can be
doubled in a few minutes even a day or two after birth (9) by placing
an infant in an environmental temperature not much lower than its
zone of thermal neutrality. This is of some importance to the water
economy of an infant on minimal intakes, but its major importance is
that nutrients which might have been used for growth are dissipated
in keeping the infant warm, much to the detriment of its health and
even of its survival (25).

The insensible loss of water also varies inversely with the relative
humidity of the environment (20). Decreasing the loss of water by
raising the humidity would raise the skin and body temperature of an

infant if it were already in its zone of thermal neutrality, and its critical temperature would fall.

Losses of water by the bowel should be small, say 10 g/kg/day. PRATT, BIENVENU and WHYTE (26) found that the amount so lost was of this order. If minimal water requirements are in question this loss should be measured, if possible by weight, and replaced.

If the water provided by the milk of a healthy infant, 3–4 weeks old, be taken as before to be 174 g/kg/day by mouth (table 1), and 6 g be added for the water produced by metabolism, the total comes to 180 g. The infant will lose about 10 g by the bowel, and in a state of rest about 20 g/kg/day through the lungs and skin. The kidney therefore will be left to excrete 180—(20+10) =150 g/kg/day less the water retained by the growing tissues, but this will not be large. Five g/kg/day is a reasonable estimate for a 3 kg infant on its way to gain 3 kg of weight in 5 months. A small premature baby would retain more per kg/day. Growth at this rate, however, would require intakes of food and expenditures of energy well above 48 kcal/kg/day. The urine of a baby on breast milk will have a low osmolar concentration, probably less than 300 m.osm./kg, and its volume may be as high as 145–150 ml/kg/day. This may all be required for some days or weeks after birth because at this age the ability of infants to concentrate their urine is so much less that of adults. It was shown by PRATT et al. (26), however, that by the age of 4 weeks or a little more infants could produce urines as concentrated as those of adults. The mean osmolar concentration in their series was 1200 m. osm./kg of urine water so that the volume of the urine might be allowed to fall to 38 ml/kg/day without unduly altering the composition of the internal environment and endangering the child's life. The mean figure actually obtained by PRATT et al. (26) was only 25 ml/kg/day, but see also PRATT and SNYDERMAN (27). An infant in this age range (see table 3) should, therefore, maintain itself

Table 3. *The turnover of water by an infant 3–4 weeks old getting only 50 kcal/kg/day and minimal intakes of water under basal conditions at 34°C and 45% relative humidity. All the figures are expressed/kg/day.*

Intake		Output	
By administration	68 ml	By the lungs and skin	20 ml
		By the bowel	10 ml
Oxidation of the hydrogen in organic molecules	6 ml	By the kidney	44 ml

in water balance even if it did not grow on intakes of water by mouth or vein as small as 62 or let us say 70 ml/kg/day. Table 3 summarises the turnover of water by such an infant 3–4 weeks old on minimal intakes under basal conditions at 34 °C and a relative humidity of 45%.

One more matter requires consideration. No child would grow on intakes of food providing only 48 kcal/kg/day. If satisfactory growth is to be obtained an intake providing 150 kcal/kg/day would be more realistic. Table 4 shows that the metabolism of these amounts of

Table 4. *The minimal water requirements and turnover of a healthy growing infant 3–4 weeks old, getting 150 kcal/kg/day at 34°C and 45% humidity. All the figures are expressed/kg/day.*

Intake		Output	
By administration	115 ml	By the lungs and skin	58 ml
		By the bowel	10 ml
From oxidation	17 ml	By the kidney	60 ml

N.B. About 5 ml H_2O/kg. day should be getting incorporated into the growing tissues.

nutrients would provide 17 ml of metabolic water and necessitate the excretion of 58 ml by the lungs and skin. It need not alter the output in the stools, but it would increase the waste products to be excreted by the kidney and, therefore, the amount of water required to excrete them, and it would make it advisable to raise the amount of water to be administered to 110 or 120 ml/kg/day.

It is worth a thought that the difference between the desirable intake of water (174 ml/kg/day) and the smallest intake now suggested as being compatible with healthy growth (115 ml/kg/day), say 60 ml/kg/day in round numbers, is the margin of safety provided by nature for the intestinal upsets and other misadventures that few children in their natural surroundings could have escaped.

b. *Sodium*

The minimal requirements for sodium are not known, but if 75% of the intake from breast milk is normally excreted – see above – the child would probably do well on half those obtainable from this source, say 0.7 m eq/kg/day, for the losses by the skin are minimal. Abnormal losses from the bowel would have to be replaced.

7

PRACTICAL CONSIDERATIONS

The magnitude of the figures just discussed show that the amount of water to be administered must far exceed the water of metabolism even if this were to be doubled by a cool environment. The bad effects of the increased metabolism are due to the rise in the requirements of organic nutrients to maintain body temperature and consequently a fall in the amount of those available for growth.

The losses of water and sodium by the skin and lungs are obligatory but those of sodium are small. The losses of water are by no means small if minimal water requirements are under consideration.

There are 4 ways of keeping an eye on the progress and well being of infants such as the ones under discussion.

1. The weight of the baby must rise if the child is to grow, but a rapid rise should be suspected as it may indicate oedema due to the administration of too much water or too much sodium.
2. The osmolar concentration of the serum is a guide to this but:-
3. The determination of the serum Na is probably better.
4. If minimal fluid intakes and outputs are desirable, the osmolar concentration of the urine must be followed and probably not allowed to rise above 400 m. osm./kg water in the first week or two of life and 900 m. osm./kg over the age of 3 weeks.

REFERENCES

1. National Academy of Sciences, (1968) *Recommended dietary Allowances.* 7th ed. Publication 1694, Washington D.C.
2. Department of Health and Social Security Reports on Public Health and Medical Subjects, (1969) *Recommended Intakes of Nutrients for the United Kingdom,* No. 120, H. M. Stationary Office, London.
3. FOMON, J. F., (1967) *Infant nutrition.* Saunders, Philadelphia and London.
4. MCCANCE, R. A. and WIDDOWSON, E. M., (1967) *The composition of foods.* Medical Research Council. Special Report Series. No. 297. H. M. Stationary Office, London.
5. DROESE, W., STOLLEY, H., SCHLAGE, C. and WORTBERG, B., (1973) Significance of the salt level in food for infants and children. In: J. C. Somogyi (ed.), *Nutrition and technology of foods for growing humans.* Bibliotheca 'Nutritio et Dieta' 18, 215.
6. SLATER, J. E., (1961) Retention of nitrogen and minerals by babies 1 week old. *British Journal of Nutrition* 15, 83.
7. MCCANCE, R. A. and WIDDOWSON, E. M., (1957) Hypertonic expansion of the extracellular fluids. *Acta Paediatrica* 46, 337.
8. BRÜCK, K., (1961) Temperature regulation in the newborn infant. *Biologia Neonatorum* 3, 65–119.

9. HILL, J. R. and RAHIMTULLA, K. A., (1965) Heat balance and the metabolic rate of newborn babies in relation to environmental temperature; and the effect of age and of weight on basal metabolic rate. *Journal of Physiology* 180, 239.
10. DAVIDSON, S. and PASSMORE, R., (1966) *Human nutrition and dietetics* 3rd ed., p. 15 et seq. Livingstone, Edinburgh.
11. LEES, M. H., YOUNGER, E. W. and BABSON, S. G., (1966) Thermal requirements of undergrown human neonates. *Biologica Neonatorum* 10, 288.
12. SCOPES, J. W. and AHMED, I., (1966) Minimal rates of oxygen consumption in sick and premature newborn infants. *Archives of Disease in Childhood* 41, 407.
13. DURNIN, J. V. G. A. and PASSMPRE, R., (1967) *Energy, work and leisure.* Heineman, London.
14. JONXIS, J. H. P., VAN DER VLUGT, J. J., DE GROOT, C. J., BOERSMA, E. R. and MEIJERS, E. D. K., (1968) The metabolic rate in premature, dysmature and sick infants in relation to environmental temperature. In: J. H. P. Jonxis, H. K. A. Visser and J. A. Troelstra (eds.), *Aspects of praematurity and dysmaturity.* Nutricia Symposium, 201–209, Stenfert Kroese, Leiden.
15. HEY, E. N., (1969) The relation between environmental temperature and oxygen consumption in the new-born baby. *Journal of Physiology* 200, 589.
16. MELLANBY, K., (1942) Metabolic water and desiccation. *Nature* 150, 21.
17. McCANCE, R. A. and YOUNG, W. F., (1944) Observations on water metabolism. *British Medical Bulletin* 2, 219.
18. LADELL, W. S. S., (1965) Water and salt (sodium chloride) intakes. In: O. G. Edholm and A. L. Bacharach (eds), The physiology of human survival pp. 235–299. Academic Press, London and New York.
19. BOYD, E., (1935) *The growth of the surface area of the human body.* University Press, Minnesota.
20. HEY, E. N. and KATZ, G., (1969) Evaporative water loss in the newborn baby. *Journal of Physiology* 200, 605.
21. ZWEYMÜLLER, E. and PREINING, O., (1970) The insensible water loss of the newborn infant. *Acta Paediatrica Scandinavica Suppl.* 205.
22. FARANOFF, A. A., WALD, M., GRUBER, H. S. and KLAUS, M. H., (1972) Insensible water loss in low birth weight infants. *Pediatrics* 50, 236.
23. LITTLE, J. A., BRODSKY, W. A. and GREATHOUSE, R., (1955) The insensible weight loss of newborn and older infants. *American Journal of Diseases in Children* 90, 630.
24. BROOKE, O. G., (1973) Personal communication. To be published.
25. JOLLY, H., MOLYNEUX, P. and NEWELL, D. J., (1962) A controlled study of the effect of temperature on premature babies. *Journal of Pediatrics* 60, 889.
26. PRATT, E. L., BIENVENU, B. and WHYTE, M. M., (1948) Concentration of urine solutes by young infants. *Pediatrics* 1, 181.
27. PRATT, E. L. and SNYDERMAN, S. E., (1953) Renal water requirement of infants fed evaporated milk with and without added carbohydrate. *Pediatrics* 11, 65.

DISCUSSION

PAPER OF DR. WIDDOWSON

Prof. Visser: Thank you very much, Dr. Widdowson, that was a splendid 'warm-up' for this symposium.

Who wants to open the discussion on energy requirements? I'm sure we shall come back to them during the meetings, but who would like to begin?

Dr. Shaw: Have any measurements been made of the absorption of the nutrients in these very large intakes? Are calories being wasted in the stools?

Dr. Widdowson: Prof. McCance could answer that. He made such measurements. There are however just the normal amounts in the stools. There is no steatorrhoea.

Dr. Valaes: Has anybody studied the pattern of secretion of the growth hormone during this rapid 'catch up' growth of children, particularly those with high post-prandial oxygen consumption?

Dr. Widdowson: Studies have been made in undernourished children, but not with special reference to the post-prandial period. But Prof. Visser might help you with this.

Prof. Visser: I don't think growth hormone levels have been determined during the post-prandial period.

Prof. Bickel: I was sorry, Dr. Widdowson, that you said so little about fat cells. This of course is an important problem later on in adipose children. What happens to the fat cells as the children grow? Are they certain to become fat later?

Dr. Widdowson: Evidence suggests that fat cells do not disappear once they are formed. There is no doubt that obese adults have more fat cells than thin adults. The same is true of children. I don't think anyone has done a longitudinal study as yet, because we have not been interested in fat cells long enough to take the necessary biopsies. But evidence shows that what I have told you is correct. There has been one paper published on rats suggesting that fat cells may atrophy and disappear. But that's all.

Fat cells of course can be half full. There is no question about that. When an obese individual slims down, the fat cells become half full. Appetite however makes this individual, when given free access to food again, eat to fill up his fat cells.

Prof. McCance: We have to be a little careful about the growth hormone in undernourished children, because the concentration is quite high when they are undernourished and before they begin to grow. This was one of the surprising discoveries made two or three years ago. A follow-up study during recovery has been made, but I cannot give you the details. As far as the fat cells are concerned, there are various theories why fat cells which are not as full as they might be stimulate appetite. One is that their surface area is altered. But this is not certain.

Dr. Hommes: You touched upon a very essential point, Dr. Widdowson, when you indicated our difficulties in evaluating the calory requirements for the actual synthesis of the tissue components. I should like to draw your attention to a theory developed by Daniel Atkinson from Los Angeles, which is called the 'metabolic prize system'. He calculated the energy requirements for synthesis of triglycerides, proteins and so on, not directly in terms of calories but in terms of the ATP molecules required for the synthesis of specific bonds. If you then work out the ATP requirements in terms of kilocalories, you can calculate quite accurately how much energy is needed to effect the tissue synthesis.

Dr. Nicolopoulos: I was surprised that the baby demonstrated by Dr. Widdowson could take 300 kcal/kg/day. In our experience with babies with marasmus after infection of the intestinal tract, there was insufficient activity of intestinal enzymes. It was very hard to get them to take even 250 kcal/kg/day.

Dr. Widdowson: The babies with marasmus that took up to 300 kcal/ kg/day had not had any intestinal infections. I did point out too, you will remember, that if a baby has an infection of any kind, it is unlikely to respond in such a satisfactory way until the infection has been overcome.

Dr. Richards: Another short question for Dr. Widdowson. Part of the energy requirement is needed for the digestion of food. So one might expect that for a synthetic diet the energy requirement might be a little lower. Rose and his colleagues showed that in adults the energy requirement was apparently higher on a synthetic diet. I wonder if you would like to comment on this paradox.

Dr. Widdowson: I suggest that this depends on the composition of the synthetic diet. There are many problems not yet solved. More information would often help.

PAPER OF DR. MILLS

Prof. Visser: Thank you very much, Dr. Mills. This is a most stimulating introduction to the subject of trace elements, and it shows again that those who work with animals can make a great contribution to human nutrition.

Dr. Richards: Firstly, Dr. Mills, you said the cadmium intake must be carefully controlled. How do you do this?

Secondly, the low plasma copper levels in nephrotic syndrome and in sprue suggest that copper in plasma is normally protein-bound. What is important for normal function, the ionized fraction or the protein-bound component?

Dr. Mills: Control of cadmium intake from food can be difficult to achieve. To illustrate the magnitude of the problem, we know of one area where the cadmium content of vegetable material in an area adjacent to an industrial complex has risen to a maximum of 40 parts per million on a dry matter basis. Fortunately the industrial concerns responsible for cadmium emission have rapidly become aware of the problem and are taking steps to reduce emission. This is however extremely costly and I am not confident that satisfactory control can be achieved immediately.

With copper, zinc and chromium, we must face the fact that we cannot make an unequivocal differentation between a clinically normal and a clinically deficient animal solely on the basis of what we know about the content and distribution of these elements in the blood. There are very large genetic differences in the copper distribution in the liver and in the relationship between plasma or serum copper and clinical normality or clinical deficiency. We know of situations, again with farm livestock, where we have extremely low blood copper values and caeruloplasmin values without any clinical signs of deficiency. In other situations there can be clear chemical evidence of deficiency without dramatic changes in blood or tissue copper or zinc content. The answer to the problem of finding better parameters for the detection of trace element deficiency is to see if we can find the systems which are affected in the clinically deficient animal and to discover how we can use this information to improve diagnostic techniques. If this seems improbable, can I just emphasize that the progress that has been made towards the assessment of vitamin status in man has really been achieved by just this type of approach. We have been very content to do tissue trace element analyses, often without attempting to relate the results to the existence of metabolic lesions attributable to a deficiency or an excess of these elements. In consequence interpretation is often difficult which limits the value of this approach as a diagnostic procedure.

Prof. Bickel: I have been interested in Wilson's disease for many years. There seem to be astonishing discrepancies sometimes between the values for copper and those for caeruloplasmin. For instance in the young infant, the caeruloplasmin level is low during the first 5 or 6 months of life and then it slowly increases. In the same period serum copper seems to be high according to your figures. One has to look at the metabolism of copper together with that of caeruloplasmin. The caeruloplasmin complex is a powerful oxidase. What is the function of copper in the caeruloplasmin of deficiency of infancy? In Wilson's disease there is copper accumulation in the brain and yet the basal ganglia, where the cytochrome oxidase enzymes are so important, can't use the copper. It is the excess of copper? Is it the caeruloplasmin deficiency?

Dr. Mills: The difficulty with the caeruloplasmin level is in determining its metabolic relevance. There is an impact of disturbed iron
metabolism in severely copper-deficient subjects probably arising from
an involvement of caeruloplasmin in iron metabolism and iron release
from transferrin. It is however important to recognize that as deficiency
develops we are going to get a progressive spectrum of lesions. Anaemia and disturbances of the iron metabolism are relatively late
manifestations. Changes in cytochrome oxidase activity occur earlier
and are preceded by a decline in amine oxidase activity. Thus there
is no good single parameter at this moment for the diagnosis of a
copper-deficient subject. Low serum copper, low caeruloplasmin,
low liver copper merely tell us that a risk exists.

Dr. Steendijk: I would like to come back to your last slide. I think you
showed an increase in zinc excretion in rats with fractures. If you
fracture the bone of an animal or a human being, calcium excretion
in the urine also goes up in exactly the same way and this means bone
loss. We know there is zinc in bone. This is possibly just bone loss and
does not mean any real depletion of zinc.

Dr. Mills: Radioisotope studies by Fell and his colleagues now suggest
that this zinc comes from muscle; this view is supported by the observation that zinc excretion is paralleled by creatine excretion. Zinc
loss due to the catabolism of muscle may also arise during starvation;
moreover there appears to be an inverse relationship between plasma
zinc and food intake. Initially, when food is witheld plasma zinc often
rises. Providing the diet has an adequate protein or essential amino
acid content, re-alimentation decreases the plasma zinc content
suggesting that tissue anabolism and the incorporation of zinc into
those tissues proceeds so rapidly that the plasma pool of zinc cannot
normally be maintained against this demand.

Dr. Shmerling: Dr. Mills, you showed the radiograph of the hand of a
copper-deficient child with a reduction of bone mass and symptoms
of severe rickets. Was this rickets also due to copper deficiency or were
there any other deficiencies? We have seen a peculiar form of rickets
during long-term parenteral nutrition when a solution without copper
supplements was used.

Dr. Mills: In those trials particular attention was paid to vitamin D intake in relation to skeletal rarefaction. However an increased intake of vitamin D and calcium did not have any beneficial effects. This is also characteristic for the copper-deficient rat: it does not respond to an increased calcium or vitamin D intake. I should stress however that this skeletal rarefaction has not been observed in all cases. Again it is a question of the duration of depletion.

PAPER OF PROF. STANBURY

Dr. Fernandes: Rickets as observed in severe hepatic insufficiency is often described as being due to malabsorption of vitamin D and calcium. Maybe this rickets is due to a deficient 25-hydroxylation of cholecalciferol?

Prof. Stanbury: Precisely that explanation has been postulated by Haddad in St. Louis, who has found that a group of patients with non-specific hepatic diseases and a group with hepatic cirrhosis may have lower levels of 25-hydroxycholecalciferol in the plasma than a group of controls. I am a little unhappy about this because these patients are usually on a restricted diet and I don't think that those observations alone are sufficient to prove that point. We have found that shortly before death due to liver failure, patients still have a normal capacity for 25-hydroxylation of cholecalciferol. I think that two factors are probably more important than the actual failure of liver function. One is the dietary restriction produced by anorexia causing a reduced intake of vitamin D. Secondly it is the group of patients with obstructive jaundice in particular who develop hepatic rickets. In thesecases evidence is very strong that there is a specific failure of the intestinal absorption of vitamin D itself.

Dr. Mills: Could I possibly ask for more details about the nature of renal failure which is associated with the failure of hydroxylation at the 1-position? Can you relate this to any structural changes? What type of renal damage may be associated with this?

Prof. Stanbury: I think that it does not matter very much what the nature of the primary renal disease is. You can find this development in any form of bilateral progressive renal disease. In animals it is possible to demonstrate that when you remove both kidneys, there is literally no production of 1,25-dihydroxycholecalciferol. On the other hand if you produce uraemia by ligating both ureters, a capacity to produce the metabolite is retained. But we find that it is quantitatively less than you would get in an intact control, presumably because of non-specific damage of the ureteric obstruction.

Prof. Schretlen: Where in the kidney do you think hydroxylation takes place? We know of children with severe renal failure without rickets. Do you have any explanation?

Prof. Stanbury: We have no opinion because there just is no precise information about that point! It is known with reasonable certainty to be produced in the proximal renal tubules and that is all one can say.

But coming back to your question about children with renal failure without rickets, I presume these children also showed growth retardation. One wonders whether retardation of growth in this situation may not be important.

Dr. Valaes: I would like to present some observations on children with rickets. I am referring to our work on the sex difference in the incidence of rickets under similar conditions. You know the ratio male: female is 2 : 1 for vitamin D-deficient rickets. There are also observations from Australia. Tetany in newborn infants with low blood calcium is more frequent in males than in females. We studied amino-aciduria in children with vitamin D-deficient rickets and in their parents. With one exception, all children had amino-aciduria. During the period of healing and after complete healing, half of the children still had amino-aciduria. Almost all of the parents of the children with persistent amino-aciduria had slight amino-aciduria. Only two of the parents of the children with complete recovery had amino-aciduria.

It seems to us that there is some factor that determines the sensitivity to vitamin D. One can form a complete spectrum ranging from children with a normal intake of vitamin D, or normal production of vitamin D in the skin, and no danger of developing rickets to the children on other side where a sex-linked vitamin D-resistant rickets is situated. I wonder if you can place these facts in your hypothesis.

Prof. Stanbury: I can answer that very simply indeed by saying no. I am of course aware of these observations of yours. Perhaps having said no, which is the most honest and simplest answer, I might pass on one small piece of technical information to indicate the difficulties one is up against in trying to study aspects of vitamin D metabolism in man. When you have injected your radio-isotopic tracer and subsequently study the lipid extract from serum, the total group of triols including 1,25, 24,25 and 25,26 dihydroxycholecalciferol rarely amounts to more than 5% of your total plasma radioactivity at that time. So you really are fiddling around with a needle in a haystack, and the chance at this time of being able to pick out minute nuances of a sensitivity which is determined genetically is very small indeed. I hate to think what would be involved in even trying to detect whether there was any quantitative difference in the handling of vitamin D in males versus females. Until we have a radioimmunoassay for cholecalciferol as well as each of the three triols and can measure changes in them easily, I think there is not a hope of amplifying the answer I gave you initially, which was no.

Dr. Steendijk: I would like to take up the question of growth and renal osteodystrophy again. It is well-known that one can treat children with a very low renal function with either high doses of vitamin D or dihydrotachysterol with good results.

Prof. Stanbury: I have had exactly the same experience. The fact of course is that because the A-ring is rotated 180° the 25-hydroxylated derivative of dihydrotachysterol has its native 3-hydroxyl in a position stereically analogous to the 1-hydroxyl position in the doubly hydroxylated derivative of vitamin D_3. Thus 25-hydroxy-dihydrotachysterol is a sort of poor man's 1,25 dihydroxycholecalciferol.

As far as to the beneficial effect of vitamin D_2 or D_3 is concerned, we know that the plasma concentration of their respective 25-hydroxy derivatives increases with dose, and I believe that the beneficial effects observed are produced by those 25-hydroxy derivatives which are effective when present in amounts much greater than those required for 1,25 derivatives.

When Dr. Adams joined us, he came from that very best of all stables – namely that of McCance and Widdowson, and he brought with him the pattern of thinking as well as the techniques essential for the study of human nutrition and experimental nutrition. One of the things that he soon became interested in was the problem of renal dwarfism, which has remained unexplained, in spite of all the advances made in the study of vitamin D metabolism. Having worked with pigs, like all the experts, he immediately translated his acquired knowledge to these children. By providing them with a great increase in calories, he could promote body growth in children with renal dwarfism.

Prof. Bickel: Prof. Stanbury, could you explain how the familial vitamin D-resistent rickets fits into the picture now?

Prof. Stanbury: I think, Prof. Bickel, most clinicians would agree that the syndrome of familial hypophosphataemia differs greatly from the clinical features of vitamin D deficiency. It is therefore unlikely that a disturbance of the vitamin D metabolism plays a critical role in the pathogenesis of the former. Most people now consider the defective mineralization in this syndrome to be a consequence of hypophosphataemia, developing as a result of impaired renal tubular reabsorption of phosphate. These patients also tend to have impaired intestinal absorption of calcium, and it is conceivable that a disturbance of the vitamin D metabolism could be involved in this component of the syndrome. In this respect, it may be relevant that Arnaud and his collaborators at the Mayo Clinic found reduced serum immunoassayable parathyroid hormone in these patients. There may be therefore a functional hypoparathyroidism, secondary to the hypophosphataemia. In view of the trophic influence of parathyroid hormone on the renal formation of 1,25 dihydroxycholecalciferol, one wonders if secondary hypoparathyroidism could result in inadequate production of this metabolite and so account for the variably reduced intestinal absorption of calcium in patients with familial hypophosphataemia. Viewed in this way, the reduced intestinal absorption of calcium would be a physiological consequence of the hypophosphataemia. We are attempting to explore this possibility by studying the formation of 1,25 dihydroxycholecalciferol in these patients before and after correction of hypophosphataemia by phosphate therapy.

Prof. Bickel: I do not agree with you if you say that the phosphate loss is purely renal. We have done early experiments in Birmingham with careful balanced studies. We found that the intestinal absorption of calcium and phosphorus was reduced.

What may fit in with your suggestion of hypoparathyroidism is that these children never had amino-aciduria.

PAPER OF DR. MOLENAAR

Prof. Boldingh: In the model which you showed for α-tocopherol, is the configuration of arachidonic acid U-shaped?

Dr. Molenaar: No, it is straight.

Prof. Boldingh: There is a lot of evidence that the arachidonic acid in membrane phospholipids has a U-shaped configuration.

Dr. Molenaar: The configuration is straight, but it is of course fixed by its double bonds.

Prof. Boldingh: But is the cyclic structure of tocopherol located at the double bonds of the arachidonic acids in that model?

Dr. Molenaar: No, it is located at the surface of the bilayer, lying together with the polar groups of the phospholipids.

Prof. McCance: How many vitamin E molecules do you picture, Dr. Molenaar, in these membranes? Is there one molecule of tocopherol for every arachidonic acid molecule?

Dr. Molenaar: It depends on the kind of membrane. In erythrocyte membranes there is, according to Diplock, one vitamin E molecule for 500 arachidonic acid molecule. We calculated 1 in 50 for inner mitochondrial membranes. You should realize that in the model described by Singer with its isolated protein islands, the fatty acid molecules around these protein islands are in quite a different situation and are of another kind than the fatty acids elsewhere in the bilayer. It is quite conceivable that vitamin E is located especially in the neighbourhood of the protein islands. This would also fit in with the supposed selenium function.

Dr. Mills: I didn't get the last point. I would like to ask you about that selenium function, which was discovered by the Wisconsin group, and its role in glutathion-peroxidase. How does this tie in with the action of vitamin E in peroxidase reactions?

Dr. Molenaar: Vitamin E would protect in particular the selenium-containing proteins.

Dr. Mills: Possibly it may even go further than that. They have isolated selenium as a component of this glutathion-peroxidase enzyme. One of its functions seems to be peroxide or free peroxide elimination. Rather similar to the suggested role of vitamin E. Is this one of the keys to the problem of vitamin E? We so often see replacement of vitamin E by selenium or vice versa. Quite often a common syndrome appears to be a distinct function between vitamin E and selenium. I wonder if this clarifies the function of vitamin E anyway.

Dr. Hommes: I'll try to speculate on that. Perhaps the original hypothesis of Lucy and Diplock went a little bit further than lining up the phytyl-type side chain beside arachidonic acid. In fact they have speculated that the other group of vitamin E somehow interacts with sulphur from the non-haem iron proteins in which they assume some of the sulphur can be replaced by selenium. If this hypothesis is true, and I think it is open for experimental verification, then you have to look for an interrelationship and mutual dependency of selenium and vitamin E.

Dr. Mills: Dr. Molenaar said we have no clear evidence of the existence of vitamin E deficiency as a practical problem in man. In a recent working group of the W.H.O., the same conclusion was reached with regard to selenium. We must be cautious however. Because 10 years ago we would perhaps have said the same with regard to many commercially important animals. In the interim there has been a thorough investigation of vitamin E requirements. Even now we get some very nasty surprises. In the United Kingdom the vitamin E requirements of farm animals have been worked out carefully. On the basis of this work, recommendations have been made for the inclusion of vitamin E. And we still run into trouble. There seems to be an increase in the number of vitamin E-responsive situations, and perhaps the number of selenium-responsive situations, for reasons we don't understand. Certainly there are antagonists that are not necessarily polyunsaturated fatty acids. Some seem to be associated with the rapid rate of growth. Certainly those factors have not been identified. I'm concluding with a plea that vitamin E or perhaps the mysterious selenium should not be dismissed from our minds.

PAPER OF DR. VERGROESEN

Prof. Wretlind: May I ask you about one of your very interesting diagrams. In one of the diagrams you showed the different effects which the cis- and trans-isomers of oleic acid have on the serum cholesterol level. Is that difference significant?

Dr. Vergroesen: Yes.

Prof. Wretlind: Have you noticed any other effect of trans-acids? It is an old question. Have you investigated other trans-acids which are formed during the hydrogenation of unsaturated fats?

Dr. Vergroesen: The difference between cis- and trans-oleic acids in the presence of dietary cholesterol was certainly significant. Furthermore we know from experiments with rabbits that in the absence of cholesterol, diets high in trans-oleic acid and low in linoleic acid are atherogenic – actually as atherogenic as coconut oil. The trans-fatty acids present in this diet were obtained from hydrogenated olive oil.

Nutritionally with respect to food consumption, caloric efficiency, growth rate and macroscopical and microscopical pathology, we never observed any difference between the cis- and trans-oleic acid. They only differ with respect to their influence on blood lipid levels and their atherogenic effect.

Dr. Fernandes: On one of your slides, the effect of myristic and palmitic acid on serum cholesterol was compared with that of linoleic acid. What is known about the effects of the medium-chain fatty acids such as caproic and caprylic acids and the short-chain acids such as butyric acid?

Dr. Vergroesen: We have never tested butyric acid but from an unpublished human dietary experiment with a margarine made from C8 and C10 fatty acids, we concluded that these behave more or less as oleic acid confirming again the results of Keys et al. They increase the blood cholesterol concentration much less than the other saturated fatty acids do.

PAPER OF PROF. HEGSTED

Dr. Richards: Quite apart from the difficulties imposed by different ages and sex as well as calories and disease, we have the problems of experimental techniques. Perhaps with growing children or animals it's reasonably straight forward. But otherwise, when we try to measure the adequacy of nitrogen intake with regard to nitrogen balance, we all know it is a rough but very useful technique.

I wondered which techniques you have thought about, and which you perhaps foresee will give us the same information as that of the nitrogen balance but more accurately.

Prof. Hegsted: I wish I had an answer to that. As many of you know I have not been a great enthousiast of balance studies for quite a long time. Data almost uniformly show that the more you feed, the more positive the balance becomes. Nobody knows where the stuff is going, if the balance data are correct. And I have always thought that this is at least due to the bias of experimental methodology. There are many things which can be used for biochemical tests in protein malnutrition. As far as I know not many of them are very useful, until you have a really deficient animal. In terms of the estimation of normal protein requirements, I don't think we really have any technique.

Prof. Wretlind: I agree that it is very hard to tell which method should be used as the most ideal method. But until we get the ideal method, I would like to ask you, Prof. Hegsted, which method should we use for the time being. It is a practical problem. It doesn't help if you wait 50 years to get the right answer.

Prof. Hegsted: The best method is to estimate the slopes of the regression lines. That's true either in man or in animals. Not slopes from zero but slopes near the maintenance requirement. The slopes of these lines are indeed measures of the efficiency of utilization. I think that is the way we have to measure protein quality.

Prof. Wretlind: I agree completely with what you have shown, that a healthy adult needs a smaller amount of essential amino acid in the protein. On the other hand, from a practical point of view, all of us eat the same type of food. Would it be more useful to have a protein which causes good growth in children and to use that for the whole population?

A second question: in a patient you not only must maintain body weight but must also for instance increase body protein. What is your idea about protein in that case?

Prof. Hegsted: I think the severest test for protein quality is in growing rats. And if you are willing to agree to that, we can almost be sure the proteins which are the highest quality for rats will be of the highest quality for man. I think that some of the industrial people don't like that approach, because it places a maximum nutritional quality on protein products. They would like to keep it down for various reasons. Sometimes because they simply cannot provide that kind of quality. I don't know of any indication that high-quality protein for rats is not high-quality for man.

Prof. Jonxis: It may be true for rats but they have fur. The human has no fur. Fur is mainly protein with a high content of sulphur-containing amino acids. The need for sulphur-containing amino acids should be lower for human beings. Is the rat the right experimental animal?

Prof. Hegsted: As I said I think the quality for rats is probably an underestimation of the quality of proteins for man. Unfortunately the estimates of the requirements of sulphur-containing amino acids are worse than those of other amino acids. The estimates of the methionine requirement are terrible. It is likely that experiments with rats will not provide a correct evaluation of proteins limited in sulphur for say children. I don't have a clear idea of the magnitude of that difference. There is some evidence that methionine-cystine requirements vary with age.

8

PAPER OF PROF. MACDONALD

Dr. Fernandes: Could you elaborate more on the metabolic facts of maltose when given orally or intravenously. Is it broken down by the lysosomal neutral maltase?

Prof. MacDonald: In the literature it has been suggested that maltose can be taken into cells as maltose. This transfer is not insulin-dependent.

Dr. Eggermond: Is it possible to know the specific activity of the injected maltose. I think that may be an important problem. Trace doses can be easily metabolized. If it is a load of several grams you may have a limit in the metabolism of maltose. I think it is important to know, before we can use maltose clinically.

Dr. Shmerling: May I just add that Young and Frazer performed different experiments. In some of the experiments they used trace doses, but they also gave bulk infusions of 25 grams. I do not believe that they gave any long-term infusions of maltose. It is probable that there are lysosomal maltoses.

Dr. Widdowson: I'm interested in your comment that children might get kwashiorkor on high-fat diets. We found that in pigs. We fed them high-fat diets. We got exactly the same effects as we did with high-carbohydrate diets. We didn't find any difference between them.

Prof. MacDonald: So what I said in theory was right in practice.

Dr. Widdowson: In pigs.

Prof. MacDonald: What sort of fat did you feed them. I'm sure Dr. Vergroesen will want to know that.

Dr. Widdowson: We tried various fats, but what we finished up/with was lard.

Prof. Bickel: You said that these problems are not of great value to the paediatricians, but this is not completely true anymore. Because in some diseases now, we must know very clearly what the different sugars mean. Think of intolerances for various sugars, for instance malabsorption of disaccharides or monosaccharides; think of glucose-malabsorption, where you use fructose as the only sugar. So I think paediatricians have a great interest in sugars.

Prof. MacDonald: I didn't discuss that because it seemed to me that a substance not absorbed from the intestine would not be metabolized. But I take your point that if you have a child who can only take fructose and if he has lived on fructose all his life, then this would be a very interesting study.

Dr. Hommes: Fructose is primarily phosphorylated in the liver to fructose-1-phosphate, which is then split by the fructose-1-phosphate specific aldolase into two C3 units which go to the end of the glycolytic scheme. It largely bypasses one of the main controlling enzymes of the glycolytic scheme, phospho-fructo-kinase. This is one of the reasons it is so lipogenic.

Prof. MacDonald: Another reason might be of course that fructose forms glyceraldehyde and it could go to glycerol or glyceric acid and to glycerol-phosphate in this way.

Dr. Hommes: In this way it upsets the redox state of the cytoplasm. This has been shown in liver perfusion experiments. This may be one of the dangers of clinical application, especially in paediatrics. You get a much higher decrease in the ATP level in the liver with fructose infusions than with glucose infusions.

Prof. Zöllner: That comparison is not quite fair because if you infuse the same amounts, fructose is only metabolized in the liver and glucose is metabolized all over. Is there a certain amount of fructose which can be tolerated without all the consequences you have shown? Is there a direct effect starting from zero or is there a limiting value up to which you can give fructose without dangers, as Prof. Bickel would need for his patients?

Prof. MacDonald: I think that the question, what is the dose response of fructose, is a good one. This has not been worked out, as far as I know. I suspect that if you take small amounts of fructose, it will convert to glucose in the liver and therefore you do not have any fructose in the systemic circulation. But if you give glycerol, glycerol has very striking effects on serum triglyceride levels.

Dr. Shaw: You said you didn't know why we depend on lactose. I didn't know either I wondered about the galactose. Do you have any information on whether galactose is an essential carbohydrate?

Prof. MacDonald: I keep asking the question, why does the breast go to all the trouble of making lactose and the infant to all the trouble of having to metabolize lactose?

Prof. Zöllner: I would like to make a comment on galactose. We have studied the rate of utilization of galactose. The maximum rate is very low in the adult compared with that of fructose or glucose. It is below or around 0.5 g/kg/hour. If you go above that range, you get an ever increasing level of galactose in the blood and a beautiful galactose excretion.

Prof. MacDonald: Did you give it intravenously? I think it is important because in that case the liver is handling it under abnormal circumstances.

Prof. Zöllner: Yes.

Dr. Mills: Could I ask a question which will immediately show my ignorance. Has the effect of the type of dietary carbohydrate on the bacterial and protozoal population of the intestinal tract been studied at all? Particularly in terms of the total number of organisms. Is there any situation occurring in man where you have a degree of bacterial growth which will produce a protein of a given quality with respect to the initial quality when ingested.

In animals this is a well-known phenomenon and is influenced by the type of carbohydrate. Is there anything in it from the human point of view.

Prof. Hegsted: We have always thought this might be a factor. Some of the acute changes that you get with fructose and glucose can be produced by giving them intravenously, in other words bypassing the gut. You know it is very difficult to look at the gut flora and to get some quantitative estimations.

PAPER OF PROF. MCCANCE

Dr. Shaw: I'm not aware of any systematic measurement being made of the osmolar concentration in the urine of breast and bottle-fed infants. But there is a publication giving figures for osmolar concentration in the urine of infants attending a well-baby clinic in Sheffield. The mean osmolality of the breast-fed infants was 105 mOsm/kg water, which is what you might expect from the figures you put up on the board. The osmolality of the artificially fed infants was greater than that of plasma: 377 mOsm/kg water. The highest value was found in a 6 week-old baby: 1300 mOsm/kg water.

Prof. McCance: That is possible in a 6 week-old baby. But it would be highly undesirable.

Dr. Shaw: If you calculate the urine osmolality on the basis of an insensible water loss of 200 ml/day/for a 4 kg infant, you arrive at a figure close to 377.

Prof. McCance: Thank you very much. That is very helpful. In a baby fed on breast milk you have to estimate both the salt and water intakes, but in an artificially fed baby nobody knows except the mother what the child is receiving. If I knew the osmolar concentrations in the urine of a breast-fed baby from birth to 3 months of age, I could make all my calculations much more accurately.

Prof. Jonxis: I should like to make one remark. In this country during the 20's and 30's, the normal way of feeding a baby when there was no breast milk, was to give buttermilk – only buttermilk with some sugar and flour added. It must have had a very high concentration of salts, far more than your safety margin. As I remember, it was given to many newborns and even prematures from the first day onward and on the whole, they survived.

Prof. McCance: Yes, we know more or less what happens when you do this. The babies show a rise in serum sodium, expansion of their extracellular fluid and an increase in weight during the first few days; then they stabilize. If you change a baby from breast milk to cow's milk, the same thing happens and the baby survives with an unnecessarily large volume of extracellular fluid. Potassium is excreted satisfactorily.

Prof. Jonxis: To me it is all very remarkable; nowadays we would never feed a child like that, not even as an experiment. Still in this country, whole generations survived it for many years.

Prof. McCance: During the war, when everybody was keen on feeding amino acids to avoid all digestive problems, they decided to feed premature babies on hydrolysed proteins. The proteins were hydrolysed with hydrochloric acid neutralized with sodium hydroxide and then fed to the babies.

Prof. Bickel: But you don't know how they survived? I mean, there is danger in hyperosmolality. I have never forgotten a child that was treated by mistake with too much salt when it had diarrhoea. When the blood sodium level reached 160 mEq/1, the child became unconscious. It woke up from unconsciousness when it was given a hypotonic solution. I sometimes wonder if in the past children may have been harmed, without anyone realizing it, by high osmolalities in the blood followed by dehydration of the cells, particularly of the brain cells. You may not notice anything until much later, or you may not realize how the damage was caused.

Prof. McCance: That is perfectly true. The babies I had to deal with during the war gained weight very rapidly but did not thrive. I advised putting them back onto diluted milk. This soon put them right.

Dr. Richards: How well does the colon of an infant normally conserve sodium?

Prof. McCance: I don't know. I do not think any experimental work has been done on neonatal animals. It would be an interesting study. I think the neonatal surgeons might be able to provide us with a certain amount of information.

SYNTHETIC DIETS

SYNTHETIC DIETS IN PAEDIATRICS

J. H. P. JONXIS*

It is possible to keep the human being in a satisfactory nutritional condition on a diet consisting of L-amino acids, pure triglycerides of fatty acids, glucose, vitamins, minerals and demineralized water (Nature 105, 741, 1965). It even seems to be possible to keep a child's growthrate more or less normal on such a diet, whereby dextrin-maltose replaces glucose, over a period of years (DE GROOT).

This possibility proves that all major dietary factors necessary for normal growth and development as well as the relative amounts in which they should be administered are known. This does not preclude, however that disorders may still occur in the long run. The possibility of keeping a human being, and likely the growing child as well, in good health on a completely artificial diet offers many opportunities for observation, both long and short-term. In paediatrics initial experience with synthetic or partially synthetic diets was obtained in children with inborn errors of metabolism. During long-term observations, we were able to study the growth, development and blood chemistry of a number of children with inborn errors of metabolism, keeping our eyes open for eventual signs of nutritional deficiencies. During relatively short-term administration of synthetic diets, we were able to obtain at least some preliminary information about the absorption of several nutrients in a number of children suffering from diseases other than inborn errors of metabolism.

The administration of artificial diets to healthy children is, except perhaps over a very short period, not justified on ethical grounds. Therefore we can only observe those children in whom a synthetic diet is an essential part of the treatment of their disease. This, however, complicates the interpretation of our observations.

We have treated some children with non-ketotic hyperglycinaemia using a synthetic diet without any glycine or serine over a period of years.

* Department of Paediatrics, State University, Groningen.

There are two other groups of patients in whom we were able to study the effect of a synthetic diet. The first is the group between 8 and 13 years of age with severe intestinal problems. The patients were an eight-year-old boy with severe mucosal atrophy of the ileum due to non-gluten-sensitive coeliac disease and a 13-year-old girl with ileitis terminalis. Secondly, we have had under our care a number of young infants who had been operated on, because severe congenital malformations of the intestinal tract necessitated resection of parts of the small intestine, as well as several infants with severe dystrophy of unknown origin.

I would like to discuss the case histories, especially from a nutritional point of view, of some of the children in these groups – but first I want to consider the composition of the synthetic diet we used.

When considering the composition of a synthetic diet, we should keep in mind that in addition to sufficient calories it should also contain all necessary nutrients in adequate quantities. In relation to the caloric intake, the demands for many nutrients are higher in the growing individual than in the adult; therefore one standard diet for all age groups will result either in a mixture that is not adapted to the requirements of the rapidly growing child or in the administration of certain nutrients in proportions which are no longer needed by the adult and may be harmful. A synthetic diet that is made to meet the child's requirements can, however, be adapted to those of the adult by adding supplementary quantities of carbohydrates and fat.

In composing our synthetic diet, we first took the amino acid requirements of the growing infant into account. Like others before us, we accepted the amino acid composition of human milk protein as being optimum. However, the total amino acid nitrogen per 100 grams of dry weight of our mixture is 50% higher than that of human milk. In taking up 100 cal/kg bodyweight/day, the child receives a total quantity of amino acids which corresponds to 2.7 grams of protein with this diet, as compared with 1.6 g per 100 cal with human milk. Whereas about 50% of the calories in human milk derive from fat and about 40% from carbohydrates, the proportions in our synthetic diet are just the reverse: namely about 30% of the calories are provided by fat and 60% by carbohydrates. The reason for this is that in many patients who need a synthetic diet it is just the fatabsorption that is limited. Furthermore there are technical reasons (suspensibility of the powder) for preferring a fat percentage which is not too high. In order to improve fat absorption, half of the fat consists of medium chain fatty acids (triglycerides) and half of vegetable oil with a high percentage of doubly unsaturated fatty acids (C 18^{-2}).

Dextrin-maltose was chosen as carbohydrate. This mixture of relatively simple carbohydrates is easily broken down into glucose in the intestinal tract whereas the difficulties arising from the administration of considerable amounts of glucose can be avoided. For the composition of the diets, see tables 1 and 2.

Table 1. *Analysis of synthetic diet per 100 g.*

	powder per 100 g	
water	2.5 g	
Fat	14.5 g	
maize oil		7.2 g
MCT oil		7.2 g
lipids		0.1 g
Dextrin maltose	65.3 g	
Amino acids (N × 7,71 =)	13.5 g	
Minerals	3.3 g	
Vitamins	0.1 g	
CMC	0.8 g	
	100.0 g	
Kcal	452	

Table 2. *Analysis of synthetic diet – amino acids per 100 g.*

L–lysine	0.68 g	L–glycine	0.31 g
L–histidine	0.37 g	L–alanine	0.52 g
L–arginine	0.48 g	L–valine	0.80 g
L–tryptophane	0.29 g	L–methionine	0.72 g
L–aspartic acid	1.16 g	L–leucine	1.20 g
L–threonine	0.64 g	L–isoleucine	0.76 g
L–serine	0.72 g	L–tyrosine	0.64 g
L–glutamic acid	2.32 g	L–cysteine	0.31 g
L–proline	1.09 g	L–phenylalanine	0.49 g
Total 13.5 g/100 g			

Table 3. *Analysis of synthetic diet – minerals per 100 g.*

Na	207	mg	Mn	0.1	mg
K	620	mg	Cu	0.207	mg
Ca	207	mg	J	0.1	mg
P	160	mg	Al	0.0104	mg
Mg	26	mg	Mo	0.001–0.005	mg
SO$_4$	180	mg	Co	0.001–0.005	mg
Fe	3.1	mg	Cl	(850±50)	mg
Zn	0.5	mg	Citric acid	460	mg

For the mineral composition, we have followed with some adaptations that of human milk (table 3). Thus the calcium percentage is as low as that in human milk. The sodium content is somewhat higher at 44 mg per 100 cal, human milk contains 30 mg; potassium contents are 75 and 135 mg, respectively and chlorine contents, 45 and 180 mg, respectively. The percentage of chlorine in the synthetic diet is clearly higher than that in human milk because some basic amino acids were added as chlorides. Trace-elements were added according to available literature and the values in human milk insofar as they are known.

As for the water-soluble vitamins, the concentration per 100 cal was about twice as that of human milk. See table 4 for the fatsoluble vitamins, the vitamin D concentration being 90 E per 100 cal.

Table 4. *Analysis of synthetic diet – vitamins per 100 g.*

Vitamin A	0.35	mg	Vitamin B$_{12}$	0,4	µg
Vitamin D	400	I.E.	Vitamin E	4,0	mg
Vitamin C	25	mg	Folic acid	40	µg
Vitamin B$_1$	0,2	mg	Choline	60	mg
Vitamin B$_2$	0,3	mg	Biotine	10	µg
Niacine	2,0	mg	Inositol	20	mg
Vitamin B$_6$	0,15	mg	Ca-pantothenate	8	mg
Total: 120,45 mg					

Owing to the presence of metal ions, the vitamin C in the diluted formula is soon oxydized and further broken down. Therefore it is necessary to store the diluted mixture in a freezer or to administer it shortly after dilution. When these precautions are not taken, there is the considerable risk that most of the vitamin C will be lost before reaching the patient and vitamin C deficiency may occur, as illustrated by patient W's case history.

We started to use this type of diet in three patients with the non-ketotic form of glycinaemia. The diet given differed from the one mentioned above in that it did not contain the amino acids glycine and serine. The reason we decided to exclude glycine and serine was the consideration that in this way the high blood glycine levels of these children might drop. In this respect we were partially successful and the condition of our patients improved to some extent. This was sufficient reason to continue administration. They were given, according to their age and grade of activity, a diet with a caloric value ranging between 100 and 70 cal/kg bodyweight/day.

Patient 1, a girl of 8 months, was admitted to our hospital with a severe mental and a moderate growth retardation. Length and weight were slightly under the 5th percentile curve. Attempts to lower the blood glycine level with a low-protein diet (0.5 g/kg/day) were unsuccessful and caused, for obvious reasons, retarded weight gain. It was then decided to change over to the synthetic diet, without glycine and serine, because it offered the possibility of giving the essential amino acids in sufficient amounts. Since a certain improvement was noted, we continued to administer this diet for three years. In that period the child's length and weight increased in accordance with the normal growth curve, but she was not able to catch up the loss caused by the initial growth retardation. Her bone age followed the normal pattern of development. Since no further improvement was seen, the child was

Length and weight of toddlers (girls) Netherlands, 1965.

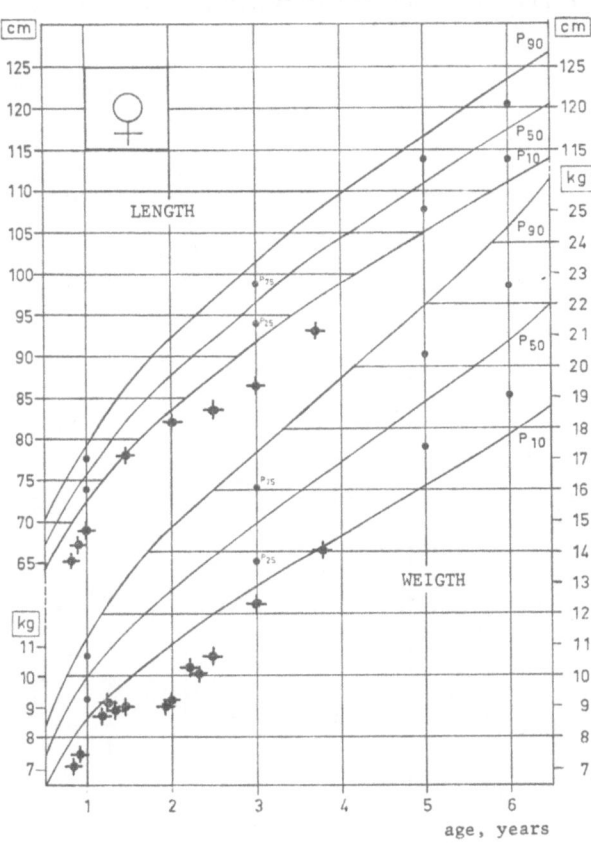

Fig. 1, patient 1.

discharged at the end of this three year period. Shortly after discharge, the child died of an intercurrent infection (fig. 1).

Her sister, patient 2, was admitted shortly after birth. Since we found that she had the same hereditary disease, treatment with the synthetic diet was already started three weeks after birth. During the first three months, the child developed reasonably and mental damage, if present, seemed to be slight. At the age of three months, her condition deteriorated perhaps in connection with an intercurrent infection. Her blood glycine level rose to such high values that we decided to proceed to peritoneal dialysis. At the age of 6 months her condition restabilized. However by then, the child was severely damaged mentally with a markedly retarded growth (see fig. 2). Since this episode her physical development has been more or less normal,

Length and weight of infants (girls) Netherlands, 1965.

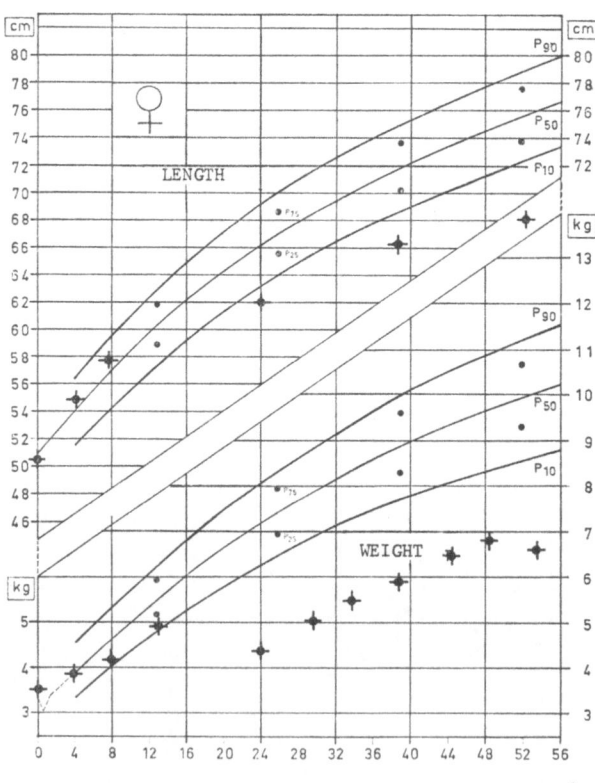

Fig. 2, patient 2.

Length and weight of toddlers (girls) Netherlands, 1965.

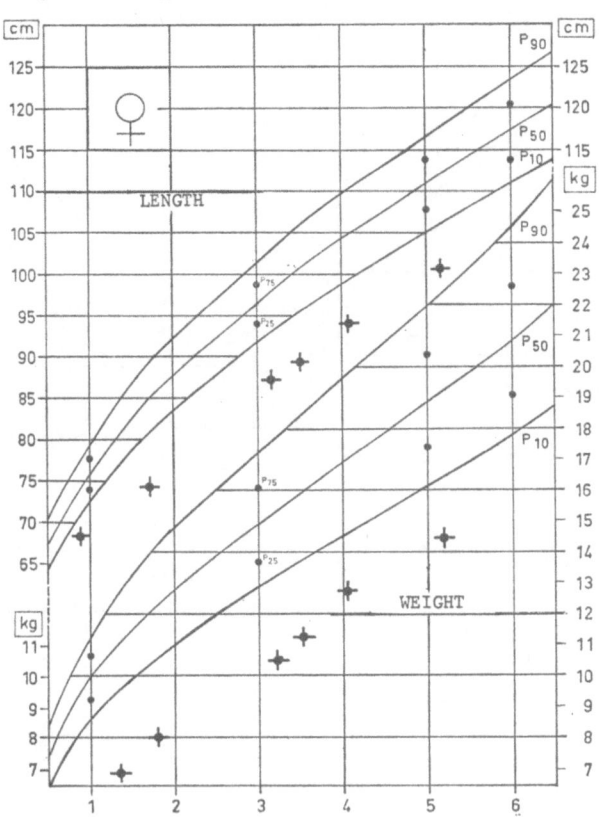

Fig. 3, patient 2.

taken into account her considerable mental defect. She is still in our clinic and is kept on the synthetic diet (figs. 2 and 3).

Patient 3 was admitted at the age of one year with the same syndrome. She was treated with the same diet for about 1½ years. During that period her physical development was normal. After an initial relatively satisfactory course, the neurological condition deteriorated rapidly at the age of 2½ years and the child died of an intercurrent infection (fig. 4).

In an attempt to improve patient 2's condition during periods of rapid mental decline, we decreased the amount of amino acids in the diet to 0.6 g/kg/day. This, however, soon caused the clinical picture

Length and weight of toddlers (girls) Netherlands, 1965.

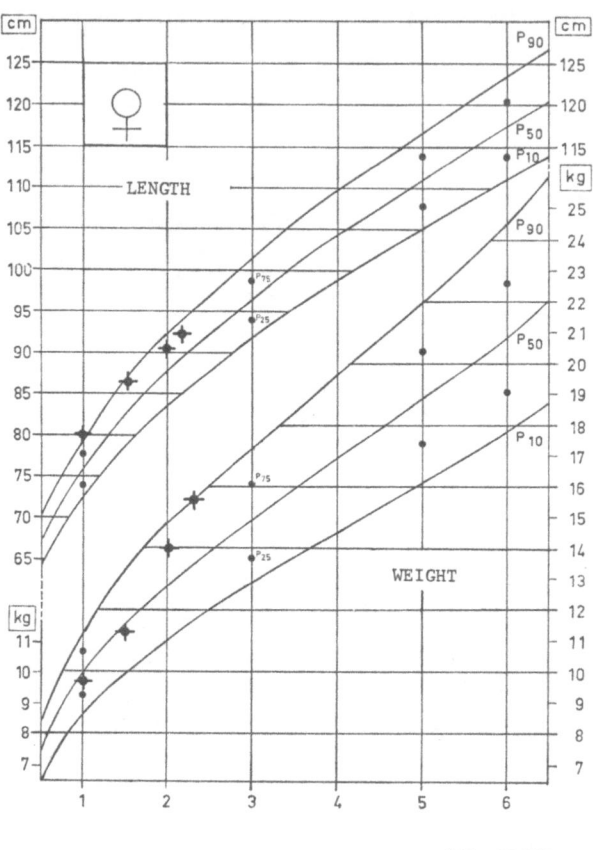

Fig. 4, patient 3.

of protein malnutrition (oedema, skin lesions) with a drop in serum protein to 4.1 g/100 ml. The symptoms of protein deficiency disappeared promptly after the amino acid administration had been increased to 1.8 g/kg/day. During a period of otherwise normal physical development, X-ray examination showed changes in the epiphysical lines which were taken as an indication of vitamin C deficiency.

The blood vitamin C level was found to be low (0.1 mg/100 ml). We then discovered that the vitamin C concentration in the synthetic diet as given to the child was very low. We believe that the reason for this shortage of vitamin C in the food was the method of storage, which caused the vitamin C content of the formula to drop to practically zero.

Any symptoms other than the above-mentioned could not be observed in these patients. Except for a slight retardation in bone age, the skeletal development was normal. This was also the case for the teeth; no caries was found nor was there any symptom of skin deficiencies in the children. Blood chemistry was performed regularly in all three patients, offering normal values for haemoglobin (14 g %), protein spectrum, total fat and cholesterol contents, calcium and phosphate levels and vitamin C level. The blood sugar values were also normal. The plasma amino acid levels of patient 2 were determined regularly. They were found to be within the normal range except for glycine and serine, if we exclude the period of protein malnutrition. This was also the case for the tubular reabsorption of amino acids except for glycine. No increased urinary level was noted in the 24-hours urine for the other amino acids. Stools were fairly frequent, although not very voluminous, and thickish.

I believe that we may conclude that in these children, one of whom has taken our synthetic diet for 3 years, the physical development has been normal to slightly retarded without signs of deficiencies, except for the periods mentioned.

Now I should like to discuss a group of somewhat older children. In the first place an 8-year-old boy, who was admitted to our hospital in a very poor nutritional condition with all the signs of protein malnutrition (serum protein content 3.8% per ml). From the case history given by the parents, it appeared that he had developed normally during his first 5 years of life. Then a coeliac disease – like picture had developed which should have responded well initially to a gluten-free diet. After some time, a relapse occurred in which there was no longer a satisfactory reponse to the gluten-free diet. Physical examination upon admission revealed that besides the common manifestations of coeliac disease, (practically total mucosal atrophy, disaccharidase activity remarkably reduced with a fat absorption of ±50%) there were however symptoms which did not fit into the picture of coeliac disease. There was a severe amino-aciduria. Determination of the tubular reabsorption of amino acids revealed serious disturbances in the reabsorption of histidine, isoleucine, leucine, alanine, valine and threonine. The reabsorption of some other amino acids, however, was found to be normal. Moreover large amounts of indican were found in the urine. Nevertheless it was not the clinical picture of Hartnup disease. The excretion of tryptophane in the urine was found to be only slightly

9

increased. We started to treat the protein malnutrition with plasma transfusions and intravenous administration of amino acids (Amino-sol[R]). Thereafter we prescribed a synthetic diet of 1500 calories per diem (body weight 18 kg, length 121 cm). This diet consisted of 240 g dextrin-maltose, 46 g medium chain fatty acids and 43 g of the amino acid mixture.

During the following 6 months, the boy received hardly any other food and his condition improved (weight increased to 25 kg). The signs of protein malnutrition disappeared, the serum protein level recovered to 6.8% whereas his initially brittle and reddish hair regained its dark brown colour and became glossy. The skin lesions disappeared also. At the end of the 6 months, it was possible to gradually put him on a more normal diet. At the moment he is still receiving a gluten-free diet. With this diet the boy is thriving, although he is surely not cured. Intestinal biopsy still reveals a partial mucosal atrophy, but a normal disaccharidase activity. The tubular amino acid reabsorption is still distinctly disturbed and the indican reaction in the urine is still markedly positive, the fat absorption being 89%.

Most probably there is here a combined defect in the amino acid transport through both the intestinal epithelium and the tubular epithelium. In view of the retarded growth in length and bone age, it seems to me likely that the syndrome already existed before his 5th year and that we may consider the acute phase as a deterioration of the already existing disturbance in the amino acid transport.

It is not clear why the boy has reacted so well upon the synthetic diet. It may be that the amino acid absorption in the most proximal part of his intestinal tract is less disturbed than in the somewhat more distal parts where amino acid absorption normally takes place.

Our second case is a 13-year-old girl. Four months before admission to our hospital, she had fallen ill with intermittent, but gradually exacerbating complaints of abdominal pains and diarrhoea. Her appetite was failing, resulting in a considerable loss of weight.

On examination we saw a not acutely ill, very emaciated girl who had lost 14 kg during the preceding months. The diagnosis of Crohn's disease determined elsewhere could be confirmed (table 5 shows the principal data gathered during treatment). The stools were frequent (3–4 times daily), loose and mucous, containing large quantities of undigested food. The markedly positive indican reaction in the urine pointed to a disturbed protein digestion. Fat absorption, however

Table 5. *Plasma amino acid levels of the patient during the different phase of treatment (in mmoles per ml).*

	Before 23-9-71	I. v. nutr. 5-11-71	14 hours of fasting 17-11-1971	Synthetic diet			
				14-12-71	3-1-72	17-1-72	6-3-72
Ornithine	0.04	0.07	—	0.05	0.02	0.06	0.08
Lysine	0.10	0.19	—	0.08	0.06	0.12	0.15
Histidine	0.05	0.10	—	0.08	0.02	0.09	0.07
Tryptophane	—	—	—	—	—	—	—
Arginine	0.03	0.05	—	0.03	—	0.04	0.04
Aspartic acid	0.01	0.03	0.02	0.02	0.01	0.01	0.01
Threonine	0.05	0.15	0.07	0.14	0.25	0.19	0.27
Serine	0.10	0.19	0.10	0.12	0.13	—	0.11
Asparagine $\}$ Glutamine $\}$	0.37	0.55	0.39	0.53	0.69	0.54	0.66
Proline	0.14	0.52	0.20	0.29	0.33	0.31	0.45
Glutamic acid	0.12	0.13	0.10	0.11	0.07	0.10	0.08
Citrulline	—	—	—	0.03	0.03	—	0.03
Glycine	0.22	0.23	0.28	0.30	0.42	0.33	0.43
Alanine	0.16	0.47	0.36	0.43	0.63	0.46	0.56
α-Amino-butyric acid	—	—	—	0.01	—	0.01	0.02
Valine	0.12	0.29	0.11	0.16	0.15	0.22	0.22
Methionine	—	0.03	0.01	0.01	0.01	0.02	0.02
Isoleucine	0.05	0.12	0.04	0.03	0.04	0.08	0.07
Leucine	0.08	0.12	0.05	0.06	0.05	0.10	0.11
Tyrosine	0.04	0.04	0.03	0.05	0.05	0.05	0.06
Phenylalanine	0.06	0.12	0.03	0.03	0.03	0.04	0.05
Half-cystine	—	0.05	0.04	0.05	0.07	—	0.04

amounted to 90% on a gluten-free diet, whereby the fat consisted
mainly of maize oil and the medium chain triglycerides C_8 and C_{10}.
In spite of this diet, the diarrhoea and anorexia continued so that the
girl lost another 7 kg during the first weeks after admission. It was then
decided to limit the amount of food taken orally and to proceed intravenous feeding, namely a 30% sorbitol solution supplemented with a 10%
fat-emulsion (Intralipid[R]) and a 7% amino acid solution (Vamin[R]).
Oral administration of food was limited to water and a concentrated
solution of glucose and dextrin-maltose (Hycal[R]) with a small amount
of medium chain fatty acids as well as mineral and vitamin mixtures.
In this way 1560 calories were administered intravenously and about
1000 calories orally per day. The indican reaction in the urine became
negative, and the number of stools decreased and became less voluminous. We managed to feed the girl mainly intravenously for 4 weeks.
This resulted in a stabilization of her weight and a slight tendency
toward increase in the serum plasma protein level (see fig. 5).

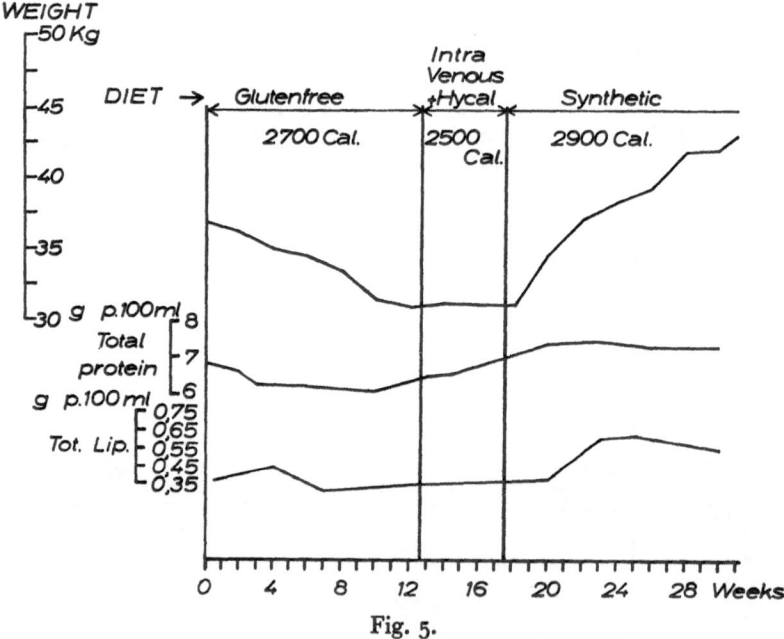

Fig. 5.

Owing to the condition of the veins however, it was impossible to
continue this treatment after these 4 weeks. Therefore we decided to
give the girl an almost completely synthetic diet. Moreover she eats
4 truffles daily, consisting of dextrin-maltose, medium chain fatty

acids and cocoa powder. In this way she received 2900 calories per day: 400 grams carbohydrates, 90 grams fat, 67 grams L-amino acids, vitamins and minerals (tables 1, 2, 3, 4). The daily mineral intake consisted of 950 mg calcium, 600 mg sodium, 1260 mg potassium, 200 mg magnesium, 15 mg iron, 2 mg copper, 6 mg zinc, 0.8 mg manganese, 0.2 mg iodine and traces of aluminium (0.002 mg), cobalt (0.008 mg) and molybdene (0.003 mg). The total amount of fluid was limited to about 2 l daily.

The results of this therapy were most satisfying. The frequency of the stools decreased, the average amount of faeces dropped to about 100 g per day. Defaecation took place once a day or on alternate days. As for the change in the blood levels of haemoglobin, calcium, phosphate, magnesium, total protein, total lipoid, cholesterol, serum iron and vitamins A, C and E, see table 6.

In 12 weeks the girl gained 10 kg in weight. In spite of the rapid weight gain, no signs of deficiencies were noted. Repeated examinations showed normal fat absorption. Roentgenograms of the intestinal tract showed a certain degree of improvement. 12 weeks after the onset of treatment with the synthetic diet, the girl was discharged in good nutritional condition. She is taking her diet at home. Today, two months after discharge, she is still in good condition and has gained another 2 kg. Since falling serum iron values and a slight drop in the haemoglobin level pointed to a certain degree of iron deficiency, we have doubled the quantity of iron in the diet. Table 5 shows the plasma amino acid levels upon admission, during the intravenous feeding and during the synthetic diet. It is clear that the levels of the essential amino acids, which were low upon admission, have become normal.

Especially at the age when growth is normally most rapid, deficiencies resulting from a partial malnutrition are probably the first to manifest themselves. Therefore use of a new nutritional formula such as the synthetic diet should be limited in this group of children to those cases in which all other feeding has failed.

This was the case in a baby who at the age of 6 months was admitted to our hospital in a state of severe malnutrition. Her birth weight had been about 2200 g. During the first two months she had developed rather satisfactorily. Thereafter, however, her growth had come to a standstill, although the stools had remained practically normal on a normal baby formula. Upon admission her weight was only 3400 g and it dropped to 3000 g in the first weeks of hospitalization. It not

Table 6. *Some data gathered during treatment.*

Time in days:	Admission to hospital 0 days	Start intravenous nutrition 96 days	Start synthetic diet 144 days	Discharge on synthetic diet 244 days	As outpatient, still on synthetic diet 313 days
Haemoglobin (g/100 ml)	11.0	11.9	11.0	11.0	10.7
Ca (mg/100 ml)	8.8	8.7	9.3	9.1	9.7
PO$_4$ (mg/100 ml)	4.8	4.3	3.4	4.5	4.0
Mg (mg/100 ml)				3.8	3.6
Total protein (g/100 ml)	6.4	6.5	7.4	7.1	6.8
Total lipoid (mg/100 ml)	269–385	344	417	498–557	
Cholesterol (mg/100 ml)	117	82	192	231	144
Serum iron (μg/100 ml)	12	81	92	55	42
Vitamin A (μmol/l)				0.85	
Vitamin C (mg/100 ml)			0.8	0.9	
Vitamin E (ml/100 ml)				1.0	

possible to make a straight diagnosis. Her abdomen was distended and her appetite was poor. It was noted that the child had cataracts on both eyes. Moreover in the urine small amounts of those disaccharides were found that were present in her formula. The pH of the faeces was normal; fat absorption was at the lower end of normal range. Intestinal biopsy showed a slight mucosal atrophy, whereas with normal percentages of lactase and saccharase those of maltase and isomaltase were found to be reduced. No abnormalities were found in the monosaccharide metabolism. After some hesitation we decided to put the child on the synthetic diet of the above-mentioned composition, but to replace dextrin-maltose with glucose. This replacement may have been the cause of her continuously loose stools which were, moreover, rather voluminous. This diet was administered for 6 months. In the beginning 100 cal per kg body weight/day were given. Soon, however, the caloric value of the diet was increased to about 160 calories per kg. It was kept at this level during the entire period of rapid growth resulting from administration of the diet.

In 6 months there was a weight increase from 3000 to 6800 gr. (fig. 6). During a period of one month, the daily gain amounted to 0.8%

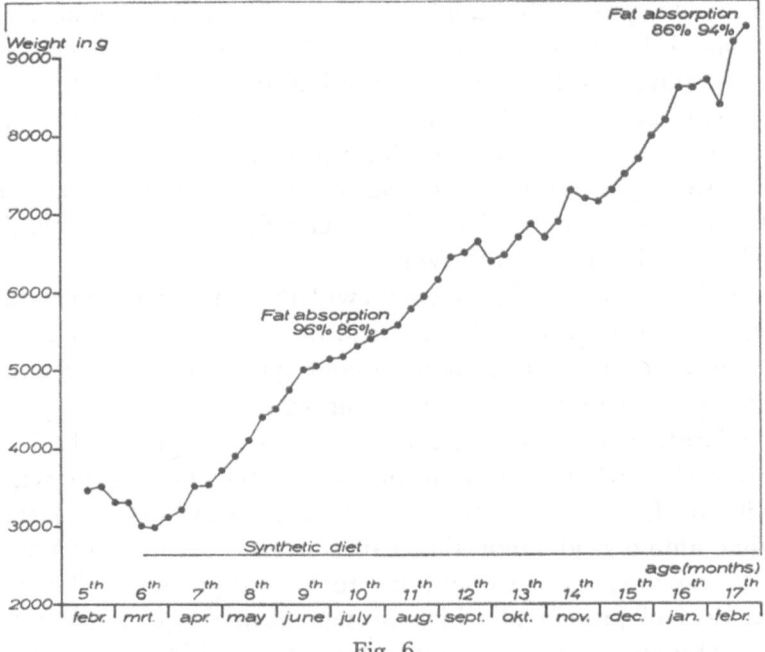

Fig. 6.

daily. No signs of deficiency were noted. There were no rickets or anaemia, the serum protein levels as well as the calcium and phosphate levels remaining normal. Occasional fat resorption determinations were done, with an average percentage of 90. The haemoglobin level did not change notwithstanding the rapid weight gain.

It is noteworthy that with the improvement in her general condition the child was able to digest disaccharides and higher carbohydrates normally. Therefore we then decided to place her again on a normal diet. Why the child improved on the diet remains unsolved.

Finally I want to discuss the administration of this diet to a newborn baby with a congenital malformation of the intestinal tract. It concerns a premature twin (birth weight 1700 g) who at the age of 3 days was operated on for ileal atresia; 10 cm of ileum was removed. During the first days after surgery, the child received 10% glucose and Aminosol[R] intravenously. 7 days after surgery (10 days after birth), this was replaced by oral feeding. In order to relieve the intestinal tract as much as possible, we chose the synthetic diet of the above-mentioned composition; 120 calories/kg body weight/day were given.

In the following three weeks, there was an increase in weight from 1800 g to 2100 g. The stools were rather frequent, but small in quantity. In spite of the rapid gain in weight, no signs of deficiencies were noted. Blood chemistry was normal, notably that of the calcium and phosphate levels. The fat absorption amounted to 91%; mainly long chain saturated and unsaturated fatty acids were excreted. There was a drop in the haemoglobin level from 13.8 to 9.9 g per 100 ml. After 3 weeks, the synthetic diet was replaced by a humanized formula with a high percentage of medium chain fatty acids (Caprilon[R]) on which the child has been thriving.

Our observations are in agreement with those mentioned in literature, namely that even young children can develop satisfactorily in length and weight on a synthetic diet without symptoms of deficiencies. A normal growth rate can also be achieved in some children with intestinal disturbances who did not thrive or lost weight on classic diets. It is not clear what the basis of this favourable effect of the synthetic diet is. One factor may be that no food proteins have to be broken down so that amino acid absorption can start in a very early phase. It should, however, be borne in mind that the organism itself secretes a great deal of protein to which protein from desquamated mucosal cells is also added. The absorption of the fat used in the synthetic diet was good in all cases.

As for the carbohydrates, it is our experience that glucose is not to be preferred, probably owing to the effect of osmotic pressure.

Since even atrophic intestinal mucosa produces maltase and iso-maltase in moderate amounts, the absorption of dextrin-maltose seldom causes difficulties. It is necessary to verify whether there is a reasonable absorption of amino acids, fats and carbohydrates in patients with any form of intestinal malabsorption who are taking a synthetic diet. Examination of the faeces for the lactic acid content, the nquatity and quality of fat, the percentages of fatty acids and calcium together with the indican reaction in the urine may provide useful information about the absorption process.

It is improbable that the good results are caused only by the absence of cellulose and otherwise indigestible or non-absorbable elements in the food and therefore their influence on the bacterial flora. Milk and baby formulas on a milk basis, and especially human milk, do not contain indigestible or non-absorbable elements either and yet some patients with malabsorption show a definite improvement on the synthetic diet but do not thrive on humanized milk formulas, even when the lactose concentration is low and the fat is composed mainly of medium chain fatty acids.

INDICATIONS FOR A SYNTHETIC DIET

In which childhood disorders of health can the synthetic diet be o therapeutic benefit?

1. In some congenital metabolic disturbances a pure synthetic diet may be necessary, for instance in maple sugar disease.
2. Severe mucosal atrophy of the small intestine may form an in-dication for the synthetic diet. In view of the very limited absorb-ing surface of the small intestine in such cases, it is important that absorption starts in the most proximal part of the small in-testine.
3. A marked reduction in the production of faeces may be of im-portance in patients with disorders of the ileum or colon.
4. I shall not discuss indications in the surgical field, especially those cases where it is important to reduce the content of the intestine as much as possible.

5. I should, however, still point out the possibilities which these synthetic diets offer for the detection of noxious factors in diets of natural composition.

It may, however, be advisable to approach the frequent and early administration of synthetic diets with reservation. Administration of homogenized food mixtures gives satisfactory results in many cases of malabsorption. Such a homogenized mixture of meat, vegetables with a low cellulose content, milk protein and carbohydrates other than lactose or saccharose should preferably contain medium chain fatty acids and should have a rather low percentage of calcium. Upon administration of such food with a minimum of indigestible elements, the enzymatic breakdown in the intestinal tract of most patients with intestinal malabsorption usually takes place so satisfactorily that only a limited absorbing surface is needed for the absorption of the nutrients.

SYNTHETIC DIET IN INTERNAL MEDICINE

S. JARNUM*

Water-soluble, chemically defined diets were developed at the National Institute of Health, U.S.A., about 15 years ago. These diets were composed of balanced proportions of L-amino acids, water-soluble and fat-soluble vitamins, mineral salts, glucose or other simple sugars as the source of carbohydrate and ethyl linoleate as the source of essential fat (1).

Later experiments with volunteers at the California Medical Faculty (2) showed that the administration of a chemically defined or elementary diet in normal man produced a number of significant changes:

Faecal elimination was strikingly diminished. After a week stool weight was greatly reduced. The frequency of bowel movements became quite low with intervals between movements of up to a week or more. Faeces became dark green to black and almost odourless; the bacterial count dropped to a figure which was only a small fraction of the normal value. Furthermore the bacterial spectrum changed at the expense of the anaerobic flora.

At the same time the subjects maintained their health and weight over an experimental period of a $\frac{1}{2}$ year.

On this basis the diet was proposed as nutrition for men in space during prolonged space flights (3). However, in practice greater interest was attached to the applicability of the diet in human disease.

Within internal medicine certain gastrointestinal diseases form the major field of application.

One can almost predict which clinical conditions may benefit from treatment with an elementary diet.

* Medical Department P, Division of Gastroenterology, Rigshospitalet, Copenhagen, Denmark.

Acknowledgements: The work was supported by grants from Christian d. X's Fond, P. Carl Petersens Fond and Statens laegevidenskabelige Forskningsfond.

Table I lists a number of gastrointestinal diseases for which an elementary diet has been recommended.

Table 1. *Elementary diet. Applications in gastroenterology*

1. Intestinal *fistula*
2. Chronic 'intractable' *diarrhoea* of unknown cause
3. *Short bowel syndrome*
4. Chronic *inflammatory bowel disease*: Crohn's disease Ulcerative colitis
5. Other *malabsorption syndromes* resistant to conventional therapy: Non-tropical sprue Blind loop syndrome

The 'medical' treatment of *internal fistulae*, whether enterocutaneous or rectovaginal, aims at reducing both the intestinal content and secretion from the fistula to promote spontaneous healing of the fistula.

Chronic diarrhoea of unknown origin may be due to unidentified micro-organisms which may succumb to the changed environment during an elementary dietary regime.

In the *short bowel syndrome* the rapid absorption of an elementary diet permits a higher net absorption of calories and amino acids.

In *chronic inflammatory disease of the intestine* the reduced intestinal content 'immobilizes' the diseased segment which, from a conventional surgical viewpoint, is always attractive in the treatment of inflammation. Furthermore the possible role of dietary antigens and noxa in the aetiology and pathogenesis of these conditions is minimized.

Finally, it seems logical to use elementary diets in the treatment of various *malabsorption syndromes*, e.g. sprue, blind loop syndrome, when the established treatment fails: gluten-free diet in non-tropical sprue, antibiotics in the blind loop syndrome.

I shall report some of the results we have obtained with an elementary diet in a limited number of patients.

METHODS

In most of the studies we used Vivasorb[R]*. It is supplied in 80 g packets, containing 300 calories and 6.3 g amino acids together with

* J. Pfrimmer & Co., Erlangen, kindly supplied samples for a large part of the study.

vitamins and electrolytes which, according to present-day knowledge, are known or assumed to be needed.

Our practical management of the elementary diet appears in table 2.

Table 2. *Elementary diet (Vivasorb®). Scheme of treatment.*

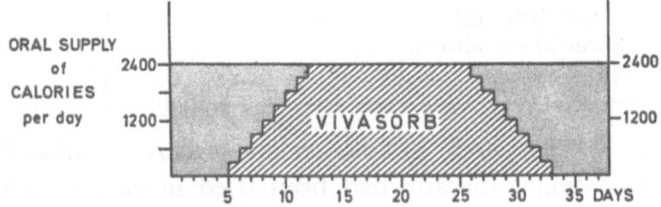

Allowed during Vivasorb regime:
1. A total of 1 liter per day to drink of:
   Water
   Diluted, clear fruit juice
   Tea without milk or sugar
   Coffee without milk or sugar
   Not allowed: Milk or skimmed milk
               Beer
               Bouillon
2. Smoking
All oral medication is withheld

We attach great importance to a gradual substitution of the elementary diet. If substitution is too fast nausea, vomiting and diarrhoea are likely to arise and the future cooperation of the patient is jeopardized. Complete substitution should not be effected in less than a week or so.

The total number of calories given as elementary diet is determined by the calculated requirement of the patient, his preceding spontaneous caloric intake and his feeling of hunger. It varied between 1800 and 2700 calories. In addition to the diet he is allowed to drink clear fluids, tea and coffee, and to smoke. Drinks containing fat or residue such as milk and most fruit juices are not allowed.

When the normal diet is reinstated it is done gradually in the same way as it was stopped. Normal diet, in most cases, means a liberal, protein-rich diet with some restriction of residues.

CASE MATERIAL

Fourteen patients were studied (table 3). Two had intestinal fistulae, one chronic diarrhoea and 3 short bowel syndrome. There were 6 patients with ulcerative colitis, one with Crohn's disease and one with sarcoidosis and a sprue-like syndrome.

Table 3. *Case material*

Intestinal fistula	2
Chronic diarrhoea	1
Short bowel syndrome	3
Chronic inflammatory disease of the intestine	
Crohn's disease	1
Ulcerative colitis	6
Sprue-like syndrome	1
Total	14

All patients were severely ill with weight loss. A common feature was that conventional therapy had been tried in vain or with unsatisfactory results in all of them.

RESULTS

Table 4. *Effects of elementary diet in fistulas and chronic diarrhoea (n=3).*

Case	Diagnosis	Duration of element.diet days	Other treatment	Result
I.O. female, 72 y.	Diverticulitis Left hemicolectomy + small intest resect. *Multiple* internal and external *fistulas*	4	Parent. nutrit. (2400 Cal. per day)	Closure of one of two external fistulas → Reoperation
I.M.J., female, 44 y.	Extensive Crohn's disease *Rectovaginal fistula*	7	Prednisone 80 mg per day	Decreasing secret., but mechanical ileus supervened → operation
E.H.O. male, 37 y.	Perforated appendicitis Appendectomy, two draining procedures for intraabd. abscesses Anuria (12 haemodialyses) Severe *diarrhoea* when oral feedings was reinstituted 6 weeks after appendectomy	10	Initial parent. nutrit.	Cease of diarrhoea within 3 days

Fistulae: In two patients with fistulae (table 4), one with diverticulitis and internal and external intestinal fistulae and one with Crohn's disease and a rectovaginal fistula, the dietary treatment was only partially succesful. Both had to be operated on.

Chronic diarrhoea: One patient with a perforated appendix was appendectomized; later 2 draining procedures for intra-abdominal abscesses were performed. He became anuric. Twelve haemodialyses were carried out before renal function recovered. Furthermore, tracheostomy and respirator treatment became necessary. When oral nutrition was resumed after 6 weeks of parenteral nutrition, severe diarrhoea developed. Its cause could not be determined. With an elementary diet, it vanished within 3 days.

Short bowel syndrome: In 3 patients with short bowel syndrome (table 5), the elementary diet turned out to be a failure.

Table 5. *Elementary diet in short bowel syndrome (n=3).*

Case	Diagnosis	Period from resection to treatment, weeks	Duration of element. diet days	Result
1. K.A.S., male, 48 y.	Mesenteric thrombosis Resection of all small intestine except 20 cm Right hemicolectomy	7	2	Increased stool volume
2. B.K. female, 21 y.	Crohn's disease Subtotal colectomy Resection of 1m ileum	2	18	Stopped because of patient's refusal
3. H.D.O. male, 39 y.	Crohn's disease Right hemicolectomy Resection of 180 cm ileum	5	21	No significant change of stool volume

In one patient stool volume increased, one patient refused to go through with the treatment, and in one patient (fig. 1) the stool volume was essentially unchanged.

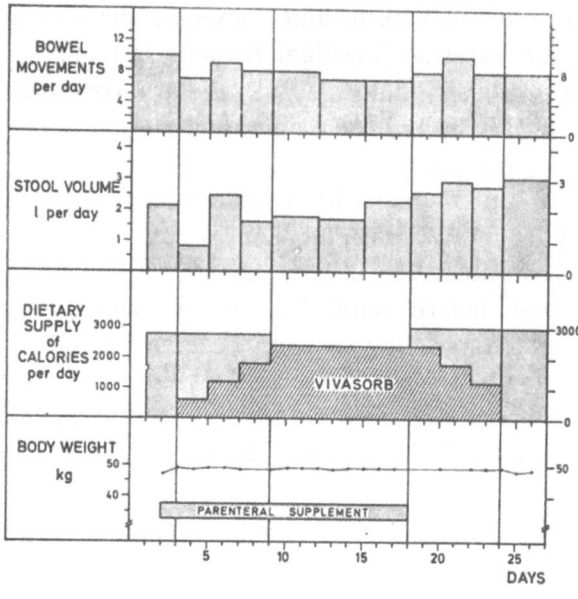

Fig. 1. Elementary diet (Vivasorb®) in *short bowel syndrome*. H.D.O., male, 39 years old. Postoperative phase following intestinal resection due to Crohn's disease. Vivasorb regime was started 5 weeks after surgery. The four vertical lines indicate the periods of Vivasorb regime, which altogether lasted 21 days. No significant change in bowel movements and stool volume occurred.

This patient (H.D.O.) was a 39-year-old male with Crohn's disease which required extensive intestinal resection. A Vivasorb regime was started 5 weeks after surgery. No significant change in bowel movements and stool volume occurred.

It should be pointed out that all three of the cases with short bowel syndrome were in the early or late postoperative phase following intestinal resection.

Chronic inflammatory diseases of the intestine (see table 6):

Altogether, 7 patients were studied.

One had extensive *Crohn's disease* and 6, ulcerative colitis.

Five of these 7 patients went into remission. All 7 had been treated with prednisone in high dosages (80–160 mg per day) for 7 to 21 days before dietary treatment. None of them responded satisfactorily to prednisone treatment alone.

The course of the patient with *Crohn's disease* is seen in fig. 2. She

Table 6. *Elementary diet in chronic inflammatory bowel disease (n=7).*

Case	Diagnosis	Duration of prednisone therapy before diet, days	Duration of elementary diet, days	Other treatment simultaneous with diet	Result
1. A.S. female, 22 y.	Crohn's disease (colon + ileum)	12	23	Prednisone Cholesty-ramine Parent. nutrit. initially	Remission Surgery cancelled
2. K.K. male, 28 y.	Distal ulcerative colitis	15	24	Prednisone Azathioprine	Remission
3. I.O., female, 44 y.	Distal ulcerative colitis	21	22	Prednisone	Remission Surgery cancelled
4. G.J. female, 42 y.	Distal ulcerative colitis	7	26	Prednisone	Remission
5. E.B. female, 44 y.	Total ulcerative colitis	8	31	Prednisone Cholesty-ramine	Remission Surgery cancelled
6. M.M.J., female, 75 y.	Total ulcerative colitis	27	13	Prednisone Azathioprine	→Perforated colon →Operation
7. T.A., male, 54 y.	Total ulcerative colitis	9	3	Prednisone Parent. nutrit.	→Perforated colon →Operation

(A.S.) was a 22-year-old female. Vivasorb was started when a 12-day high dosage course of prednisone (80 mg per day) had failed. Although she improved on the diet, her stools did not become normal until she was treated with the bile acid-binding resin, cholestyramine, despite the fact that the bile acid concentration in a duodenal aspirate follo-wing a test meal was normal (see fig. 2).

Turning to ulcerative colitis, we reserved the elementary diet for those severe cases which did not respond satisfactorily to prednisone treatment. A satisfactory response is illustrated in fig. 3, which shows the course during prednisone treatment in a 42-year-old woman with a fulminant ulcerative colitis. It is seen that body temperature became normal within 24 hours, the pulse rate within 4 days and the stools within a week after the initiation of steroid therapy.

Table 6 lists 6 cases of ulcerative colitis which did not respond or

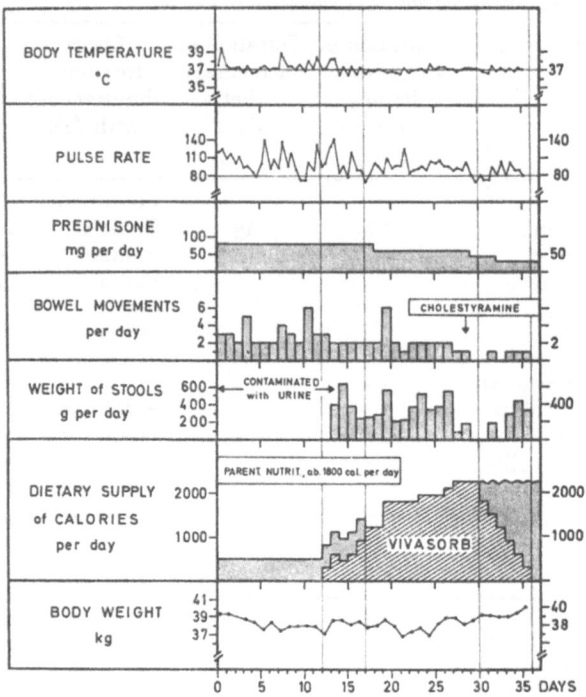

Fig. 2. Elementary diet (Vivasorb®) in *extensive Crohn's disease* (terminal ileum, right half of colon, sigmoideum). A. S., female, 22 years old. Vivasorb was started when a 12-day high dosage course of prednisone treatment (80 mg per day) had failed. During the Vivasorb regime her general condition improved. Stools became less liquid, but not until the institution of cholestyramine therapy did they become solid and normal.

responded unsatisfactorily to steroid therapy. Three of the 6 patients had *ulcerative colitis* of the distal part of the colon. They all went into remission (fig. 4, 5, 6).

In one patient (K.K., fig. 4), a 28-year-old male, prednisone in increasing doses (from 40 to 160 mg per day) brought about an incomplete remission. The stools remained contaminated with large amounts of blood and pus. After 15 days of prednisone treatment, a Vivasorb regime was initiated. Bowel movements decreased to one or two per day. Blood and pus disappeared. He was placed on azathioprine therapy as long-term treatment.

In another patient (I.O., fig. 5), a 44-year-old female with ulcerative colitis of the distal part of the colon complicated by a Stevens-Johnson's syndrome, prednisone (100 to 60 mg per day) induced only a partial remission. When it had been given for 21 days, a Vivasorb regime was added. The stools became normal and blood contamination ceased within a few days. Clinically the patient improved rapidly.

The last patient with ulcerative colitis of the distal part of the colon, (G.J., fig. 6) was a 42-year-old woman. On prednisone treatment (80 mg per day), her bowel movements decreased in frequency. However the stools remained liquid and haemorrhagic, and she was unable to urinate and defaecate separately.

After a Vivasorb regime stool volume decreased, her general condition improved and the stools became solid. No parenteral nutrition was given. Her body weight decreased. During the Vivasorb regime she became hungry, ate more and her weight remained constant.

Of the 3 patients with *ulcerative colitis* of the whole colon, 2 developed toxic megacolon and signs of intra-abdominal perforation and had to be operated on.

One patient (E.B., fig. 7), a 44-year-old, female had made no satisfactory progress after 8 days of prednisone treatment. During a

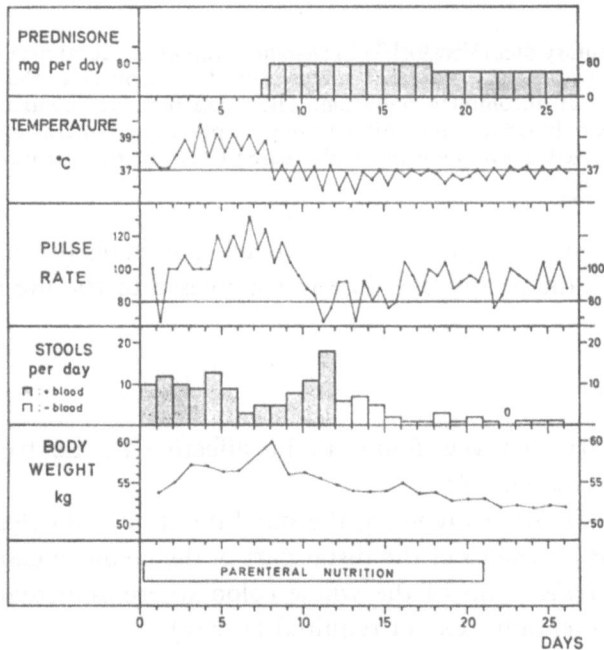

Fig. 3. Prednisone therapy in fulminant ulcerative colitis. E.H.O., female, 42 years old. Prompt effect was seen on body temperature. Blood disappeared from stools in 4 days, and stools became normal within a week.

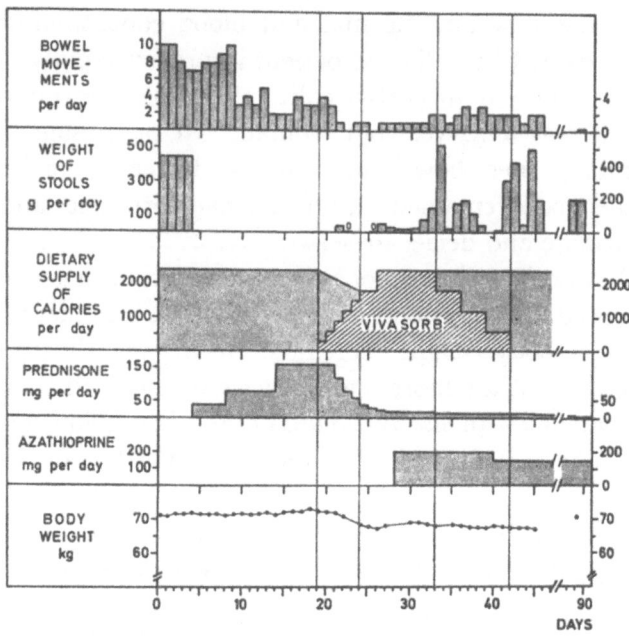

Fig. 4. Elementary diet (Vivasorb®) in *ulcerative colitis* of the distal part of the colon. K.K., male, 28 years old. Prednisone in increasing doses (from 40 to 160 mg per day) brought about an incomplete remission. The stools remained contaminated with large amounts of blood and pus. After 15 days of prednisone treatment, a Vivasorb regime was started. Bowel movements decreased to one or two per day. Blood and pus disappeared.

Vivasorb regime she gradually improved, but stools did not became normal until the prednisone dose was increased to 160 mg per day.

CONCLUSIONS

1. Elementary diet was found to be effective in the treatment of *selected, severe cases* of:

   1.1. *Crohn's disease* involving the small intestine and colon (1 case).

   1.2. *Ulcerative colitis* of the distal part of the colon (3 cases).

   1.3. *Ulcerative colitis* of the whole colon where immediate surgical intervention was not required (1 case).

      In all 5 patients with Crohn's disease or ulcerative colitis, prednisone treatment beforehand induced incomplete remission.

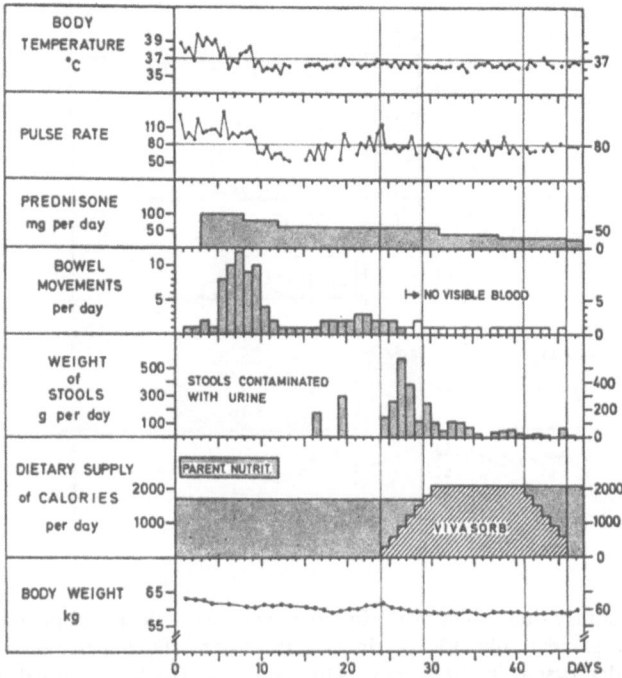

Fig. 5. Elementary diet (Vivasorb®) in *ulcerative colitis* of the distal part of the colon with Stevens-Johnson's syndrome. I.O., female, 44 years old. Prednisone (100 to 60 mg per day) induced only a partial remission. When it had been given for 21 days, a Vivasorb regime was added. The stools became normal and blood contamination ceased within a few days. Clinically, the patient improved rapidly.

1.4. *Chronic diarrhoea* of unknown origin (1 case).
2. No effect was seen in *intestinal fistula* (2 cases) nor in the postoperative phase of the *short bowel syndrome* (3 cases).
   Wheter absolute oral fasting and total parenteral nutrition is more efficient in the treatment of fistulae is still unknown.
3. When treatment with an elementary diet is undertaken, it should always be *initiated in small amounts* and *in a weak solution*. Changing over to a total elementary diet should take about a week.

REFERENCES

1. WINITZ, M., BIRNBAUM, S. M., SUGIMURA, T., & OTEY, M. C., (1960) Quantitative nutritional and in vivo metabolic studies with water-solube, chemically

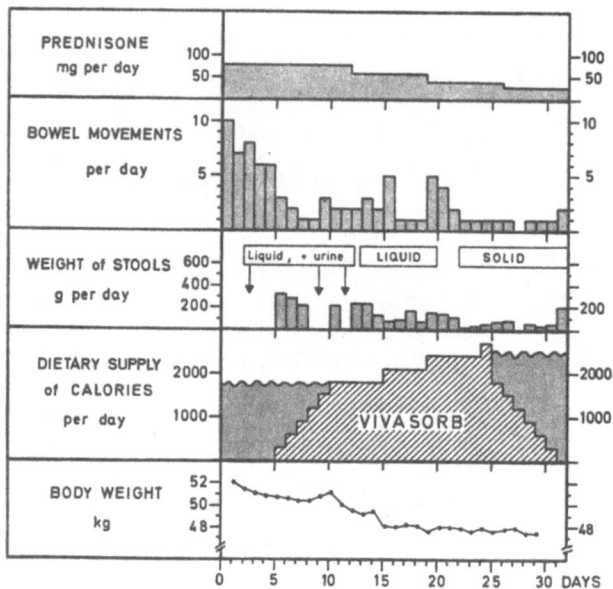

Fig. 6. Elementary diet (Vivasorb®) in *ulcerative colitis* of the distal part of the colon. G.J., female, 42 years old. On prednisone treatment (80 mg per day) her bowel movements decreased in frequency. However the stools remained liquid and haemorrhagic, and she was unable to urinate and defaecate separately. After a Vivasorb regime, stool volume decreased, her general condition improved and the stools became solid. No parenteral substitution was given. Her body weight decreased. During Vivasorb regime she became hungry, ate more and her weight remained constant.

defined diets. In: J. T. Edsell, J. P. Greenstein (eds.) *Amino Acids, Proteins and Cancer Biochemistry*, p. 9. Memorial Symposium. Academic Press, New York.

2. WINITZ, M., & ADAMS, R. F., (1971) Chemically defined diets. A new approach to metabolic nutrition. In: K. Lang, W. Fekl & G. Berg (eds.), *Balanced Nutrition and Therapy*, p. 46. Georg Thieme, Stuttgart.

3. WINITZ, M., GRAFF, J., GALLAGHER, N., NARKIN, A., & SEEDMAN, D. A., (1965) Evaluation of chemical diets as nutrition for man-in-space. *Nature*, 205, 741.

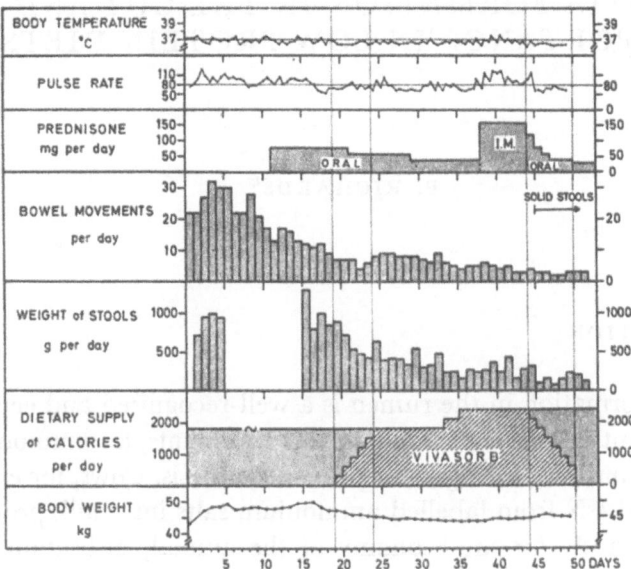

Fig. 7. Elementary diet (Vivasorb®) in *total ulcerative colitis* of the whole colon. E.B., female, 44 years old. After 8 days of prednisone treatment she had made no satisfactory progress. During a Vivasorb regime she gradually improved, but stools did not become normal until prednisone dosage had been increased to 160 mg per day.

AMMONIA FORMATION IN THE GUT AND ITS IMPORTANCE IN LOW PROTEIN DIETS

P. RICHARDS*

INTRODUCTION

Ammonia formation in the rumen is a well-recognised and economically important facet of the metabolism of ruminants, for ammonia is an acceptable source of nitrogen for protein synthesis. Cows, for example, incorporated ^{15}N from labelled ammonium salts into milk protein (1) and, significantly for the economy of the animal, utilisation of ammonia nitrogen was increased when dietary nitrogen was scarce (2). Not only is ruminal ammonia derived from dietary protein and nitrogen salts, but urea, which diffuses into the rumen, is hydrolysed to ammonia and carbon dioxide according to the reaction – $CO(NH_2)_2 + H_2O = 2NH_3 + CO_2$.

Hydrolysis of urea by bacterial ureases has assumed great commercial importance. Because urea is efficiently converted to ammonia it provides a cheap and useful dietary supplement. An estimated 422,000 metric tons of urea were consumed by cattle in 1965–66 in the United States (3). Not only did urea improve the cattle-raisers' profits, but it spared natural resources: the nitrogen contained in the urea was equivalent to the nitrogen contained in about 3 million tons of soybean meal (3).

I have recently reviewed the evidence that monogastric animals also have the capacity to use ammonium salts or urea as a source of nitrogen for aminoacid synthesis (4). Man is no exception; both infants (5, 6) and adults (7–13) utilised ammonia or urea nitrogen and utilisation was greatest when dietary protein intake was restricted (fig. 1). Although both ammonium salts and urea were effective sources of nitrogen, ammonium salts were the most efficient, an ob-

* Department of Medicine, St. George's Hospital Medical School, Hyde Park Corner, London S.W.I. This research was supported by grants from the Medical Research Council and the British Nutrition Foundation Ltd.

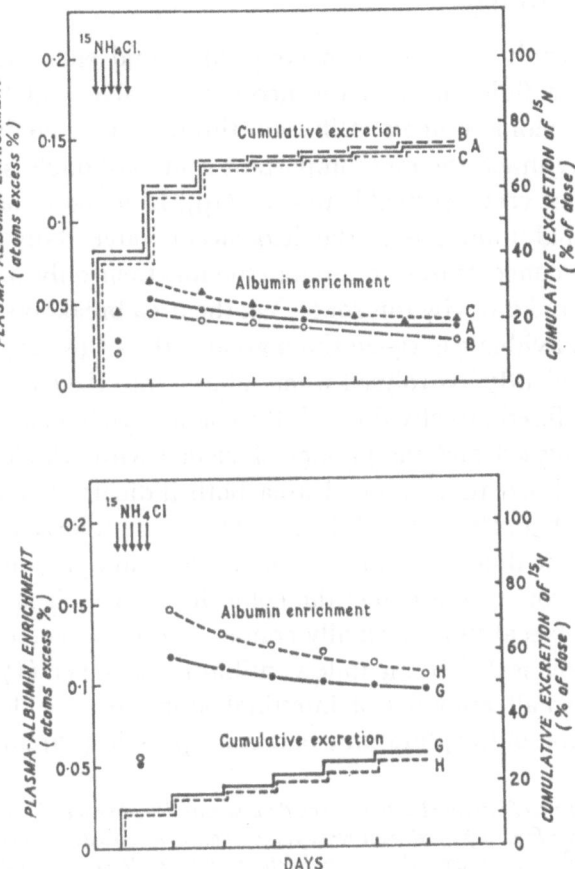

Fig. 1. The cumulative excretion of ¹⁵N after oral ¹⁵NH₄Cl, and the plasma enrichment of 3 healthy adults (A, B, C) on a normal diet and of 2 healthy adults (H, G.) studied 3 weeks after starting a 3–4 g. nitrogen diet. During protein restriction the excretion of ¹⁵N is greatly reduced and enrichment of plasma albumin increases (4).

servation which is explained by the fact that urea nitrogen is only utilised if urea is first converted to ammonia (9). Urea is not metabolised in animals raised in a germ-free environment (14) and its metabolism is greatly impaired by antibiotics (15–18). We can therefore conclude that conversion of urea, an end-product of protein metabolism, into a potentially useful nutrient is a function of commensal intestinal bacteria. The colon is the only site of substantial bacterial activity within monogastric animals. A small amount of mucosal urease is found which may not be bacterial in origin, but its contribution to urea hydrolysis is insignificant (18).

UREA METABOLISM

Urea is uniformly distributed in body fluids and enters the colon in small intestine fluid through the ileo-coecal valve and by diffusion through the colonic mucosa. Diffusion through the colonic mucosa is quantitatively much the more important route although, surprisingly, the colon is not very permeable to urea (19). If no more than 1 litre of small intestinal fluid passes the ileo-caecal valve daily and has a normal urea concentration of 40 mg/100 ml, then only 0.4 g of urea will be delivered daily by this route. Yet the urea breakdown measured in healthy individuals is 15–20 times greater than this (15). Urea is in fact more efficiently hydrolysed when infused into the circulation than when it is perfused directly through the colon (19). The large quantity of urea hydrolysed and the greater efficiency with which circulating urea is hydrolysed than luminal urea both indicate that most of the urea which is hydrolysed has diffused through the colonic mucosa from blood and tissue fluids, and that it is hydrolysed at a juxtamucosal site. By whatever route urea enters the colon its hydrolysis is remarkably complete for faecal fluid normally contains no urea; even in uraemia little or no urea is detectable unless antibiotics are given (17) (table 1).

Although small amounts of intestinal ammonia are derived from peptic digestion of the glutamine of dietary protein (20) and doubtless

Table 1. *The effect of intestinal antibiotics on the concentration of urea and ammonia in faecal dialysate from a patient with renal failure (blood urea concentration 160–185 mg/ 100 ml; 27–31 mmol/l). An antibiotic mixture containing bacitracin, colomycin, neomycin and nystatin was given from days 1–6 inclusive (from 17). Normal subjects: mean and 95% range, shown in upper part of the table.*

Day	Specimen	Urea (mmole/l)	Ammonia (mmole/l)	pH
		0	11.2	6.96
			2.9–44	5.92–8.00
1	1	0	16.4	—
	2	31.9	2.3	6.86
3	3	29.8	2.2	5.94
	4	28.1	2.5	5.88
4	5	24.1	9.7	5.32
5	6	7.0	35.6	5.84
6	7	16.3	16.6	6.55
8	8	26.1	11.2	6.54
	9	14.2	12.5	7.38
10	10	0	34.0	—

also from bacterial deamination of aminoacids in the colon, ureolysis is the only substantial source of intestinal ammonia. Ammonia is so well absorbed from the colon that in health only 1–2 mmole of the 150 mmole of ammonia liberated daily appears in the stool (21). The balance of evidence at present supports the view that ammonia is absorbed from the colon by non-ionic diffusion (22), facilitated by a paired non-ionic diffusion of NH_3 and CO_2 with continuous regeneration of each non-ionic species at the expense of the ionic member of each buffer pairs as follows (23, 24):-

$$NH_4^+ + HCO_3^- = NH_3 + CO_2 + H_2O.$$

The carbon dioxide is derived both from ureolysis and from bicarbonate secreted into the colon.

Ammonia is absorbed into the portal vein which, as expected, contains an ammonia concentration as much as thirteen times greater than systemic blood (25); derivation of this ammonia from bacterial activity in the colon is confirmed by the observation that the portal ammonia concentration is reduced by treatment with antibiotics (25) and portal and systemic blood ammonia concentrations are equal in

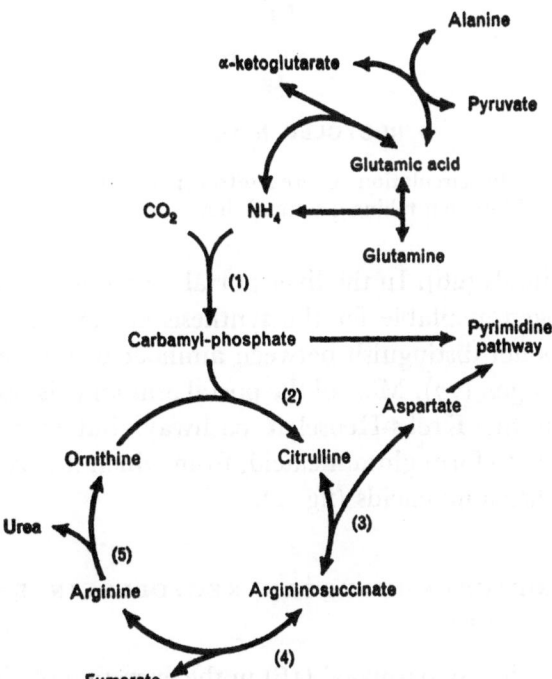

Fig. 2. Pathways of ammonia metabolism in the liver.

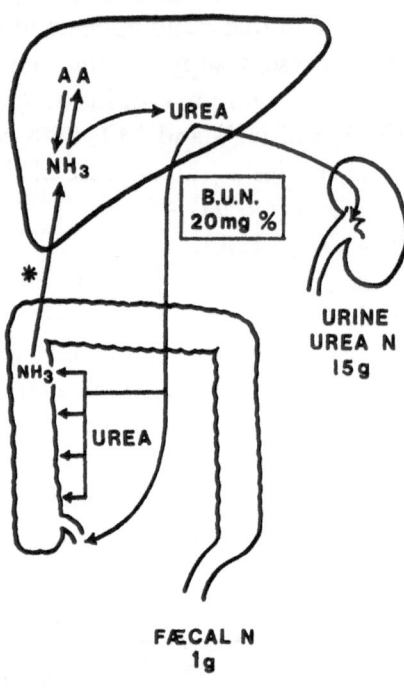

DIET 16g N
(100g PROTEIN)

Fig. 3. Enterohepatic circulation of urea nitrogen as ammonia in an individual with normal renal function taking a normal diet.

germ-free animals (26). In the liver portal ammonia enters a common pool of nitrogen available for the synthesis of aminoacids and urea; the liver does not distinguish between aminoacid nitrogen and portal ammonia nitrogen (27). Most of the portal ammonia is resynthesised to urea through the Krebs-Henseleit pathway, but some reacts with α-ketoglutarate to form glutamic acid, from which it may be transaminated into other aminoacids (fig. 2).

QUANTITY OF UREA-NITROGEN RECYCLED IN HEALTH AND IN RENAL FAILURE

There is thus a 'delay pathway' (16) in the excretion of nitrogen which may have nutritional potential. Figure 3 represents the enterohepatic circulation of urea nitrogen in a normal subject on a normal diet, the value of x, the recycled nitrogen, is 3–4 g in 24 hours (15). If hydrolysis of urea increased in proportion to the blood urea concentration (which is proportional to the body urea pool) substantial quantities of urea nitrogen would be recycled in people with renal failure. Figure 4

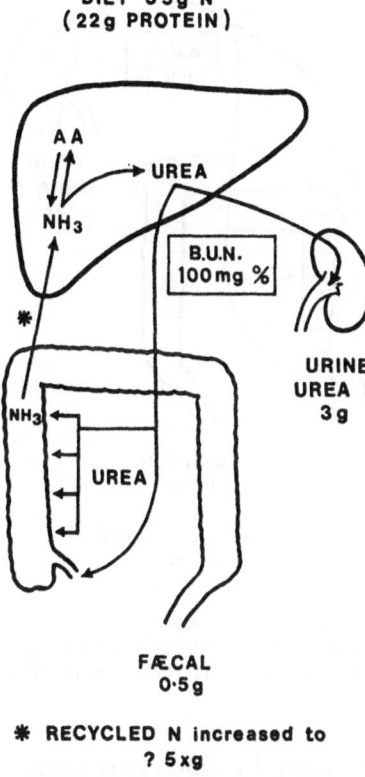

DIET 3·5g N
(22g PROTEIN)

A A

→ UREA

NH₃

B.U.N.
100 mg %

URINE
UREA N
3 g

*

NH₃ ←

UREA

FÆCAL
0·5g

* RECYCLED N increased to
? 5xg

Fig. 4. Enterohepatic circulation of urea nitrogen as ammonia in an individual with chronic renal failure taking a low-protein diet. If urea hydrolysis increases in direct proportion to the blood urea concentration 5 times more nitrogen will be recycled daily.

represents the dynamic state in a patient with chronic renal failure who is in nitrogen balance on a low protein diet; if urea hydrolysis is directly proportional to the blood urea concentration 5 times more urea nitrogen would be recycled than in the healthy individual represented in figure 3. The converse is also likely to be true, namely that very little urea nitrogen would be recycled in protein-deprived individuals. This situation is represented in figure 5. Thus when dietary

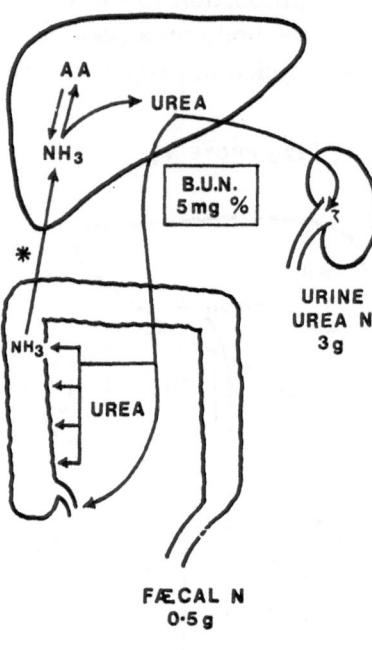

DIET 3·5g N
(22g PROTEIN)

Fig. 5. Enterohepatic circulation of urea nitrogen as ammonia in a healthy individual taking a low protein diet. The amount of urea nitrogen recycled is only about one twentieth of the amount recycled by the uraemic individual taking the same diet.

nitrogen is scarce, a situation in which maximum reutilisation of waste nitrogen is most desirable, recycling of urea nitrogen falls to about one quarter of its normal level. The low turnover may partly be offset by greater efficiency of reutilisation of the nitrogen which is recycled (9) (fig. 1).

The concept that urea nitrogen is recycled in proportion to the size of the body urea pool is of such basic importance to any discussion of the nutritional potential of endogenous ammonia that we must examine the evidence in some detail. Urea metabolism in man has been investigated independently by four groups of workers using a similar method. Urea breakdown was calculated as the difference between urea synthesis (measured by the fall in plasma specific activity after an intravenous injection of ^{14}C-labelled urea) and the amount of urea excreted in the urine. Urea synthesis normally exceeds urea excretion because some urea is hydrolysed, its nitrogen is liberated as ammonia and it is resynthesised into urea. In uraemia the synthesis of urea greatly exceeds excretion, indicating a larger enterohepatic recycling of urea nitrogen. In health an average of 7.2 g of urea was metabolised thus liberating 3.4 g of nitrogen for recirculation to the liver. Measurements of urea metabolism in uraemic individuals by DEANE et al. (28), by JONES et al. (16) and by WALSER (20) show that in spite of a wide scatter of results urea breakdown is directly proportional to the size of the body urea pool (fig. 6). The upper regression line is calculated from the data of DEANE et al. (28) and represents a highly significant correlation ($r = 0.68$ $p < 0.001$) between urea breakdown and pool size. Although the data of ROBSON et al. (30, 31) also show a significant correlation between urea metabolism and pool size expressed by the lower regression line in Figure 6 ($r = 0.54$ $p < 0.02$), a systematic

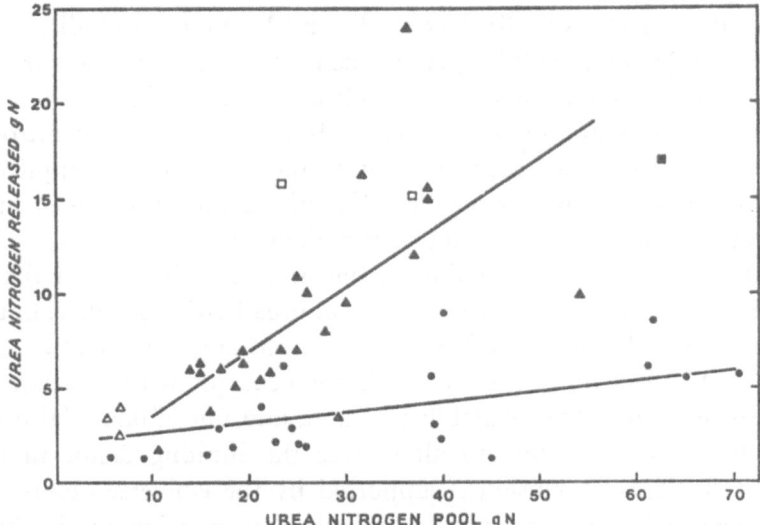

Fig. 6. Relationship between urea hydrolysis and the body urea pool in man. The upper regression line is calculated from the data of DEANE et al (28) and the lower regression line is calculated from the data of ROBSON et al (3).

△ healthy individuals studied by WALSER and BODENLOS (15)
■ one uraemic individual studied by WALSER (29)
▲ uraemic patients studied by DEANE *et al.* (28)
● uraemic patients studied by ROBSON *et al.* (30)
□ uraemic patients studied by JONES *et al.* (16)

difference is apparent between ROBSON's data and the findings of the others. It is important to note this discrepancy because on the basis of ROBSON's low figures for urea breakdown in uraemia an eminent authority has recently stated that 'although it is widely held that urea breakdown is increased in absolute terms in uraemic patients, the available data, considered *in toto*, do not establish this conclusion unequivocally' (32). Few of ROBSON's uraemic patients metabolised as much or more urea than the healthy individuals studied by WALSER and BODENLOS (15). All but three of the uraemic patients studied by the other groups of investigators metabolised more urea than normal. The difference between the findings of ROBSON and those of DEANE is all the more surprising because all DEANE's patients were treated with antibiotics at the time of the study; the antibiotic regime used would not have eradicated urease-producing micro-organisms, but it would be expected to reduce total urease activity: in the event, any reduction seems not to have been sufficient to interfere significantly with the hydrolysis of urea.

The data of DEANE (28), JONES (16) and WALSER (29) indicate that when the blood urea nitrogen concentration was in the range of 50–100 mg/100 ml from 5–23 g of nitrogen was released from urea and recycled as ammonia – a very substantial amount of nitrogen, which at greatest amounted to about 7 times the nitrogen supplied by the conventional low-protein diet. The proportion of the pool metabolised was variable. Reference to 6 patients studied by DEANE et al. (28) before and after reduction of the urea pool by diet or dialysis shows that as the pool falls the amount of urea hydrolysed falls, but the proportion of the pool metabolised remains at approximately 20–40% (fig. 7). The fact that urea metabolism fell sharply within 24 hours of dialysis indicated that availability of urea and not of bacterial urease (which hardly had time to alter) was the limiting factor in urea hydrolysis. This conclusion is supported by the converse observation that bacterial urease activity increased in proportion to the blood urea (fig. 8).

INTESTINAL AMMONIA AND LIVER FAILURE

Reduction of ammonia formation in the gut is therapeutically valuable in cirrhotic patients in whom, with little doubt, ammonia is one of the factors causing hepatic encephalopathy (34). Several measures have

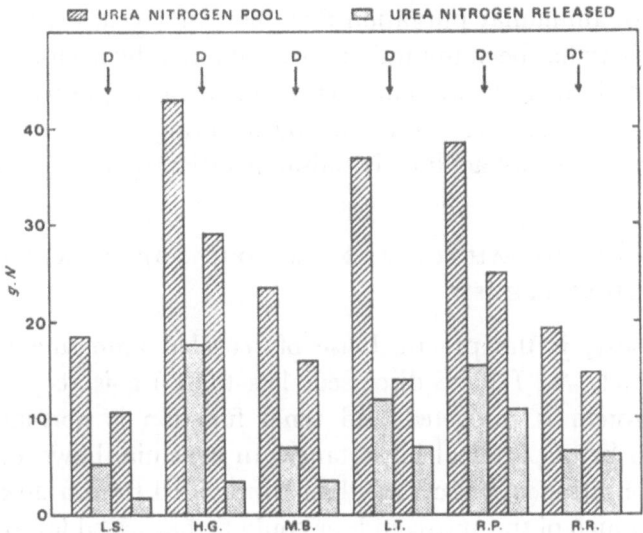

Fig. 7. Urea nitrogen pool and urea nitrogen released as ammonia in 6 uraemic individuals before and after treatment with dialysis (D) or diet (Dt). [plotted from the data of DEANE *et al.* (28)].

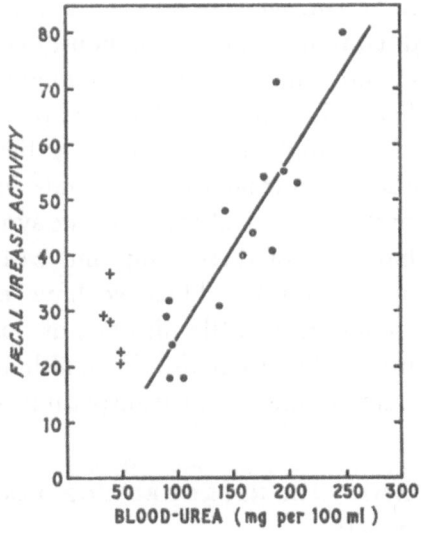

Fig. 8. The relationship between faecal urease activity (expressed as μeq. ammonia released per minute per g of dry faeces) and the blood urea concentration (33).

been used: a low-protein diet reduces the urea pool and thus limits the recycling of ammonia; purgation may increase faecal urea excretion; urease activity has been minimised by antibiotics, by acetohydroxamic acid, and by inducing antibodies to urease; and absorption of ammonia from the colon has been impaired by lowering the luminal pH by colonising with lactobacilli or by administration of lactulose (35).

UTILISATION OF AMMONIA NITROGEN FOR NON-ESSENTIAL AMINOACID SYNTHESIS

What, if any, is the practical use of recycled ammonia nitrogen? Unfortunately, as I have discussed, less than 1 g is recycled when dietary protein is restricted and renal function is normal: this is unlikely to be of practical importance. In uraemia, however, several times more nitrogen is recycled than is provided from a 20 g protein diet: how much of this nitrogen is or could be harnessed for aminoacid synthesis? From studies of the incorporation of ^{15}N-ammonia nitrogen into albumin we calculated a disappointing total incorporation of ammonia nitrogen into body protein of 1–2 g, and this may be an overestimate. However, although it represents only about 10% of the total available nitrogen it amounts to a substantial proportion of the minimal non-essential nitrogen requirement (4). The diet of all individuals studied contained adequate non-essential and essential nitrogen. How much more ammonia nitrogen might have been utilised if the diet were deficient in nitrogen? The best prospect of harnessing ammonia nitrogen fully might be to provide a diet deficient in both non-essential and essential nitrogen but adequate in all other respects (9). Whatever the precise chemical causes of the symptoms of uraemia the fact remains that most of these symptoms can be minimised by reducing dietary protein intake. Thus we have every incentive to devise a diet which contains as little nitrogen as possible, even to the extent of a protein-free diet to maintain health in end-stage renal failure without recourse to dialysis or transplantation.

UTILISATION OF AMMONIA NITROGEN FOR ESSENTIAL AMINOACID SYNTHESIS

We have shown that man can synthesise several essential aminoacids adequately. Rose (36) predicted that the essential part of essential aminoacids was their carbon skeleton and, as so often, he was correct. Phenylalanine, valine and tryptophan can be adequately synthesised from their α-ketoacid analogues (37–42) (fig. 9). In work published a month ago WALSER et al. (32) have gone much further and have shown a remarkably efficient and sufficient nitrogen metabolism on a diet which supplied 1.8 g of nitrogen daily, together with the α-ketoacids of valine, leucine, isoleucine, methionine, phenylalanine,

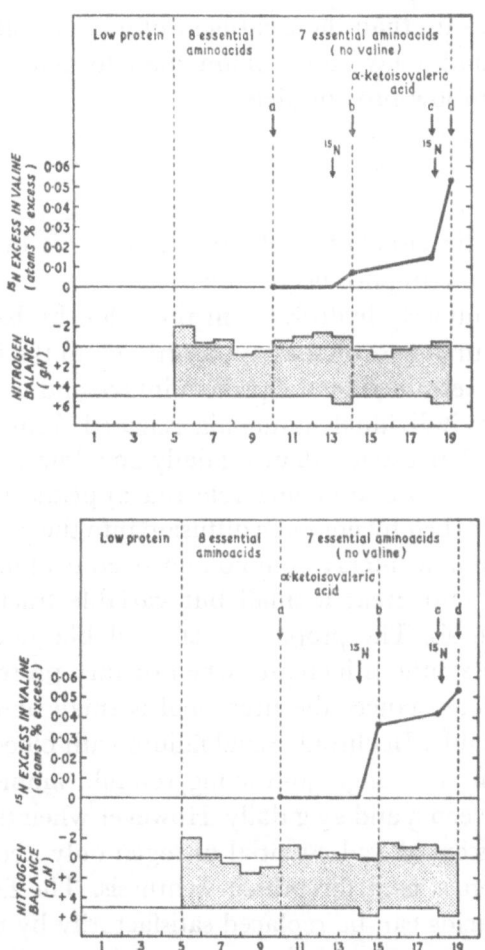

Fig. 9 ¹⁵N excess in valine from hydrolysate of plasma albumin, and the nitrogen balance of two young women who received 2 g, of the sodium salt of α-ketoisovaleric acid for 5 days when taking a valine-free diet. Nitrogen balance improved and the incorporation of ¹⁵NH₄Cl increased when the ketoacid was given (41).

and in one case also tryptophan and histidine. No accumulation of ketoacids was found and no signs of toxicity were evident. The serum urea nitrogen of one individual increased by only 20 mg/100 ml during one month although he was virtually anuric.

It should not too readily be assumed that this result was achieved through greater reutilisation of ammonia nitrogen, rather than by a fundamental resetting of protein turnover. If resetting rather than reutilisation is the key to this remarkably efficient metabolism, a much wider field opens up than the treatment of uraemia. But that horizon extends far beyond today's topic of ammonia formation in the gut and its importance in low-protein diets.

SUMMARY

The enterohepatic circulation of urea nitrogen is described and its possible nutritional importance is discussed.

Urea is continuously hydrolysed in the colon by bacterial ureases. The amount of urea hydrolysed is proportional to the body urea pool, which is itself determined by the protein intake and by renal function. Thus in healthy individuals ammonia released from urea falls from 3.5 g on a normal diet to less than 1 g daily on a low protein diet. Only a small fraction of the ammonia released appears in the stool, the remainder is absorbed by nonionic diffusion into the portal circulation. Portal vein ammonia enters a common nitrogen pool in the liver: most is resynthesised into urea; a small but variable fraction is used for aminoacid synthesis. The proportion of available ammonia nitrogen used for protein synthesis increases when dietary protein is restricted, but in these circumstances the urea pool is small and less ammonia nitrogen is available. In chronic renal failure with blood urea nitrogen concentration in the range 50–100 mg/100 ml., ammonia formation increases to between 5 and 23 g daily. However when the diet contains adequate non-essential and essential nitrogen only about 10% of this recycled nitrogen is used for protein synthesis. The fact that several essential aminoacids can be replaced satisfactorily by their α-ketoacid analogues makes an extremely low nitrogen diet feasible. Initial work with such diets indicates either that reutilisation of nitrogen becomes very efficient or that nitrogen turnover is reset at a remarkably low level.

Endogenous ammonia is probably of no practical nutritional importance during protein deprivation unless renal function is impaired. Its full nutritional potential in chronic renal failure has yet to be explored.

REFERENCES

1. LAND, H. and VIRTANEN, A. I., (1959) Ammonium salts as nitrogen source in the synthesis of protein by the ruminant. *Acta Chemica Scandinavica*, 13, 489.
2. VIRTANEN, A. I. and LAND, H., (1959) Synthesis of aminoacids and proteins from ammonium salts by ruminants. *Suomen Maatalonstieteellisen Seuran Julkaisuja*, 94, 7.
3. McPHERSON, A. T., (1970) Protein from synthetic ammonia – routes for producing high quality protein for human consumption. *Indian Journal of Nutrition and Dietetics*, 7, 171.
4. RICHARDS, P., (1972) Nutritional potential of nitrogen recycling in man. *American Journal of Clinical Nutrition*, 25, 615.
5. SNYDERMAN, S. E., HOLT, L. E., DANCIS, J., ROITMAN, E., BOYER, A. and BAYLIS, M. E., (1962) 'Un-essential' nitrogen: a limiting factor in human growth. *Journal of Nutrition*, 78, 57.
6. NICHOLSON, J. F., (1970) The metabolism of ingested ammonia 15N by premature infants. *Pediatric Research*, 4, 398.
7. GIORDANO, C., (1963) Use of exogenous and endogenous urea for protein synthesis in normal and uremic subjects. *Journal of Laboratory and Clinical Medicine*, 62, 231.
8. GIOVANNETTI, S. and MAGGIORE, A., (1964) A low nitrogen diet with proteins of high biological value for severe chronic uraemia. *Lancet*, 1, 1000.
9. RICHARDS, P., METCALFE-GIBSON, A., WARD, E. E., WRONG, O. M. and HOUGHTON, B. J., (1967) Utilisation of ammonia nitrogen for protein synthesis in man, and the effect of protein restriction and uraemia. *Lancet*, 2, 845.
10. GIORDANO, C., DE PASCALE, C., BALESTRIERI, C., CITTADINI, D. and CRESCENZI, A., (1968) Incorporation of urea 15N in amino acids of patients with chronic renal failure on low nitrogen diet. *American Journal of Clinical Nutrition*, 21, 394.
11. READ, W. W. C., McLAREN, D. S., TCHALIN, M., and NASSAR, S., (1969) Studies with 15N-labelled ammonia and urea in the malnourished child. *Journal of Clinical Investigation*, 48, 1143.
12. FÜRST, P., JONSSON, A., JOSEPHSON, B. and VINNARS, E., (1970) Distribution in muscle and liver vein protein of 15N administered as ammonium acetate to man. *Journal of Applied Physiology*, 29, 307.
13. TRIPATHY, K., KLAHR, S., and LOTERO, H., (1970) Utilisation of exogenous urea nitrogen in malnourished adults. *Metabolism*, 19, 253.
14. LEVENSON, S. M., CROWLEY, R. E., HOROWITZ, R. E., and MALM, O. J., (1959) The metabolism of carbon-labelled urea in the germ-free rat. *Journal of Biological Chemistry*, 234, 2061.
15. WALSER, M. and BODENLOS, L. J., (1959) Urea metabolism in man. *Journal of Clinical Investigation*, 38, 1617.
16. JONES, E. A., SMALLWOOD, R. A., CRAIGIE, A. and ROSENOER, (1969) The enterohepatic circulation of urea nitrogen. *Clinical Science*, 37, 825.
17. WILSON, D. R., ING, T. S., METCALFE-GIBSON, A., and WRONG, O. M., (1968) In vivo dialysis of faeces as a method of stool analysis. III. The effect of intestinal antibiotics. *Clinical Science*, 34, 211.

18. SUMMERSKILL, W. H. J. and WOLPERT, E., (1970) Ammonia metabolism in the gut. *American Journal of Clinical Nutrition*, 23, 633.
19. WOLPERT, E., PHILLIPS, S. F., and SUMMERSKILL, W. H. J., (1971) Transport of urea and ammonia production in the human colon. *Lancet*, 2, 1387.
20. MELVILLE, J., (1935) Labile glutamine peptides, and their bearing on the origin of ammonia set free during the enzymic digestion of proteins. *Biochemical Journal*, 29, 179.
21. WRONG, O. M., METCALFE-GIBSON, A., MORRISON, R. B. I., NG, S. T., and HOWARD, A. V., (1965) In vivo dialysis of faeces as a method of stool analysis. I. Technique and results in normal subjects. *Clinical Science*, 28, 357.
22. DOWN, P. F., AGOSTINI, L., MURISON, J. and WRONG, O.M. (1972) The inter-relations of faecal ammonia, pH and bicarbonate:evidence of colonic absorption of ammonia by non-ionic diffusion. *Clinical Science*, 43, 101.
23. ROSENFELD, J. B., ABOULAFIA, E. D. and SCHWARTZ, W. B., (1963) Influence of non-ionic diffusion on absorption of NH_4 and HCO_3 from the bladder. *American Journal of Physiology*, 204, 568.
24. SWALES, J. D. TANGE, J. D. and WRONG, O. M., (1970) The influence of pH, bicarbonate and hypertonicity on the absorption of ammonia from the rat intestine. *Clinical Science*, 39, 769.
25. SILEN, W., HARPER, H. A., MAWDSLEY, D. L. and WEIRICH, W. L.,(1955) Effect of antibacterial agents. *Proceedings of the Society for Experimental Biology and Medicine*, 88, 138.
26. WARREN, K. S., and NEWTON, W. L., (1959) Portal and peripheral blood ammonia concentrations in germ-free and conventional guinea-pigs. *American Journal of Physiology*, 197, 717.
27. HOUGHTON, B. J., (1968) In: G. M. Berlyne (ed.), Nutrition in Renal Disease, p. 107. Livingstone, Edinburgh.
28. DEANE, N., DESIR, W., and UMEDA, T., (1968) The production and extrarenal metabolism of urea in patients with chronic renal failure treated with diet and dialysis. *Proceedings of the European Dialysis and Transplant Association*, 4, 245.
29. WALSER, M. (1970) Use of isotopic urea to study the distribution and degradation of urea in man. In: *Urea and the kidney*. Excerpta Medica International Congress Series, 195, 421.
30. ROBSON, A. M., (1964) *Urea Metabolism in Chronic Renal Failure*. (MD. Thesis), Newcastle-Upon-Tyne, England.
31. ROBSON, A. M., KERR, D. N. S. and ASHCROFT, R., (1968) Urea metabolism in chronic uraemia. In: G. M. Berlyne (ed.), Nutrition in Renal Disease, p. 71. Livingstone, Edinburgh.
32. WALSER, M., COULTER, A. W., DIGHE, S. and CRANTZ, F. R., (1973) The effect of Keto-analogues of essential amino acids in severe chronic uremia. *Journal of Clinical Investigation*, 52, 678.
33. BROWN, C. L., HILL, M. J. and RICHARDS, P., (1971) Bacterial ureases in uraemic man. *Lancet*, 2, 406.
34. SHERLOCK, S., (1958) Pathogenesis and management of hepatic coma. *American Journal of Medicine*, 24, 805.
35. EDITORIAL, (1971) Urea metabolism in man. *Lancet*, 2. 1407.
36. ROSE, W. C., (1937) The nutritive significance of the aminoacids and related compounds. *Science*, 86, 298.
37. RICHARDS, P., BROWN, C. L., HOUGHTON, B. J. and THOMPSON, E., (1971) Replacement of two essential aminoacids by ketoacids in the diet of healthy and uraemic men. *Clinical Science*, 40, 11P.
38. RICHARDS, P., BROWN, C. L., HOUGHTON, B. J. and THOMPSON, E., (1971)

Synthesis of phenylalanine and valine by healthy and uraemic men. *Lancet*, 2, 128.

39. RUDMAN, D., (1971) Capacity of human subjects to utilise keto analogues of valine and phenylalanine. *Journal of Clinical Investigation*, 50, 90.

40. GALLINA, D. L., DOMINGUEZ, J. M., HOSCHOIAN, J. C., and BARRIO, J. R., (1971) Maintainance of nitrogen balance in a young woman by substitution of α-keto-isovaleric acid for valine. *Journal of Nutrition*, 101, 1165.

41. GIORDANO, C., PHILLIPS, M. E., DE PASCALE, C., DE SANTO, H. G., FÜRST, P., BROWN, C. L., HOUGHTON, B. J., and RICHARDS, P., (1972) The utilisation of the ketoacid analogues of valine and phenylalanine in health and uraemia. *Lancet*, 1, 178.

42. RICHARDS, P., BROWN, C. L., and LOWE, S. M., (1972) Synthesis of tryptophan from 3-indolepyruvic acid by a healthy woman. *Journal of Nutrition*, 102, 1547.

THE USE OF CHEMICALLY
DEFINED ELEMENTARY DIETS IN SURGERY

R. K. J. KOUMANS*

When WINITZ and co-workers reported the results of long-term feeding of volunteers with a Chemically Defined Elementary Diet (C.E.D.), they indicated its potential use as nutrition for men in space. (1, 2).

Indeed the characteristics of elementary diets – complete nutrition and resorbtion, lack of faecal residue as well as compact form and good storage stability – are clearly advantageous for prolonged space flights. However lack of palatability has as yet made them unacceptable organoleptically to astronauts, though their use may have to be reconsidered for very long sojourns in space.

On the other hand the potential value of C.E.D.'s in medicine has become readily apparent as a result of their remarkable physiological properties:

1. Complete Nutrition:

The 15 volunteers in the Vaccaville experiment (3), fed exclusively C.E.D. for 22 weeks, were able to continue normal active life without any signs of nutritional deficiency. These results were subsequently confirmed by McKEAN (4, 5, 6), who reported adequate nutritional support and weight and height gains in mentally retarded phenyl-ketonuric children, nurtured for up to 30 months on a C.E.D. without occurrence of undesirable side effects.

2. Complete resorbtion:

Elementary diets, which require little or no digestion, are completely resorbed in the upper intestinal tract. This results in a reduction of faecal residue, as reflected by an average initial weight loss of 1.5 kg

* Department of Surgery, Zuiderziekenhuis, Rotterdam, The Netherlands.

in the first few days of elementary nutrition. This loss in weight is rapidly restored after returning to conventional foods.

Lack of faecal residue results in:

3. Diminished faecal production:

Small amounts of faeces are passed every few days, averaging 50 grams per day.

4. Changes in intestinal microflora:

Within a few days of elementary nutrition, a reduction in gut micro-flora populations becomes apparent in a quantitative as well as a qualitative sense (2, 7, 8). WINITZ and co-workers report the elimination of minor bowel residents after 13 days on C.E.D., leaving major residents (E. Coli, Bacteroides and enterococci) at population levels reduced by a factor 10^5. A similar reduction in bacterial populations was obtained within 4 days by administration of an enema 24 hours after initiation of the diet.

These changes are attributable to the elimination of faecal residue, depriving the intestinal microbes of their natural nutrients and habitat.

5. Diminished secretion of bile and pancreatic juice:

Ingestion of elemental nutrients apparently renders pancreatic and enteric enzymes as well as bile salts virtually superfluous. In fact, circumstantial evidence indicates a reduced stimulation of bile and pancreatic secretions (9, 10). These observations however need further investigation and confirmation.

Since the clinical introduction of elementary diets as a therapeutic adjunct in extreme short bowel syndrome (11), evidence has rapidly accumulated concerning their beneficial effects in a wide variety of pathological conditions in surgery. These include fistulae of the alimentary tract (8, 9, 12, 13, 14, 15, 16), Crohn's Disease (9, 13, 17, 18), ulcerative colitis (9, 17), short bowel syndrome (9), etc.

Their therapeutic effectiveness can be ascribed to easy digestibility (malabsorbtion, short bowel syndrome), suppression of faecal residue and intestinal microflora (enteric fistulae, inflammatory diseases of the bowel) and reduction of pancreatic and biliary secretions (pancreatitis, bile fistulae, etc.). A common denominator however in most of these conditions is a chronic catabolic state. It seems reasonable therefore to explain its main mode of action on the basis of its high nutritive value and ease of access for a starving organism. Thus metabolic conditions can be rendered optimal so that natural healing tendencies can take their course.

CLINICAL EXPERIENCE

We have used C.E.D.* to therapeutic reasons in different clinical conditions, including fistulae of the intestinal tract, malabsorbtion after irradiation, Crohn's disease, etc. In addition we have started to use this diet to prepare the bowel for abdominal surgery. We were able to study 20 patients (table 1) with regard to clinical results and changes in intestinal microflora patterns and body weight as well as serum protein and albumin levels.

Table 1. *Clinical application of C.E.D. in 24 patients.*

Bowel preparation:		
Surgery of the colon:		13
– malignancy	5	
– benign lesions	7	
– irradiation reaction	1	
Colon bypass		1
Total enterolysis		1
Resection and closure of enteric fistulae		1
Extensive bowel resection + resection colo-jejunal fistula		1
		17
Therapeutic:		
Enterocutaneous (enterovaginal) fistulae		5
Massive intestinal bleeding (Crohn's disease)		1
Skin maceration following ileostomy		1
		7
Total number of the patients		24

THERAPEUTIC USE OF C.E.D.

In all 7 patients in this group, results were satisfactory as the initial therapeutic objectives were attained within 2–4 weeks of elementary nutrition (table 2). Four patients had enterocutaneous fistulae following an appendicular abcess (1), irradiation (1) and colon surgery (2).

* Vivonex

Table 2. *Results of the therapeutic use of C.E.D. in 7 patients. *A large cecocutaneous fistula, following a peri-appendicular abcess, healed rapidly and faecal drainage had stopped on C.E.D., when elementary nutrition had to be discontinued because of lack of supply. A small mucocutaneous fistula persisted that eventually required surgical excision.*

Disease	Number of patients	Duration of C.E.D. (weeks)	Results
Bowel fistulae	4	2–4	healing of fistulae*
Anastomotic leakage after left hemi-colectomy	1	3	spontaneous healing (colostomy prevented)
Massive recurrent intestinal bleeding	1	5	blood loss stopped after initiation of C.E.D.
Ileostomy (prevention of skin maceration)	1	1	skin maceration after discontinuation of C.E.D.

One patient had both a rectocutaneous and a rectovaginal fistula subsequent to a low anterior resection for carcinoma of the rectum. All fistulae healed spontaneously.

A patient with anastomotic leakage after left hemicolectomy was scheduled for construction of a diverting colostomy when a trial with C.E.D. was initiated, resulting in a cure. Thus nutrition with C.E.D. may act as a 'medical by-pass' of diseased bowel segments in selected cases.

A patient with severe exacerbation of Crohn's disease, in a poor nutritional state and with copious intestinal blood loss requiring multiple transfusions weekly was treated with C.E.D. Within a few days gross bleeding had ceased entirely, though occasional guiac positive stools persisted. No further blood transfusions were required. After 5 weeks of elementary diet the nutritional state was essentially normalized and she successfully underwent extensive jejunoileal resection with closure of a colojejunal fistula.

Finally a patient with familial polyposis of the colon, necessitating total colectomy, received a postoperative course of C.E.D. to facilitate healing of his ileostomy. Only small amounts of viscous faecal material were produced and healing was uneventful. As C.E.D. was replaced by a bland diet, skin maceration developed which gradually abated with conventional treatment. This observation may lend additional support to the alleged reduction of.digestive enzyme secretion with elementary nutrition.

PREPARATION OF THE BOWEL WITH C.E.D.

17 patients received a 5-day course of C.E.D. (1800 Cal/day) to prepare the bowel for abdominal surgery. Operations included partial colectomies for benign (7 patients) and malignant (5 patients) disease, colon by-pass for oesophageal carcinoma and bowel resections for enteric fistulae subsequent to irradiation and for Crohn's disease (table 1). At no time were pre-operative antibiotics administered and no additional mechanical bowel preparation was prescribed, except for a routine cleansing enema 24 hours after initiation of the elementary diet. The bowel upon operation was virtually devoid of faecal matter, except in one instance of subtotal occlusion by an extensive carcinoma of the ascending colon. This patient subsequently developed a wound abcess necessitating incision and drainage. Other septic complications occurred in two patients with low anterior resections: a patient with sigmoid resection and closure of colostomy and one with resection of enterocutaneous fistulae following pelvic irradiation (table 3). The observed rate of septic complications in this limited number of patients is comparable to previous complication rates in our department, when vigourous mechanical cleansing, sulphathalidine and neomycine were used, and concurs with the frequencies reported in large series of patients after mechanical and antibiotic bowel preparation (19, 20, 21, 22).

At the Massachusetts General Hospital 32 patients undergoing colon surgery, including 5 colon by-pass operations for oesophageal ob-

Table 3. *Septic complications following surgery in 5 out of 17 patients after bowel preparation with C.E.D.*

Complication	Initial disease	Operation	Remarks
Wound sepsis (minor)	Anastomotic stenosis after sigmoidectomy + colostomy	Resection of stenosis Closure of colostomy	Hospital discharge not deferred
Wound abcess	Carcinoma of rectum	Low anterior resection	Drainage of abcess
Wound abcess	Carcinoma of cecum	Right hemi-colectomy	Obstructing tumour
Enterocutaneous and enterovaginal fistulae	Carcinoma of rectum	Low anterior resection	Spontaneous healing after 4 weeks C.E.D.
Recurrence of enterocutaneous fistulae	Enterocutaneous fistulae post-irradiation	Excision of fistulae	Spontaneous healing after 3 weeks C.E.D.

struction, received a 4–7 day course of C.E.D. to prepare the bowel for surgery. No pre-operative antibiotics were administered and no significant septic complications were observed. When hemicolectomies were performed, the specimen was sliced open and scraped clean. Residual matter never exceeded 5 gm per specimen (23).

BACTERIOLOGICAL STUDIES

At the start of C.E.D. administration as well as on the day before surgery, both qualitative and quantitative bacterial cultures of faeces were performed. In patients receiving C.E.D. for therapeutic purposes, these cultures were repeated once a week as well as 3 days after returning to conventional nutrition. No other food or beverages were allowed, except for water or tea without sugar or milk.

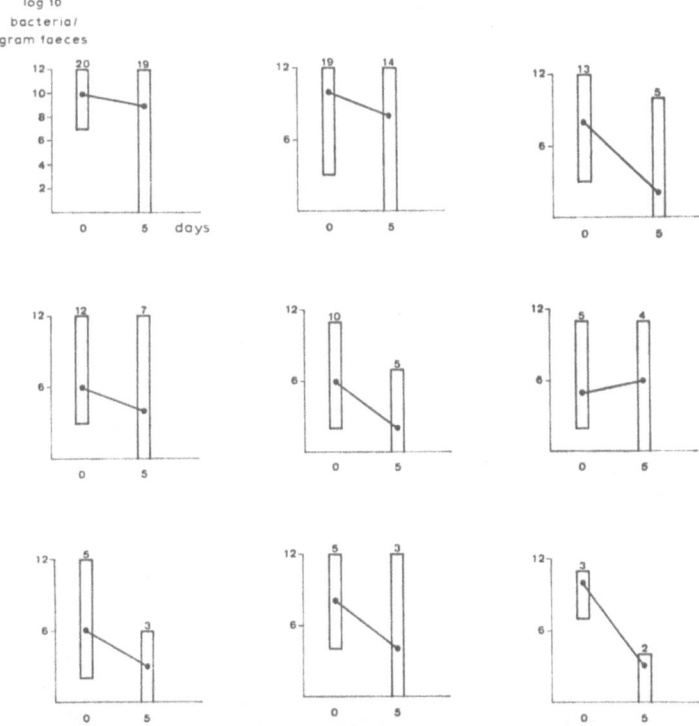

Fig. 1. Quantitative and qualitative changes in faecal microflora in 20 patients. The number above each column indicates the total number of patients from whom the particular organism was recovered. The length of the column represents the range in bacterial counts, while the black dot indicates the average number of bacteria.

Within 5 days marked changes occur in the intestinal flora (fig. 1).

While major residents, Bacteroides and E.coli, remain essentially unaffected, enterococci and most minor residents are reduced numerically by a factor 10^3–10^5; in many instances some species disappear altogether. These changes become more pronounced with prolonged elementary nutrition. However the total number of bacteria is barely influenced and reduction in microflora populations is less spectacular than was expected on the basis of the original studies in healthy volunteers (7).

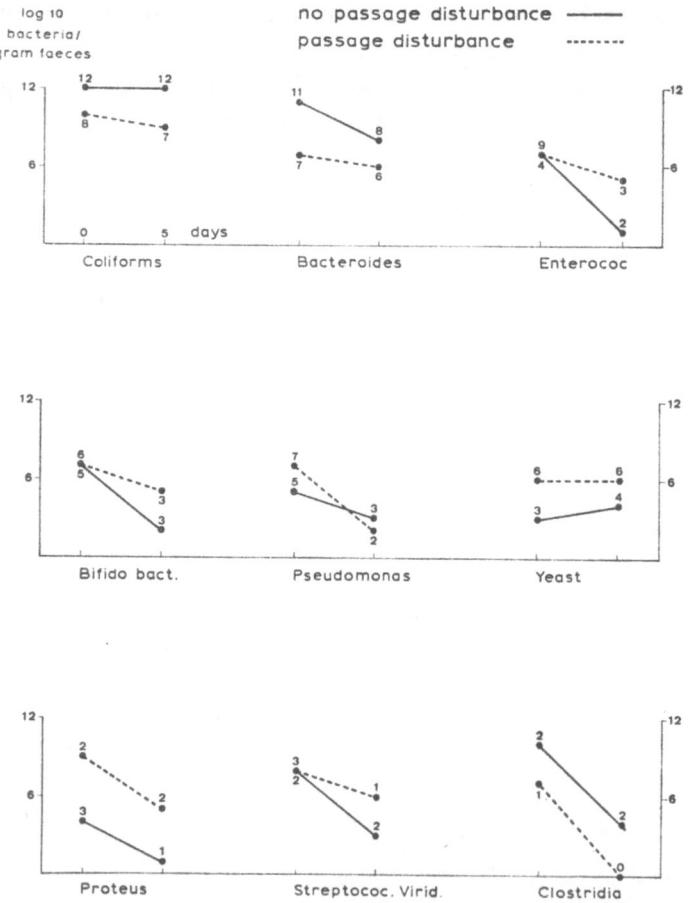

Fig. 2. Qualitative and quantitative changes in faecal microflora in 20 patients, grouped according to the presence or absence of disturbances in intestinal passage. Black dots indicate the average number of bacteria recovered. The accompanying numbers refer to the total number of patients from whom the particular organism was recovered in each category.

Surprisingly functional impairment of the bowel appears to have little effect on the reduction of intestinal microflora, as division of our patients into those with and those without disturbed intestinal passage did not reveal appreciable differences between the two groups. (fig. 2).

NUTRITIONAL STATE

With pre-operative elementary nutrition no significant loss in body weight occurred although a slight initial loss of weight, attributable to a reduction in faecal residue, was often noted.

Serum protein and albumin levels remained essentially unaltered. In those patients receiving elementary nutrition for prolonged periods, similar results were obtained. It should be noted however that in these patients, hyperalimentation was not attempted and a base line intake of 1800 Cal/day was in most instances maintained. With increasing experience we now tend to administer larger amounts of C.E.D., up to 1800–2000 Cal/m² body surface area, which are better suited to the patient's need.

PRE-OPERATIVE C.E.D. VERSUS CONVENTIONAL BOWEL PREPARATION WITH LAXATIVES AND ANTIBIOTICS

The discussion around the merits of pre-operative attempts to sterilize the bowel with antibiotics has not yet been concluded (24, 25, 26, 27). This is in essence due to the fact that no antibiotic or combination of antibiotics has yet been found that guarantees adequate bowel sterility. With the existing antibiotic regimes, on the other hand, the risk of bacterial overgrowth, the occurrence of resistant strains of pathogens and the transmission of R-factors become potential hazards, while an increased incidence of suture line implantation of tumour cells after antibiotic pretreatment has convincingly been demonstrated (28, 29).

Furthermore there can be little disagreement that mechanical cleansing is the mainstay of effective bowel preparation.

Without adequate reduction in faecal residue, intestinal antibiotic pretreatment is worthless. Since a short course of C.E.D. effectively cleans the bowel, its use appears profitable in bowel surgery while concomitant aselective suppression of endogenous microflora may be regarded as an added advantage.

Finally pre-operative bowel preparation with elementary diets permits the patient to meet his normal metabolic requirements until the day of the operation and existing catabolic states can be reversed. With conventional bowel preparation that includes laxatives and dietary restrictions, adequate nutrition is severely compromised.

TRINKLE et al. as well as MIKAL demonstrated significant metabolic disturbances, loss of electrolytes, dehydration and a negative nitrogen balance (30, 31, 32).

In the debilitated and elderly patient, these disturbances can make pre-operative correction of fluid and electrolyte losses imperative (26). It is obvious that these untoward effects are not encountered with the use of elementary diets. Those who insist on antibiotic bowel 'sterilization' may combine elementary diets with the antibiotic regime of their choice.

INDICATIONS FOR USE OF C.E.D. IN SURGERY

From a clinical point of view, elementary diets can be effective in three different ways:

1. by providing complete nutrition which is easily resorbed;
2. by decompression and cleansing of the bowel, and
3. in 'by-passing' diseased or surgically compromised bowel segments.
The indications for use in surgery (table 4) are directly related to these physiological properties, which place elementary diets somewhere between total parenteral alimentation and conventional nutrition.

Obviously these characteristics make C.E.D. a useful adjunct in the treatment of many different conditions and further investigation and evaluation are needed to define its ultimate place in medicine. On

Table 4. *Main indications for the use of chemically defined elementary diets in surgery*

1. *Preoperative*	– surgery of the colon
	– abdominal operations, requiring an empty bowel
2. *Postoperative*	– protection of bowel anastomoses
3. *Therapeutic*	– enteric fistulae malabsorbtion, short bowel syndrome
	– inflammatory disease of the intestinal tract Crohn's disease colitis etc.
	– hyperalimentation

the other hand a 'space diet' is neither a miracle drug nor a panacea for all ailments of the digestive system; furthermore, its valuable properties should not permit relaxation in surgical discipline, carelessness in prevention of contamination or sloppy surgical technique.

On the basis of the results and experience obtained thus far, it can be stated that elementary diets have opened new perspectives in the treatment of metabolic disorders and functional and inflammatory diseases of the intestinal tract, as well as in the field of abdominal surgery.

REFERENCES

1. WINITZ, M., GRAFF, J., GALLAGHER, L., NARKIN, A., SEEDMAN, D. A., (1965) Evaluation of chemical diets as nutrition for man in space. *Nature*, 205/4973, 741.
2. WINITZ, M., ADAMS, R. F., (1971) Chemically defined diets. A new approach to metabolic nutrition. In: K. Lang, W. Fekl, G. Berg, (eds.), Balanced nutrition and therapy, Thieme, Stuttgart, p. 46.
3. WINITZ, M., SEEDMAN, D. A., GRAFF, J., (1970) Studies in metabolic nutrition employing chemically defined diets. I Extended feeding of normal human adult males. *Amer. J. Clin. Nutr.* 23, 525.
4. Mc KEAN, CH. M., (1970) Growth of phenylketonuric children on chemically defined diets. *Lancet*, i, 148.
5. Mc KEAN, CH. M., (1971) The long-term effects of chemically defined diets on ambulatory phenylketonurics and bedridden, severely retarded patients. In: K. Lang, W. Fekl, G. Berg (eds.), Balanced nutrition and therapy. Thieme. Stuttgart. p. 66.
6. Mc KEAN, CH. M., (1971) Effects of totally synthetic, low phenylalanine diet on adolescent phenylketonuric patients. *Arch. Dis. Childhood*, 46, 608.
7. WINITZ, M., ADAMS, R. F., GALLAGHER, N., NARKIN, A., SEEDMAN, D. A. (1970). Studies in metabolic nutrition employing chemically defined diets: II Effect on gut microflora populations. *Amer. J. Clin. Nutr.*, 23, 546.
8. KOUMANS, R. K. J., (1972) Ruimtevaartdieet en darmchirurgie. *Ned. T. v. Geneesk.*, 116, 1040.
9. STEPHENS, R. V., RANDALL, H. T., (1969) Use of a concentrated, balanced, liquid elemental diet for nutritional management of catabolic states. *Ann. Surg.* 170, 642.
10. BROWN, R. A., THOMPSON, A. G., McARDLE, A. H., GURD, F. N., (1970) Alteration of exocrine pancreatic storage enzymes by feeding on an elemental diet: a biochemical and ultrastructural study. *Surg. Forum.*, 21, 391.
11. THOMPSON, W. R., STEVENS, R. V. RANDALL, H. T., BOWEN, J. R., (1969) Use of the 'Space Diet' in the management of a patient with extreme short bowel syndrome. *Amer. J. Surg.* 117, 449.
12. BODE, H. H., HENDREN, W. H., (1970) Healing of faecal fistula initiated by synthetic low-residue diet. *Lancet*, i. 954.
13. PINCUS, I. J., CITRON, B. PH., HAVERBACK, B. J., (1971) Nutritional Support of gastro-intestinal problems with Vivonex-100. In: K. Lang, W. Fekl, G. Berg (eds.), Balanced nutrition and therapy. Thieme, Stuttgart, p. 77.

14. BURY, K. D., STEPHENS, R. V., RANDALL, H. T., (1971) Use of a chemically defined, liquid, elemental diet for nutritional management of fistulas of the alimentary tract. *Amer. J. Surg.*, 121, 174.
15. DUKE JR, J. H., (1971) A dietary therapy for rectovaginal fistula. In: K. Lang, W. Fekl, G. Berg (eds.), Balanced nutrition and therapy. Thieme, Stuttgart p. 130.
16. GRUNDY, D. J., (1971) Small bowel fistula treated with low-residue diet. *Brit. Med. J.*, 1, 531.
17. BERG, G., WAGNER, H., WEBER, L., (1972) Bilanzierte ballastfreie Ernährung bei Darmerkrankung. *Deutsche Med. Wch. schrt.*, 21, 826.
18. JONXIS, J. H. P., DE GROOT, C. J., BOELKENS, M. TH. E., SCHILTE, P. P. M., (1973) De behandeling van een meisje met een ernstige maag-darmstoornis met een zogenaamd synthetisch dieet. *Ned. T. v. Geneesk.*, 117, 184.
19. GORDON, H. E., GAYLOR, D. W., RICHMOND, D. M., CLARKE, J. S., FINEGOLD, S. M., (1965) Operations on the colon: The role of antibiotics in preoperative preparation. *California Med.*, 103, 243.
20. RUBBO, S. D., HUGHES, E. S. R., BLAINEY, B., RUSSEL, J. S., (1965) Role of preoperative chemoprophylaxis in bowel surgery. *Antimicrob. Agents Chemother.*, 5, 649.
21. HERTER, F. P., SLANETZ, C. A., (1967) Influence of antibiotic preparation of the bowel on complications after colon resections. *Amer. J. Surg.*, 113, 165.
22. AZAR, H., DRAPANAS, T., (1968) Relationship of antibiotic to wound infections and enterocolitis in colon surgery. *Amer. J. Surg.*, 115, 209.
23. BURKE, J. F., (1973) Personal communication.
24. TYSON, R. R., SPAULDING, E. H., (1959) Should antibiotics be used in large bowel preparation? *Surg. Gynec. Obstetr.*, 108, 623.
25. NICHOLS, R. L., CONDON, R. E., (1971) Preoperative preparation of the colon. *Surg. Gynec. Obstetr.*, 132, 323.
26. HERTER, F. P., (1972) Preparation of the bowel for Surgery. Surg. Clin. N. Amer. 52, 859.
27. NYGAARD, K., RONGLAN, E., MIDTVEDT, T., (1972) Preoperative antibiotic treatment in surgery of the large intestine. *Acta Chir. Scand.*, 138, 415.
28. VINK, M., (1954) Local recurrence of cancer in the large bowel: the role of implantation metastases and bowel disinfection. *Brit. J. Surg.* 41, 431.
29. VINK, M., (1964) Surgical aspects of neoplastic disease of the large bowel (1964). *Dis. Colon & Rectum*, 1, 396.
30. TRINKLE, J. K., FISHER, L. J., KETCHAM, A. S., (1963) Metabolic effects of preoperative intestinal preparation. *Surg. Forum*, 14, 360.
31. TRINKLE, J. K., FISCHER, L. J., KETCHAM, A. S., BERLIN, N. I., (1964) The metabolic effects of preoperative intestinal preparation. *Surg. Gynec. Obstetr.*, 108, 623.
32. MIKAL, S., (1965) Metabolic effects of preoperative intestinal preparation. *Amer. J. Proctol.*, 16, 437.

SYNTHETIC DIETS IN THE TREATMENT OF INBORN ERRORS OF METABOLISM

H. BICKEL, H. SCHMIDT AND L. SCHÜRRLE*

A few of the many inborn errors of metabolism can be treated with special diets which aim at correcting the metabolic disturbance. This paper is limited to some errors of amino acid and carbohydrate metabolism, in which certain foods have to be replaced by synthetic substitutes or omitted altogether. The therapeutic principle for amino acid disturbances is to give the amino acids concerned in reduced quantities, preventing their metabolic accumulation before the enzyme block which seems to be the principal damaging factor in most of these diseases. Since all natural protein sources contain the entire amino acid spectrum, special protein substitutes without the amino acids involved are essential to complete the optimum protein requirement. This principle was practiced for the first time in 1953 when phenylalanine-free protein hydrolysates were used successfully in phenylketonuria; it then became a model for the treatment of other amino acid disturbances (1). Today protein hydrolysates and synthetic amino acid mixtures are commercially available from various manufacturers.

Phenylketonuria, histidinemia, homocystinuria and maple syrup urine disease can be successfully influenced with such diets. The biochemical disorder can be corrected and the clinical symptoms improved. In cystinosis and tyrosinosis trials lasting several years indicate that the diets seems to be ineffective; in some cases, the trials are still inconclusive. A more detailed account of the diets and the supplements will be given for these amino acid disturbances, followed by a short description of the dietary management of some inborn errors of carbohydrate metabolism.

PHENYLKETONURIA

In phenylketonuria, the deficiency of phenylalanine hydroxylase in

* University Childrens Hospital Heidelberg

the liver leads to an accumulation of phenylalanine, phenylpyruvic acid and other phenolic compounds which results in severe brain damage. It has been proven that an adequate diet restricted in phenylalanine is successful, normalizing the excessive phenylalanine concentration in the blood and other biological fluids and thus avoiding the generally severe brain damage of this disease (2). It must be emphasized that only early treatment within the first 8 weeks of life guarantees normal development (figure 1, 2). Nevertheless dietary therapy should also be initiated in older children, because limited and sometimes important improvement can still be achieved and further deterioration will be prevented (figure 3). Although no definite answer can be given as to when the diet can be discontinued,

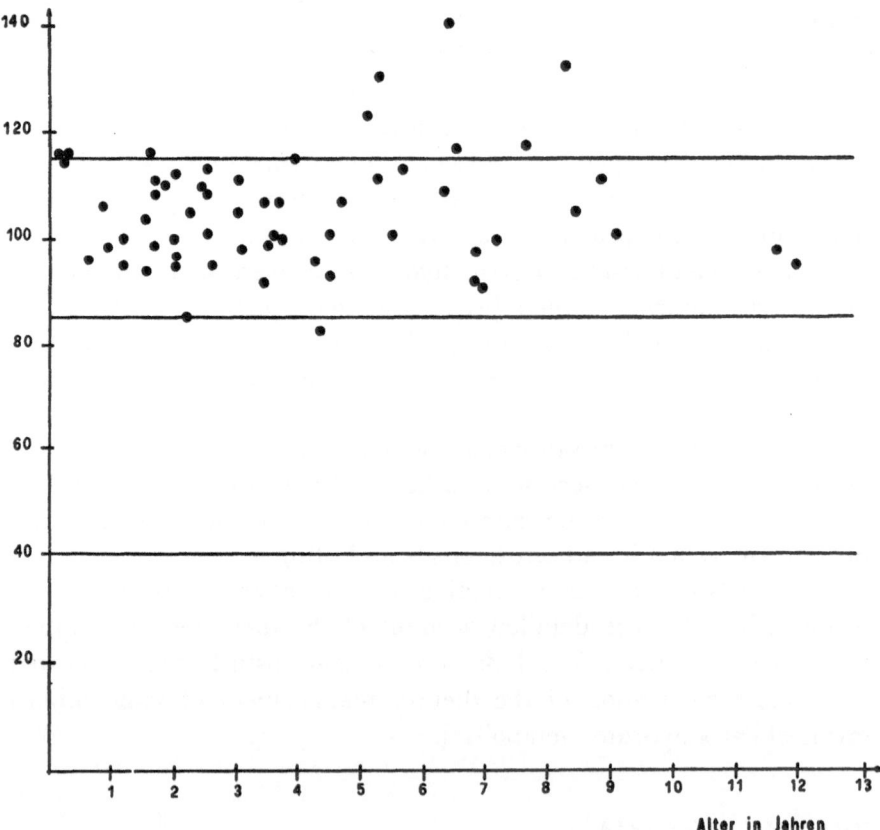

Fig. 1. Latest DQ/IQ values in 60 phenylketonuric children whose treatment was started within the first 2 months of life. DQ=Development quotient, IQ=Intelligence quotient.

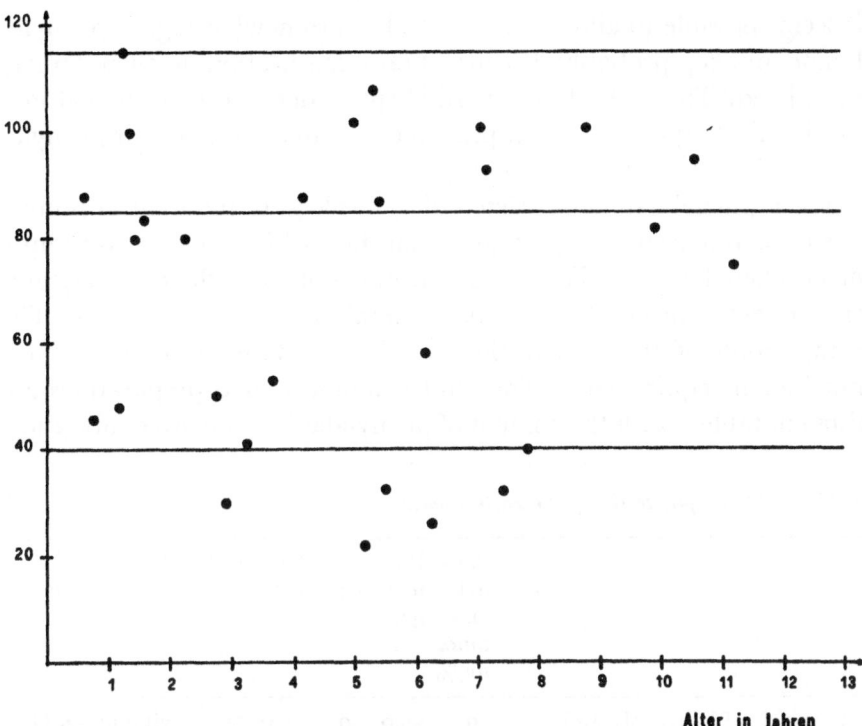

Fig. 2. Latest DQ/IQ values in 28 phenylketonuric children whose treatment was delayed, starting between the 3rd and 12th month of life.

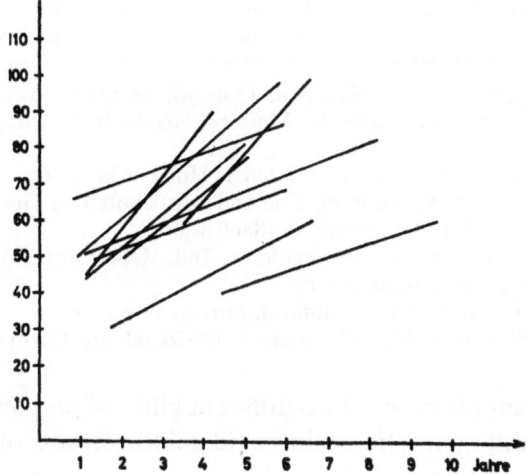

Fig. 3. DQ/IQ progression of phenylketonuric children with delayed start of treatment but excellent dietary control, ensuring near-normal phenylalanine blood levels between 2–4 mg%.

it seems possible to allow 8–10 year-olds a somewhat higher phenylalanine intake, probably because brain maturation is then largely
completed. These children are still kept under frequent clinical and
biochemical supervision. Our present goal is to maintain their phenylalanine blood level below 20 mg%.

For a phenylalanine-restricted diet, 50–80% of the natural protein
has to be replaced by a protein preparation which contains very little
or no phenylalanine. The loss of natural protein in the diet may give
rise to deficiencies of vitamins, minerals and trace elements. The
composition of the preparation should therefore meet all of these
nutritional requirements. The most commonly used preparations are
listed in table 1 with the content of phenylalanine, nutritive substances

Table 1. *Special preparations for phenylketonuria*

	Phe-nyl-ala-nine, mg%	Pro-tein, g%	Fat, g%	Ch, g%	Calo-ries	Necessary supplements
Albumaid XP[1] (hydrolysate)	0	35.0	0	50.0	350	vitamin D, C
Aponti PKU Diät[2] (hydrolysate)	0	35.0	0	50.0	350	vitamin D, C
Cymogran[3] (hydrolysate)	10	30.0	9	42.7	400	all vitamins
Lofenalac[4] (hydrolysate)	80	15.0	18	57.0	450	–
Minafen[5] (hydrolysate)	20	11.5	31	46.0	540	vitamin A, C, D
Aminogran[3] (amino acid mixture)	0	90.0	0	0	370	all vitamins
P-AM[6] (amino acid mixture)	0	80	0	0	330	vitamin D, C

[1] Scientific Hospital Supply (SHS), 38 Queensland Street, Liverpool L7 35G,
England; distributed in Germany by Maizena Gesellschaft mbH, 2 Hamburg 1,
Maizenahaus.
[2] Aponti Kindernährmittel GmbH, 5 Köln 1, Holzmarkt 59–65.
[3] Allen & Hanburys Ltd., London, England; distributed in Germany by Glaxo
Pharmazeutika, 2060 Bad Oldeslohe, Postfach 1460.
[4] Mead Johnson Laboratories, Evansville 21, Ind., USA; distributed in Germany
by Lappe Arzneimittel, 5060 Bensberg.
[5] Trufood Ltd., London Road, Guildford, Surrey, England.
[6] Maizena Gesellschaft mbH, 2 Hamburg 1, Maizenahaus, Germany

and necessary supplements. Two different kinds of preparation, protein
hydrolysates and synthetic amino acid mixtures, are on the market.
The hydrolysates listed are derived from the milk protein, casein, and
from ox serum protein. The protein source determines the amino acid
pattern and to some extent the mineral content.

Within the last few years the production of reasonably priced synthetic amino acid mixtures has become possible. With these preparations we have the choice of any desired composition.

We now have had 20 years of overall experience with diets based on hydrolysates. With individual treatment lasting 9 years, growth and gain in weight proceeded normally. There were no other clinical or biochemical signs of nutritional deficiencies when the intake of phenylalanine and other food components was well-adjusted (3–5). Within the last four years it has also become possible to administer synthetic amino acid mixtures to a smaller group of patients. During a two-year period 22 patients fed with synthetic amino acid mixtures have been closely observed at our hospital (6). A specimen diet sheet is reproduced in table 2. Clinical supervision over the entire period of treatment with these mixtures revealed no obvious symptoms of deficiencies. Gains in growth and weight proceeded undisturbed, and no abnormalities in amino acid, protein and mineral metabolism of the bones were found.

Table 2. *Phenylketonuria; 4 years, 17 kg body weight*

	Protein, g		
45g P-AM	36.0		
Natural protein			
Cream	1.8	15 mg phenylalanine	per kg BW/day
Vegetables, potatoes, fruits	3.3	2.4 g protein	
Corn starch bread	0.8		
Corn starch, sugar			
Oil, fats			

Comprehensive studies of the acid-base and electrolyte status were carried out in 64 patients on diets containing hydrolysates and amino acid mixtures (7). Depending on the preparation, more or less marked imbalances became apparent. Metabolic acidosis was observed when the preparations contained amino acids in the form of hydrochloride salts or when the proportion of sulphur-containing amino acids was too high.

Physiologically acid production is higher in infants than in older children and adults. This explains why diets with an extra acid load resulted in marked acidosis and in infants could even cause clinical symptoms such as anorexia and vomiting. We conclude that when

Table 3. *Recommendations concerning acid base balance in phe restricted diets*

1. URINARY SULPHATE correlates well with the methionine and cystine in the diet. In protein hydrolysates the methionin and cystine content must be considered. In synthetic amino acid mixtures methionine and cystine should not exceed 1 mM S/kg/day.

2. ABSORBED CATION EXCESS
Na+K should exceed Cl content.
HCl salts of arg, his, lys should be avoided.
Both a high intake of Ca and P and a high Ca:P ratio promote H⁺ excretion.
In synthetic amino acid mixtures P should not exceed Ca.

Considering all factors influencing acid base balance, renal nae in phe restricted preparations should lie within normal limits of 0.5–2 mEq/kg/day.

synthetic diets replace most of the food intake, they must be well-balanced not only with respect to the amino acid pattern but also the electrolyte composition. Table 3 lists some conclusions derived from our acid-base studies which should be considered when setting up synthetic diets. On the basis of these conclusions, the formulae of some of these products have been improved.

For the intake of protein, carbohydrate, fat and calories, we adhere to the international recommendations for healthy children. The tolerated phenylalanine intake is generally 200–400 mg/day and is relatively higher for young than for older children. This small amount is usually administered in the form of vegetables, potatoes, fruits and milk. Other foods of high protein content like meat, fish, cheese, eggs, normal bread and cake are eliminated because of their high phenylalanine content. These nutrients have to be replaced by amino acid preparations, low protein foods and special cornstarch products. Table 4 gives a list of sources for low protein products.

HISTIDINEMIA

In histidinemia the enzyme defect blocks the transformation of histidine into urocanic acid, which leads to brain damage in some patients. Though the brain damage is not as severe and frequent as that caused by phenylketonuria, we agree with Thalhammer (8) that a prophylactic histidine-restricted diet should be introduced within the first months of life. A histidine-restricted menu differs from

Table 4. *Low protein products; sources of supply*

Special bread, Wafers, Zwieback	N. Würsching, Mathildenstr. 26 6141 Einhausen (FRG)
Damin (breadmix)	Maizena Gesellschaft mbH 2 Hamburg 1, Maizenahaus (FRG)
Protein-free bread- and cakemix	Kvarn AB Tre Kronor, Stockholm; in Germany: H. Wiechert & Co., Postfach 930248, 2102 Hamburg 93; in Austria: H. Wiechert & Co., Getreidegasse 24, A-5020 Salzburg
Rite diet bread	Welfare Foods (Stockport) ltd. Stockport, Cheshire, SK 1 3HE in Germany: Greifen-Apotheke 7815 Kirchzarten, Bahnhofstr. 6
amin-ex, bisquits	LIGA Fabrieken N.V., Postbus 27, Roosendaal, Holland; in Germany: LIGA Nahrungsmittel GmbH, 403 Ratingen, Postfach 1472
Aproten products	Carlo Erba S.p.A., Milano, Italy; in Germany: Rademann Diätprodukte GmbH, Postfach 45, 638 Bad Homburg
Aglutella noodles Cookies, bisquits, wafers	Ditta Federico Salza, Via Sottoborgo 46, 56100 Pisa, Italy

the phenylketonuria diet only in the composition of the amino acid preparation, i.e. it is free of histidine instead of phenylalanine. As to the effectiveness of this diet, it is too early to draw any definite conclusions. Thalhammer who has the most experience in Europe claims that so far his patients have developed normally (9).

MAPLE SYRUP URINE DISEASE

It is much more difficult to successfully treat maple syrup urine disease. This disorder involves three essential amino acids: leucine, isoleucine and valine. The development of the syndrome with the peculiar maple syrup odor, opisthotonous, asphyxia and convulsions manifests itself during the first days of life on a normal milk formula. Without treatment brain damage rapidly progresses leading to death within the first weeks or months of life. Therapy should therefore be initiated at the earliest possible moment (10, 11).

Table 5 shows a diet for a 7-month-old child. This diet is largely synthetic, consisting mainly of an amino acid mixture free of the branched-chain amino acids, vitamins and minerals. Carbohydrates

Table 5. *Maple syrup disease; 7 months, 6.4 kg BW*

	Protein, g		
20 g L-amino acid mixture, incl. vitamins + minerals	16.0		
Natural protein			
500 g whey			
20 g cow's milk			
2 g dry yeast	2.7	55 mg leucine	
30 g potatoes		25 mg isoleucine	per kg BW/day
		40 mg valine	
30 g corn oil		2.9 g protein	
20 g corn starch			
90 g dextrose			
162 mg leucine			
93 mg valine			

and fats must be administered in their pure form. The diet contains only traces of natural protein, usually administered in the form of whey, milk and yeast. This is done to meet any possible deficiencies which may result from such a synthetic diet. We have in the past observed two patients who died within their first year due to nutritional deficiencies of unknown origin. Since then, however, a number of patients could be kept alive with the aid of such diets. Height and weight lie in the lower normal range, and there is only slight mental retardation.

One of the difficulties of the treatment is the constant fluctuation in the tolerance for the three amino acids involved, which requires frequent plasma aminograms as shown in figure 4. Infections lead to rapid metabolic imbalances. A suitable preparation is manufactured in Germany by Maizena under the name ILV-AM.

HOMOCYSTINURIA

Clinically homocystinuria is characterized by a Marfan-like syndrome with skeletal changes and lenticular ectopia, mental retardation and thromboembolic complications often resulting in the death of these patients. The biochemical disturbance involves the metabolism of methionine. Through the deficiency of cystahionine synthesis in the liver, methionine is not transformed into cystine. Methionine, homocystine and mixed disulfides accumulate in blood and urine.

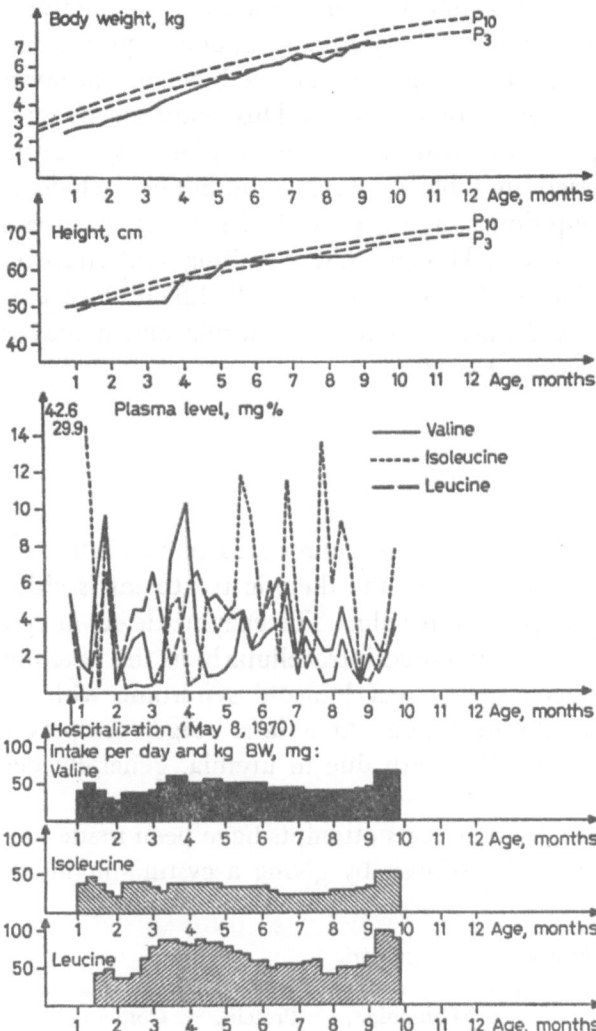

Fig. 4. The course of the disease in a patient with maple syrup urine disease during the first year of life, showing the increments in body weight and height, the plasma level and the daily intake of valine, isoleucine and leucine (mg/kg/day). Note the remarkable variation in plasma levels of the branched-chain amino acids despite frequent monitoring by plasma column chromatography and consequent adjustment of the diet.

In approximately half of the patients, a biochemical normalization occurred after treatment with large amounts of pyridoxine, the cofactor of cystathionine synthesis (12, 13). This group of patients shows some rest activity of this enzyme, which is activated by pyridoxine. Patients without any enzyme activity do not respond to pyridoxine supplementation. In these cases one can achieve biochemical normalization by restricting the methionine intake. This again means that the diet has to be complemented with special preparations low in or free of methionine, as listed in table 6. Further additions include choline, as a methyl group donor, and cystine, which becomes an essential amino acid in this disease. Though some promising results have been achieved, an evaluation of this treatment is still difficult because the natural course of the disease is somewhat chronic and it may develop only slowly over several years.

CYSTINOSIS AND TYROSINOSIS

In the last two disorders of amino acid metabolism to be discussed, cystinosis and tyrosinosis, the dietetic treatment is either ineffective or has not yet proven its value. The enzyme defect in cystinosis is still unknown. Cystine is stored intracellularly in the lysosomes. Proximal tubular damage leads to a Fanconi syndrome with dwarfism and vitamin D-resistant rickets. At a later stage, complex renal failure develops and finally death due to uremia, generally before puberty is reached.

During the last ten years attempts have been made to influence the natural course of cystinosis by giving a cystine-methionine-restricted

Table 6. *Preparations for homocystinuria*

	Methionine, mg%	Protein, g%	Content	Necessary supplements
Albumaid X Met.[1]	40	30	ox serum hydrolysate	vitamin C, D
CM-AM[2]	0	75	amino acid mixture	vitamin C, D
Sobee powder[3]	310	22	soy product	–

[1] Scientific Hospital Supply (SHS), 38 Queensland Street, Liverpool L7 35G, England; distributed in Germany by Maizena Gesellschaft mbH, 2000 Hamburg 1.
[2] Maizena Gesellschaft mbH, 2000 Hamburg 1, Maizenahaus.
[3] Mead Johnson Laboratories, Evansville 21, Ind., USA; distributed in Germany by Lappe Arzneimittel, 5060 Bensberg.

diet on the basis of a lentil powder preparation first, later by supplying mixtures of pure amino acids.

The effect of this treatment has been evaluated in 21 patients from Heidelberg and other medical centers (14)*. The period of observation ranges from 8 months to 7 years, averaging 2 1/2 years, during which time we followed kidney function, the course of rickets, the vitamin D requirement and growth. In the long run one must admit that the course of the disease was not influenced by the diet but remained progressive. Initial improvement was repeatedly observed but must be attributed to intensive symptomatic therapy and not to specific dietary management of the patients.

In tyrosinosis the metabolic disorder is also still obscure. Most authors believe now that tyrosinemia and, in some cases methioninemia, are secondary phenomena of a liver disease of unknown origin. For this reason the rationale of dietary treatment with restriction of phenylalanine and tyrosine has become questionable. In our own experience healing of rickets, normalization of phosphate in serum and increased tubular phosphate reabsorption were seen during dietary tyrosine restriction, but there was no direct influence on other symptoms such as liver dysfunction and thrombocytopenia (15).

Halvorsen followed four Norwegian patients with tyrosinosis for 5 to 10 years; the improvements in renal phosphate reabsorption, amino-aciduria, rickets and neuromuscular functions were greater in the two patients on dietary treatment than the two patients treated solely with vitamin D. There was no improvement of liver function in either of these patient groups (16).

INTOLERANCE AND MALABSORPTION OF CARBOHYDRATES

The disorders of carbohydrate metabolism which lend themselves to dietetic treatment are hereditary galactosemia, fructosemia and the malabsorption of sucrose, lactose and glucose-galactose. The principle of their treatment is uniform and simple: the sugar involved must be excluded from the diet (17).

In such acute and severe diseases as galactosemia and fructosemia,

* Contributions have been gratefully received from D. Alagille, C. Gentil and Odière (Bicêtre, France), R. Grüttner and Christine Goetze-Bender (Hamburg), M. Seip (Oslo, Norway), F. van Sprang and S. Wadman (Utrecht, the Netherlands), H. R. Wiedemann, Marianne Bontemps and U. Goll (Kiel).

where the patients are threatened by liver cirrhosis, hypoglycemia, brain damage and cataract formation, every effort must be made to start the diet as early as possible, under ideal conditions, it should be continued for the patient's lifetime. There is no clear proof that sufficiently effective alternative pathways will develop to compensate for the enzyme block.

The excellent, live-saving results of a galactose-free diet, unfortunately administered after a delay of 3 months to a patient with galactosemia, are seen in figure 5. In the treatment of galactosemia diet composition poses no real problems. Industry has provided us with complete formulae for infants (table 7). Later no special prepa-

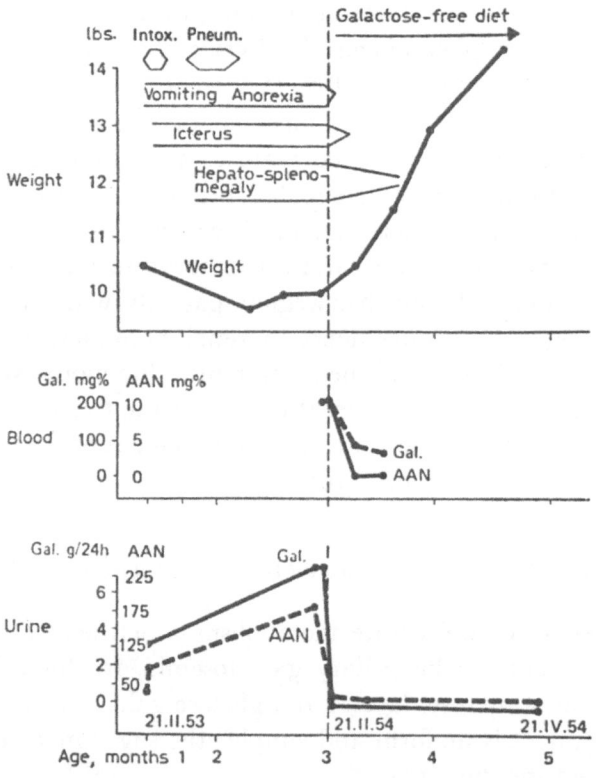

Fig. 5. Course of the disease in a patient with idiopathic galactosemia. In the first three months of life, decrease in weight, attacks of gastroenteritis, vomiting, anorexia and pneumonia. Persistent jaundice and hepatosplenomegaly, increased concentrations of galactose (Gal.) and amino acids (AAN) in blood and urine. All these symptoms normalized under a galactose-free diet started at 3 months; the subsequent gain in weight was excellent.

Table 7. Special preparations for carbohydrate malabsorptions

	Producer	Protein source	Carbohydrate	Indications	Substitutions
Al 110	Nestlé[1]	Na caseinate	glucose	all CH malabsorptions, except glucose-galactose malabsorption	0
MBF	Gerber[2]	hearts of beef	saccharose, starch	galactosaemia, lactose malabsorption	0
Lambase	Gerber[2]	hearts of lambs	maltose, dextrine, starch	galactosaemia, lactose malabsorption	0
Nutramigen	Mead Johnson[3]	casein	saccharose, starch	galactosaemia, lactose malabsorption	0
CHO-free	Borden[4]	soybean ox serum	traces	all CH malabsorptions	carbohydrate
Albumaid complete	SHS[5]	hydrolysate	0	all CH malabsorptions	carbohydrate, fat, vitamins, minerals

[1] Nestlé: Deutsche Nestlé GmbH, Postfach 3609, 6 Frankfurt 1.
[2] Gerber; distributed in Germany by Deutsche Maizena Werke, 2 Hamburg 1.
[3] Mead Johnson Laboratories, Evansville 21, Ind., USA; distributed in Germany by Lappe Arzneimittel, 5060 Bensberg.
[4] Borden Inc., Pharmaceutical Products, New York, N.Y. 10017, USA; distributed in Europe by Diadal N.V., 1890 Opwijk, Belgium.
[5] Scientific Hospital Supply (SHS), 38 Queensland Street, Liverpool L7 35 G, England; distributed in Germany by Deutsche Maizena Werke, 2 Hamburg 1.

rations are necessary but care must be taken in using commercial foods, since they may contain unknown quantities of lactose.

It is much more difficult to set up a fructose-free diet, since fructose is present in most carbohydrate-containing foods (18). A completely fructose-free diet is rather monotonous and unpalatable for the child, except in early infancy when it consists chiefly of milk. However the composition of manufactured baby foods as printed on the label has to be checked since the amount of sucrose is often omitted.

Another group of disturbances are caused by defective absorption of carbohydrates, resulting in diarrhoea. Lactose and sucrose-isomaltose malabsorption are due to a deficiency of disaccharidases. As the child grows older, the bowel may develop greater tolerance for the non-absorbed sugar so that the dietary regime can be relaxed to some extent. In sucrose-isomaltose malabsorption, sucrose has to be avoided and replaced by adequate monosaccharides. Starch is usually tolerated in small quantities. In lactose malabsorption the diet corresponds to that for galactosemia. In glucose-galactose malabsorption the only sugars tolerated are fructose and, because of their slow absorption, small amounts of sorbitel and xylitol. All polysaccharides must also be avoided.

We realize that the dietary treatment of inborn errors of the amino acid and carbohydrate metabolism is a somewhat secondary, cumbersome way to correct the metabolic disturbance. The direct approach of enzyme replacement is at present not yet available but may well become a preferable possibility in the future for management of these patients.

SUMMARY

For some important inborn errors of metabolism the only effective treatment is to prescribe a synthetic diet whereby the composition is such that the metabolic disturbance is corrected. The diet generally aims at preventing the metabolite accumulation before the enzyme block, as this seems to be the principal damaging factor in most of these diseases.

This paper is limited to some errors of amino acid and carbohydrate metabolism in which dietary treatment has proven to be successful or is at present being explored. For hereditary disorders of lipid and other metabolic pathways, synthetic diets have so far been of little or no value. The therapeutic principle for amino acid disturbances is to give the amino acids involved in reduced quantities which however also limits the total natural protein intake. To ensure normal growth the deficit must be covered either by some intact natural protein which has a low concentration of the corresponding amino acid or by a mixture of pure essential and nonessential amino acids made up to the required pattern or by amino acid mixtures derived from hydrolysis of proteins.

Data are presented giving the composition of some preparations used in these diets, and suggestions are made concerning further substitution of vitamins and minerals. A more detailed account of the diet and its success are given for the following diseases: phenylketonuria, homocystinuria, histidinemia, maple syrup urine disease, tyrosinosis, cystinosis.

The different carbohydrate intolerances are due to a variety of causes whereas the therapeutic principle for all of these disorders is identical, namely deletion of the disaccharides or monosaccharides concerned. The success of this treatment is well-established. No special food preparations are needed for sucrose malabsorption and fructosemia, whereas they are an essential part of the diet in galactosemia as well as in lactose and glucose-galactose malabsorption.

Various preparations are described. Formulae free of certain or all carbohydrates are now available and are important not only for treatment but also for diagnosis of these conditions.

REFERENCES

1. BICKEL, H., GERRARD, J., and HICKMANS, E. M., Influence of phenylalanine intake on phenylketonuria. *Lancet ii*, 312 (1953).
2. BICKEL, H. and KAISER-GRUBEL, S., Über die Phenylketonurie. Psychometrische Erfolgsbeurteilung der phenylalaninarmen Diät bei phenylketonurischen Kindern. *Dtsch. med. Wschr.* 96: 1415 (1971).
3. SCHMIDT, H., Clinical aspects of the treatment of phenylketonuria; in BICKEL, HUDSON and WOOLF: *Phenylketonuria and some other inborn errors of amino acid metabolism*, p. 232 (Thieme, Stuttgart 1971).
4. SCHMIDT, H., Nutritional aspects of the phenylalanine-restricted diet; in BICKEL, HUDSON and WOOLF: *Phenylketonuria and some other inborn errors of amino acid metabolism*, p. 237 (Thieme, Stuttgart 1971).
5. SCHÜRRLE, L. and BICKEL, H., Practical dietetics; in BICKEL, HUDSON and WOOLF: *Phenylketonuria and some other inborn errors of amino acid metabolism*, p./240 (Thieme, Stuttgart 1971).

6. Lutz, P., Schmidt, H., Schürrle, L., and Bickel, H., Die Behandlung der Phenylketonurie mit Gemischen synthetischer Aminosäuren im Vergleich zu Eiweißhydrolysaten. *Kongreßbericht des XIII. Internationalen Kongresses für Pädiatrie,* Wien 1971, vol. V/1, p. 41.

7. Manz, F. and Schmidt, H., Acid-base status in dietary treatment of phenylketonuria. *Abstract European Soc. Paed. Res.* Oct. 1–4, 1973. Ped. Res. (in press).

8. Thalhammer, O., Scheibenreiter, S., und Pantlitschko M., Über die Häufigkeit der Histidinämie. Erfahrungen mit der Massentestung an 48 000 Neugeborenen (with detailed list of references). *Mschr. Kinderheilk.* 119: 357 (1971).

9. Thalhammer, O., Personal communication (1973).

10. Snyderman, S. E., The therapy of maple syrup urine disease. *Amer. J. Dis. Child.* 113: 68 (1967).

11. Snyderman, S. E., Maple syrup urine disease; In Bickel, Hudson and Woolf: *Phenylketonuria and some other inborn errors of amino acid metabolism,* p. 283 (Thieme, Stuttgart 1971).

12. Barber, G. W. and Spaeth, G. L., The successful treatment of homocystinuria with pyridoxine. *J. Pediat.* 75: 463 (1969).

13. Carson, N. A. J., Homocystinuria (cystathionine synthetase deficiency). Trial of treatment with oral pyridoxine and a normal diet; in Carson and Raine: *Inherited disorders of sulphur metabolism,* p. 284 (Churchill/Livingstone, Edinburgh/London 1971).

14. Bickel, H., Lutz, P. and Schmidt, H., The treatment of cystinosis with diet or drugs. In J. D. Schulman: *Cystinosis.* DHEW: Publication No. (NIH) 72–249, *U.S. Gov. Printing Office, Washington* 1973, p. 199.

15. Nützenadel, W., Lutz, P. and Bickel, H., Tyrosinose. Primäre und sekundäre biochemische Veränderungen. *Z. Kinderheilk.* 113: 193 (1972).

16. Halvorsen, S., The long-term effects of a phenylalanine-tyrosine restricted diet in hereditary tyrosinemia. Abstract *European Soc. Paed. Res.* Oct. 1–4, 1973. Ped. Res. (in press).

17. Cornblath, M. and Schwartz, R., Disorders of carbohydrate metabolism in infancy; in *Major problems in clinical pediatrics,* vol. 3 (Saunders, Philadelphia/London 1966; reprinted 1967).

18. Dako, D. Y., Trautner, K. und Somogyi, J. C., Der Glukose-Fruktose- und Saccharosegehalt verschiedener Früchte. *Schweiz. med. Wschr.* 100: 897 (1970).

DISCUSSION

PAPER OF PROF. JONXIS

Prof. Bickel: You know the work of Matthews, which showed that sometimes peptides, at least in animal experiments, seem to be absorbed better than pure amino acids. I know that in phenylketonuria Dr. Snyderman has many reservations about giving pure amino acids instead of hydrolysates which may still contain some peptides. What do you think about this work? Is it really not so that giving amino acids all in one dose, i.e. swallowing a ready-made form, may cause absorption problems?

Prof. Jonxis: I'm rather astonished about our results, but they are good. There is no increased excretion of amino acids in the urine. We did have the feeling that because we gave such a load of amino acids in a feeding, it could bypass the liver and cause high levels in the blood. But we did not find high blood levels. In the past we have done some experimental work with peptides and the results were not as good as with pure amino acids.

Prof. Schretlen: You gave a synthetic diet to the boy and the girl. The children had normal weight curves. What about the height curves of these children. Were these patients also dwarfed before treatment?

Prof. Jonxis: I showed you the data of the patients with non-ketotic hyperglycinaemia. Their growth was retarded in length and weight. The other patient with severe diarrhoea had a normal increase in length, but there was no catch-up growth.

Dr. Fernandes: You showed two slides of skin lesions. May I suggest that these lesions are not signs of protein deficiency but of linoleic acid deficiency. What is your opinion of this?

Prof. Jonxis: I don't think it was a linoleic acid deficiency because we gave the same amounts of linoleic acid before and after healing of the skin lesions. The only change was a greater amount of protein.

The other child was admitted with brittle hair; we don't know exactly what causes this abnormality. The whole condition seemed to be caused by protein deficiency but we can't prove this. Maybe other factors like linoleic acid deficiency were also involved.

Dr. Corstens: In recent literature some papers have appeared about the incidence of metabolic acidosis in parenteral hyperalimentation with pure amino acids. We have had the same experience in adults. You didn't find that metabolic acidosis. Do you have any explanation?

Prof. Jonxis: No, we didn't see metabolic acidosis. The amount of hydrochloric acid in our diet was not high. I think the large amount of hydrochloric acid in such diets might be the cause of metabolic acidosis in these cases.

Dr. Hekkens: Perhaps I may comment on your last remarks about the paradox you have seen. It has been shown that there is a remarkable reduction in the excretion of all the fluids into the intestinal lumen during a synthetic diet. The reduction is more than 50% or even 75%. This means it works in two ways. You don't need to reabsorb and you don't need to synthesize as much. I think that could be one of the reasons why this type of diet is accepted so well by the patients. Another point perhaps is that your diet does not include any peptides. In sprue some peptides or other substances are toxic for the intestinal wall. With synthetic diets you don't give substances that are immunologically active.

Prof. Eekels: May I ask about the aspects of the stools?

Prof. Jonxis: The stools are different. In the patients with hyperglycinaemia, the quantity of stools was small and they were not well-formed. In the child who received glucose, we observed large quantities of loose stools with a low pH due to fermentation.

PAPER OF DR. JARNUM

Dr. Koumans: I think I completely agree with Dr. Jarnum: that the diet should be started with a diluted concentration and then slowly built up stepwise. I don't understand why you use the same method for discontinuation of the diet. Why don't you just switch over to a bland diet or another diet after elementary feeding?

Dr. Jarnum: Psychological reasons. It is much easier for a patient to accept the treatment if it is introduced gradually. Similarly the gradual reintroduction of a normal diet means an easily accepted prolongation of the treatment for a few days.

Prof. Muller: I quite agree with Dr. Jarnum that this sort of treatment might save patients. We have had some very good experiences with vivonex or vivasorb. However in some cases we got into trouble after two or three weeks. Patients developed very severe diarrhoea, so that we had to stop the synthetic diet. Did you run into this problem?

Dr. Jarnum: We had to stop the synthetic diet in several cases. In those cases however the diarrhoea started very early. We did not observe diarrhoea as a late complication.

Prof. Muller: One other remark. Twice we found we had better results with this regimen than with absolute oral fasting. I don't know why.

Dr. Jarnum: We had two cases who showed the opposite. They couldn't stand the diet, but they tolerated a complete intravenous feeding very well for a long period.

Dr. ten Thije: I noticed that you had two cases of toxic megacolon during therapy. I wonder whether you blame the regimen for that and in which way. I would like to ask you to speculate upon the common denominator of success or failure. What is the common denominator if the patient is going to benefit from it or not. Could you tell us something about that?

Dr. Jarnum: I wish I could. Of course the two patients did not have a toxic megacolon when we started treatment. From the start there was dilatation of the colon so that it was feasible that they might develop a toxic megacolon in a few days. It had nothing to do with the diet.

Prof. Jonxis: Could you tell us something about the composition of your diet?

Dr. Jarnum: I didn't give any specific figures. The fat content is very low, only essential fatty acids like linoleic acid. The carbohydrates, which provide most of the calories, are glucose and oligosaccharides formed by hydrolysis of polysaccharides from mais.

Prof. Jonxis: And the mineral composition of your diet?

Dr. Jarnum: On a full regimen with 2100 calories per day you supply about 100 mmoles of sodium and 90 mmoles of potassium.

Dr. Hekkens: There is another disease in which you can use this type of diet very satisfactorily. In patients with pancreatitis, where you have inadequate digestion, it is also possible to use this diet. We have had very good results in one patient with pancreatitis and a large infiltrate. He went home after 6 weeks of treatment. With regard to the duration of the diet treatment, perhaps the diet period used by Dr. Jarnum is a little bit short. In literature you find that patients with enterocolitis are treated for 6 weeks with parenteral feeding before remission occurs. Perhaps the time required for healing under treatment with a synthetic diet will be on the same order. We have treated patients for a rather long time. Sometimes we got results; other times it was of no value and no help. So I think the selection of the patient will be a problem. We have had patients with fistulas and they improved but only after at least two or three weeks, and never in a very short time. Sometimes you see an improvement but we have found that closure of fistulas takes two or three weeks.

Dr. Schmerling: There is another indication in paediatrics for an elementary diet. This is the 'meconium ileus equivalent' in adolescents with cystic fibrosis. There the results are astonishing because the patients no longer have abdominal pain immediately after the diet is started and the general improvement is good.

On a home-made elementary diet, we saw closure of the fistulas in one patient with perforated appendicitis within a week.

Dr. Ricour: We have used the elementary diet in 35 infants with short bowel syndrome or fistulas. The results are very good after 1 to 6 months on the specific diet. There are two important factors. The osmolar load that is administered in a short period of time into the stomach or duodenum. And the rate of infusion of water and fat. What is your opinion?

Dr. Jarnum: I'm very amazed and impressed by the case report of Dr. Hekkens on the patient with pancreatitis. When we cannot manage to feed our patients with chronic pancreatitis with enzyme supplements, we use a low fat diet with a supplement of MCT. We fed one patient with pancreatitis with elementary nutrition and that was not a success. With regard to the duration of treatment in enterocolitis, I do not agree with Dr. Hekkens for several reasons. These patients can't tolerate this type of diet for more than a few weeks. It has been impossible for us to persuade these patients to continue. When they start to improve, they want to go back to an ordinary diet. The role of the physician should be to treat the patients such that they can live normally. I have no doubt that the elementary diet represents progress in this treatment, because you can induce a remission when ordinary treatment with prednisone and salazopyrine is insufficient.

On the other hand I think it is very important to combine treatment because this will ensure that within the shortest possible time the patient can return to normal life.

We were talking about the treatment of fistulas. Maybe our treatment was too short: only two weeks. I think it is very difficult to predict which fistulas will close. We have treated several cases of fistulas with total parenteral feeding for weeks or months and had several failures.

Dr. Ricour, I wish we could treat adults like you treat children. I have no doubt that administration of a special diet through a duodenal tube for 6 months will produce formidable results. But that is quite impossible in adults. I would not be able to motivate them for that.

Dr. Veeger: We have treated adult patients for a very long time with a liquid diet via duodenal tubes.

Dr. Stauffer: On one of your slides, you discussed a patient with only 20 cm of small intestine left. Did this patient survive?

Dr. Jarnum: This patient survived and is now in good condition more than three years after the intestinal resection; he is on permanent parenteral nutrition.

Dr. Wilson: I would like to ask Dr. Jarnum if he has had any experience with elementary diets in portal systemic encephalopathy. It seems to me that you get extremely good absorption of your amino acids in the first part of the small bowel. In addition there is a decrease in the excretion of proteins and other fluids into the bowel during the course of your treatment. And thirdly bacterial overgrowth in the colon diminishes during this period. A very good method for treating portal systemic encephalopathy might be to provide essential amino acids in this manner.

Dr. Jarnum: We made no bacterial cultures or studies of the colon flora in patients with chronic inflammatory disease. I'm sure you have a point there.

Using labeled protein we have been able to demonstrate that you reduce protein loss with your elementary diet in ulcerative colitis.

PAPER OF DR. RICHARDS

Prof. Kluthe: Dr. Richards, you showed us that the nitrogen excretion was 0.5 g in patients and in normal individuals on a low protein diet. Is this a measured value?

Dr. Richards: The faecal nitrogen excretion was measured. With one exception it varied on a low protein diet from 0.5 to 0.7 g daily. Measurements were generally made with 5-day stool collections and the faecal excretion was averaged for the whole experiment.

Prof. Kluthe: We were astonished to see that the daily nitrogen excretion was higher in our patients on a low protein diet than those on a normal protein diet. Our values were about 1.7 g nitrogen a day.

Dr. Richards: That is higher than I have found either in uraemic patients or normal individuals. The highest in an uraemic patient on a 4 g protein diet was 1.1 g. Did your patients have diarrhoea or loose stools? Both our patients and the students tended to get diarrhoea on the synthetic diet but were controlled with codeine.

Prof. Kluthe: Our patients had normal stools and normal absorption. In my opinion it depends upon the type of nutrients: mushrooms instead of meat and so on, foods containing unresolvable nitrogen.

Dr. Richards: Our diet had very little residue.

Dr. Wilson: Are there any toxic effects to be expected from a-keto acids.

Dr. Richards: None have been described. Whether or not you may expect them is open to discussion.

Dr. Wilson: What about urea nitrogen retention. The urologists could help us by implanting ureters in the bowel. This seems to me to be an extremely good model for the study of the incorporation of keto acids in a clinical situation.

Dr. Richards: I investigated people with simple protein restriction or deficiency and examined their use of endogenous non-amino nitrogen. I should hesitate to implant ureters into the colon simply to give them a little more endogenous nitrogen!

Dr. Wilson: Have you ever tried reducing blood urea in patients with uraemia by acidifying their colonic contents, for instance, with lactulose.

Dr. Richards: I'm not so much concerned about reducing blood urea as making nutritional use of what urea nitrogen there is. The fact that the blood urea drops is of secondary importance. What I want to do is to become independent of dietary nitrogen.

Dr. Hekkens: Didn't you show on one of your first slides that the hydrolysis of urea to ammonia is diminished by antibiotics?

Dr. Richards: Yes, it is.

Dr. Hekkens: If you give a chemical diet, you know that you also reduce the bacterial content of the bowel. Did you find any reduction or increase in urea excretion?

Dr. Richards: Faecal nitrogen was generally not higher than normal. It is therefore unlikely that much urea was wasted in the stool. We did not determine whether there was any significant change in the urease activity in the stools.

Dr. Hekkens: But you didn't find an increase in urea excretion instead of ammonia excretion.

Dr. Richards: We did not measure urea excretion. We found that faecal nitrogen excretion was about normal.

Dr. Wilson: So you would not expect faecal nitrogen to increase. I think primarily the blood urea is catabolised by the colonic urease. You should look at the urinary urea excretion.

Dr. Richards: Urinary urea in the uraemic patient could of course not increase substantially. It would result in an increase in blood urea.

PAPER OF DR. KOUMANS

Dr. Ricour: What is the composition of vivonex? What is the osmolality of your solution? How do you give this diet, by mouth or by gastric tube?

Dr. Koumans: The composition of vivonex does not differ essentially from the original glucose-based elementary diet, as described by Winitz and co-workers.

The osmolality of a standard vivonex solution (80 g in 250 ml water) depends on the flavour used. The beef broth-flavoured diet, which is unsweetened, has an osmolality of 650 mOsm/kg. The other sweetened flavours have osmolalities in the range of 1200 mOsm/kg. Recently an unflavoured vivonex diet has become available with an osmolality of 500 mOsm/kg.

Where variety in flavours is of no importance, it is our policy to administer the low osmolality diet; in tube feedings, this implies the use of the unflavoured product.

Concerning your third question: for most of our patients, we did not need a gastric tube to administer adequate elementary nutrition. As a rule we explain to our patients why we give the diet and what we intend to achieve in giving it.

We have never had to discontinue the diet or resort to tube feedings because of its lack of palatability, except sometimes in children and of course in the mentally ill.

Dr. Jarnum: I completely agree with your conclusion that the elementary diet is no panacea and is indicated only in severe situations. I would just like to mention that there is a slight difference between your preparation and the one we used. We have also tried vivonex and I think the palatability of the vivasorb preparation is a little bit more acceptable.

Some have claimed that you can prepare the bowel even more efficiently if you evacuate the bowel with a phosphate instillation before starting the diet. I would like to know whether you do this.

Dr. Koumans: The original procedure was to give a phosphate-buffered enema. We just use a water enema to clean the colon, one day after the initiation of elementary nutrition

Dr. Schmerling: The difference between your results and those of Winitz, regarding the reduction in bacterial flora in the gut, might be explained by a difference in carbohydrate composition. Winitz and co-workers have shown that the changes in microflora populations vary with the type of carbohydrate incorporated in the diet. Vivonex has glucose as well as oligosaccharides. This might make the difference.

Dr. Koumans: Winitz observed the most significant alterations in gut microflora populations with a glucose-based diet. While vivonex is also glucose-based as far as its hexose content is concerned, it contains a substantial amount of oligosaccharides as a source of carbohydrates. I think you made a point in raising the question that this difference in carbohydrate composition might affect the influence of the diet on bowel bacteria.

Dr. Stauffer: Among your indications for the use of an elementary diet in the postoperative phase, you mentioned the protection of bowel anastomoses. Do you now use these diets as a routine procedure following bowel surgery? What is your exact indication?

Dr. Koumans: We do not yet use elementary diets routinely following bowel surgery. We have however given it occasionally when we felt that a valid indication existed, as was the case in the patient who required an ileostomy and in the patient with leakage after left colon resection.

Dr. Stauffer: I think this is very important because the danger exists that it would become fashionable to also give the diet when it is not necessary.

Prof. Muller: You said this diet is not a panacea but there is another approach. Of course we try to heal every fistula with this diet. But we also know that most fistulas will heal by themselves if you just wait another week.

Regarding Dr. Stauffer's question, I think that there is an indication following colon surgery. If you look at colon resections, especially the low anterior resections, you will find an anastomotic breakdown in about 40–60% of the cases. Luckily most patients survive. Most of them do not even show clinical signs, but some do and in those patients you might have to perform a colostomy. It might be that this diet, especially when it becomes cheaper, would offer very good protection of fresh anastomoses in all colon surgery.

Dr. Koumans: I certainly agree with this. Elementary feeding might be very useful postoperatively in patients with low anterior resections.

Dr. Veeger: It was stated that you should start the diet with a low concentration and a small quantity and then increase administration in a few days, perhaps a week, to the normal amount of about 1800 kcal. You give a diet preoperatively for 5 days, but do you give the whole diet during this period? If you don't, you are undernourishing the patient; if you do, you give the whole amount from the first day.

Dr. Koumans: If we give the elementary diet as bowel preparation, we start straight away with 1800 kcal/day. We decided to do this as we thought that the possible occurrence of diarrhoea, though interfering with nutrition, would enhance the effectiveness of the bowel preparation. We found however that these patients somehow do not develop diarrhoea.

Dr. Veeger: Many of our patients don't tolerate a full dosis immediately. You don't see diarrhoea in your patients at all?

Dr. Koumans: We have had some problems with diarrhoea in children and patients in a severe catabolic state who received the diet for therapeutic reasons. In those two categories diarrhoea can easily be provoked and you may have to watch your step.

In these patients the diet is initiated along the same lines that Dr. Jarnum indicated. We start with low osmolalities and then gradually increase the amounts. Once diarrhoea sets in, you may find yourself forced to start all over again and to proceed with even more caution.

PAPER OF PROF. BICKEL

Dr. Schmerling: Would you dare to speculate on the problems of enzyme replacement?

Prof. Bickel: When I started to study inborn errors of metabolism I asked Prof. Bücher in Marburg – many years ago – if there would be the possibility of replacing an enzyme. At that time I was very amazed that he did not say that is never possible. I always thought it would be very difficult to get enough enzyme by extraction or by synthesis. You can't give it by the enteral route but you have to inject it. There are some possibilities like transplantation of liver to provide enzymes. Another possibility is to give cultured cells, which you might be able to reimplant in the patient. This is a very tricky subject. As you know it has been tried to give infusions of normal leucocytes in mucopolysacchasidosis with no success in the long run. It has been tried to give aryl sulfatase A to patients with metachromatic leucodystrophy, but this did not have any effect on brain enzyme concentration. The

Shope virus has been tried in argininaemia, probably without any success.

Prof. Visser: There have been differences of opinion on the question how long one has to continue the diet in phenylketonuria. What is your position on this today?

Prof. Bickel: It is an important and difficult question. We are just trying now to evaluate this. There have been all kinds of opinion. Some people, like the group in Los Angeles, don't dare to take off their children at all from the diet as long as ever possible and go on even after puberty if patients and parents co-operate. Others have been very brave taking them off diet at 3 or 4 years. Unfortunately there were no follow-up reports of their patients. I heard personally that one or two of these patients did not do too well after taking off the diet. The problem is probably linked with the fact that the biochemical lesion seems to interfere with myelinisation of the brain. But this is not the only effect. Myelinisation of the brain is more or less completed at puberty. There is still some myelinisation going on in certain areas of the brain after puberty but myelinisation is more or less complete at the age of 8 or 10 years, and head circumference more or less at its maximum. If the pathogenesis is mainly one concerning myelinisation, that would be the age at which the brain is maturated so far as to tolerate more phenylalanine. We have now taken 25 cases off the diet. Most of those cases have not started the diet from infancy on. All patients have carefully been followed for two or three years. Most of those patients have not changed their intellectual behaviour when at the age of 8 or 10 years they were put on a diet somewhat restricted in protein, not a completely free diet. However, we had some very bad surprises. Three children lost about 15 I.Q. points on such a liberalized diet even at that age. So we had to put them on the diet again. I'm still uncertain and unable to give a final answer to your question. We follow-up these patients with EEG, psychometric measurements etc. As soon as we notice that they are going a little bit downhill we put them on the diet again. But this happened only a few times sofar. In Utrecht there is some experience with EEG registration when the patients are again on a normal diet.

Dr. van Sprang: We tried to take children off the diet under control of

EEG but sofar we have not enough registrations. It was very disappointing that a child, being treated from birth, on the age of 4 years had a very abnormal EEG after phenylalanine load.

Dr. de Groot: There is some discussion, Prof. Bickel, about the care for the heterozygotic mother. In cases of galactosaemia it is advised to treat the pregnant mother with a galactose-free diet. What is your opinion about that.

Prof. Bickel: Again this is an important point. When successfully treated female patients grow up they may become pregnant and than the trouble starts again. I'm only aware of some experience in phenylketonuria. It has been shown beyond doubt that nearly all children born to phenylketonuric mothers who are not treated during pregnancy, suffer brain damage and other malformations, e.g. of the heart. Those children are not phenylketonuric themselves, they are damaged by the milieu interieur during pregnancy. It is recommended to give those phenylketonuric mothers very early in pregnancy a phenylalanine restricted diet just as during their childhood. I know of two cases where this has been done and the children have been born normally. I'm not yet aware about experience in galactosaemia but I could well imagine that the foetus may also be damaged.

A galactosaemic child of a mother heterozygotic for galactosaemia has at birth in his umbilical blood an increased level of galactose-1-phosphate. There is some discussion if even not in this situation the child has already been slightly damaged in utero. If the pregnant mother herself is galactosaemic this might be a serious danger to the foetus. Though I have no personal experience nor knowledge of such cases in the literature, I would certainly recommend to give a galactose-free diet during such a pregnancy especially because it is not a difficult diet to give. You have just to avoid milk and galactose-containing products from the food.

Dr. Hommes: May I come back, Prof. Bickel, to the question of termination of the diet again. This is of course related to the mechanism responsible for the cerebral damage. Especially in phenylketonuria phenylpyruvic acid has been pin-pointed as a toxic agent, although many of the enzymes which are inhibited like hexokinase need a concentration of phenylpyruvic acid which is much higher, about

10 m molar, and this simply does not occur in vivo. Recently Land and Clark (Bioch. Journal 134, 539 and 545, 1973) have demonstrated that the dihydrolipoyl transacetylase, that is an enzyme of the pyruvic dehydrogenase complex converting pyruvate to acetyl-CoA, is inhibited by phenylpyruvic acid at a concentration of 0.1 m molar. This is a concentration, which you may expect in phenylketonuria. This interferes with the synthesis of acetyl-CoA and therefore with myelinisation and so on. If you stop treatment then you get again an increase in this phenylpyruvic acid and also inhibition of the brain pyruvic dehydrogenase complex. Most of the myelin has already been deposited in the structures. The turnover of myelin is low, but it is not completely zero. Therefore on theoretical grounds you should continue the treatment.

Prof. Bickel: Nobody knows what damages the brain of the phenylketonuric patient. There are other interesting theories, for instance that the phenylalanine itself may do harm to the brain. There has been the work of Davison in London, who has shown that even in very young rats you can reduce the incorporation of labeled sulfur into the myelin with phenylalanine blood levels which are in the range of a phenylketonuric patient and even lower. This is of course one of the most interesting pathogenetic experiments, that have been done during the last few years. There is a whole list of further pathogenetic suggestions but I think the one you mentioned is very interesting. In this connection it may be significant that brain damage only seems to set in when phenylalanine blood levels rise at levels above 10–12 mg/ 100 ml. Only at such phenylalanine levels does phenylpyruvic acid appear to be formed in measurable amounts.

There is one important point which I omitted before: I think we must distinguish between long-term damage due to demyelinisation and acute pharmacological toxic effects. The acute experiment has been performed very early in the first patient ever treated and has recently been repeated in America. If you give a patient with phenylketonuria an acute dosis of l-phenylalanine, e.g. the double daily intake, the child shows very soon toxic reactions, consisting in hypersalivation and extrapyramidal symptoms, atoxia and drowsiness. This acute pharmacological effect is disappearing completely if the patient is put on the diet again.

PARENTERAL NUTRITION

GENERAL ASPECTS OF PARENTERAL NUTRITION

A. WRETLIND*

A. INTRODUCTION

A prerequisite for life in man as well as all other living organisms is adequate nutrition. A daily supply of energy and nutrients is necessary to maintain a patient in an optimum state of nutrition and to offer the best resistance to illness and trauma, such as infections, burns, surgery, etc. If normal oral nutrition is difficult or impossible to maintain, essential nutrients may be provided by either tube feeding or the intravenous route. Intravenous feeding should be resorted to only when oral feeding and tube feeding are impossible.

Intravenous nutrition may be regarded as an alternative to oral feeding. From this point of view it is desirable that the same quantity and form of nutrients be supplied intravenously as are transferred normally to the blood from the intestine after adequate oral feeding. The amounts of energy and nutrients supplied should be adjusted to meet the basal requirements and also to compensate for increased losses and previous deficiencies.

It has cost considerable time and much hard work to acquire our present knowledge in the field of parenteral nutrition. This medical achievement is mainly the result of research completed during the most recent decades. In principle, the intravenous supply of the nutrients required does not cause any difficulties. In order to maintain or restore the normal composition of the body and to obtain normal growth in infants by intravenous nutrition, it seems to be sufficient to supply the nutrients or groups of nutrients given in table 1. However, there are still numerous problems to be studied in connection with intravenous nutrition. The future trends in this field will be to investigate these problems and to find the best methods for keeping patients in a good nutritional state when they cannot be fed enterally.

* Nutrition Unit, Karolinska Institutet, Stockholm, Sweden

Table 1. *Nutrients essential for complete intravenous nutrition.*

Fluid	Water
Sources for synthesis of body proteins and for energy	Amino acids Carbohydrates Fat
Minerals	Sodium Potassium Calcium Magnesium Iron Zinc Manganese Copper Chlorine Phosphorus Fluorine Iodine
Water-soluble vitamins	Thiamine Riboflavine Niacin Vitamin B_6 Folacin Vitamin B_{12} Pantothenic acid Biotin Ascorbic acid
Fat-soluble vitamins	Vitamin A Vitamin D Vitamin K_1 Tocopherol

Reviews on intravenous nutrition and the nutrients required under various conditions have been published by THORÉN (1), WILKINSON (2), REISSIGL (3), ALLEN and LEE (4) and WRETLIND (5), among others.

B. TREND TOWARDS COMPLETE INTRAVENOUS NUTRITION

Glucose and other carbohydrates have been used as energy sources for a long time. The infusion of blood and serum – initially intended to support blood circulation – was also found to be of some nutritional value to the patient, as the proteins in these fluids were broken down and the free amino acids could be used for specific protein synthesis. Fundamental progress was achieved in the thirties, when ELMAN (6) used amino acid mixtures in the form of enzymatic protein hydrolysates.

Amino acids and carbohydrates may be sufficient as energy sources for total parenteral nutrition. However to supply the necessary calories in a reasonable volume of fluid, hypertonic sugar solutions have to be used. The latter cause severe damage to peripheral veins and can therefore only be given via a central vein catheter, preferably in the superior vena cava. With fat emulsions as part of the energy source, it is easy to supply the required amount of energy. The advantage of fat emulsions is that a large amount of energy can be given in a small volume of isotonic fluid. They can be administered via a peripheral vein without causing thrombophlebitis.

If a patient is assumed to require nutrients intravenously for only a few days while he should not or cannot eat, then usually only water, some electrolytes, glucose and amino acids are given. This must be regarded as incomplete intravenous nutrition. Such an inadequate supply of nutrients over a period does not necessarily mean that signs of deficiences will occur. On the other hand, it seems more rational to always give complete intravenous nutrition. In this way, deficiency symptoms and nutritional complications will be avoided in those cases where the parenteral nutrition has to be maintained for a long period of time, whatever the reason.

When all nutrients absorbed from ordinary adequate oral food are given intravenously, this is termed *Complete Intravenous Feeding*. According to DUDRICK et al (7, 8) the energy requirement may be easily satisfied by glucose and amino acids with a concomitant supply of all other nutrients, but no fat ('*Hyperalimentation* according to DUDRICK'). Because of the hypertonic solutions used, such an intravenous alimentation can only be administered via a central vein catheter (figure 1). Complete intravenous nutrition, which includes fat, may be given via either a peripheral vein or a central vein catheter. The trend is toward complete intravenous nutrition.

Intravenous nutrition which supplies nutrients by the intravenous route only is called *Total Intravenous Nutrition*. In some cases the oral intake is insufficient; this indicates *Supplementary Intravenous Nutrition* with all, or some special, nutrients.

Total and supplementary intravenous nutrition should be ncluded in the regular hospital feeding programme to ensure that every patient receives an adequate daily amount of nutrients. In this way it

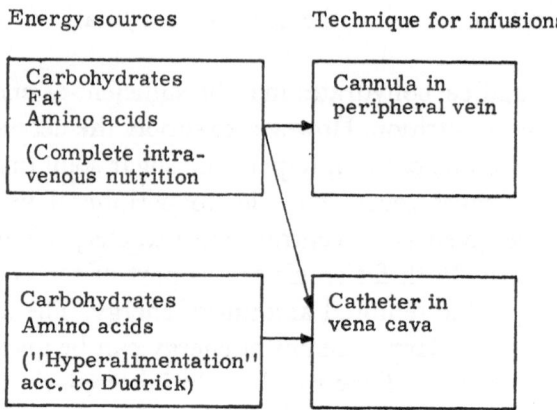

Fig. 1. Methods for intravenous nutrition with alternative mixtures of nutrients.

will be possible to maintain a patient in a good nutritional state when he *will not*, or *should not* or *cannot eat*, or *cannot eat enough*.

C. AMINO ACIDS

1. *Amino acid metabolism*

When food protein is given by mouth, amino acids are partly metabolized in the liver. ELWYN (9) found that in rats, after a meal rich in protein, 57 percent of the ingested amino acids were oxidized to urea, 23 percent passed into the general circulation, 6 percent were used for synthesis of plasma proteins and 14 percent were retained temporarily as liver protein. It must be pointed out that ELWYN's results refer to a *large* intake of protein.

An abundance of amino acids entering the liver causes an increase in the amount of catalyzing enzymes. HARPER (10) reports increased concentrations of threonine-serin dehydratase and glutamic acid-oxaloacetate aminotransferase. Tyrosine aminotransaminase is also stimulated, as shown by FISHMAN *et al* (11). An increased metabolic activity has also been shown by SOLIMAN and HARPER (12), who found a high concentration of $^{14}CO_2$ in the expired air after a meal containing amino acids labelled with ^{14}C. The diurnal variations in tyrosine-amino-transaminase reported by FISHMAN *et al* (11) and by WURTMAN (13) are certainly an expression of amino acid-induced activity. The enzyme induction seems to be a very fundamental biological reaction, which is well-known to microbiologists since it occurs readily in unicellular organisms. The complicated interaction of multiple transaminases in cells and mitochondria is quite well reviewed by MUNRO (14).

Amino acid metabolism in the liver is selective. Leucine, isoleucine and valine are not broken down, but pass into the general circulation to be metabolized mainly in muscles and kidneys (15). The liver seems to serve as a buffer to protect other organs from the effect of excessive concentrations of amino acids.

2. *Utilization of amino acids and nitrogen balance*

It has been shown that adequate intravenous protein nutrition can be maintained by amino acid mixtures which have the proper composition for optimum utilization. The nutritional value of the various amino acids is summarized in Table 2.

The protein-synthesizing system needs eighteen to twenty amino acids in order to produce the various proteins in the body. Eight of the

Table 2. *Nutritional value of amino acids in intravenous alimentation*

Isoleucine Leucine Lysine Methionine Phenylalanine Threonine Tryptophan Valine	Essential in all conditions
Arginine	Essential for optimum utilization of amino acid mixtures and for detoxification
Cysteine-cystine	Essential for the foetus and necessary for the maintenance of normal plasma level of cystine in adults.
Histidine	Essential for infants and in uraemia
Tyrosine	Essential for prematures
Alanine Glutamic acid Proline	Necessary for optimum utilization of amino acid mixtures
Aspartic acid Glycine Serine	Source of nonspecific nitrogen

amino acids cannot be synthesized by the adult body and are called essential amino acids (table 2).

The capacity of the body to synthesize arginine is limited. Thus arginine must be included in amino acid mixtures for intravenous nutrition in order to obtain optimum utilization of the other amino acids supplied. Moreover, arginine counteracts the toxic effects which are produced when glycine is used in larger amounts.

Cystine is, according to STURMAN et al (16), an essential amino acid for the foetus and immature human. This was indicated by the lack of cystathionase activity in the liver of the foetus and immature infant. In these cases, there was also an increased level of cystathionine in the liver. The results show that the synthesis of cystine or cysteine from methionine must be blocked. STEGINK and DEN BESTEN (17) administered amino acid solutions without cysteine to eight healthy men through catheters in the superior vena cava and through nasogastric tubes. When the solutions were given intravenously, the plasma cystine concentration dropped markedly. When feeding was switched to the enteral route, the concentration rose but returned to baseline when cystine was added to the diet. These studies indicate that the synthesis of cysteine from methionine is limited, even in the adult subject.

For infants histidine has also been found to be an essential amino acid (18). Investigations by BERGSTRÖM et al (19) have indicated that histidine also seems to be necessary for an optimum utilization of amino acid mixtures in patients with uraemia (19).

The phenylalanine hydroxylase system is not fully developed in prematures. This means that phenylalanine cannot be converted to tyrosine. An intravenous supply of an amino acid mixture with phenylalanine, but without tyrosine, results in a decrease in the tyrosine concentration in serum. Thus amino acid solutions used for intravenous nutrition of prematures and infants should contain tyrosine as well as phenylalanine (20).

JÜRGENS and DOLIF (21) and DOLIF and JÜRGENS (22) have shown that the utilization of intravenous amino acid preparations is greater if alanine, proline and glutamic acid are also included in the amino acid mixture. In connection with this, it may be of interest to consider that SCHLAPPNER et al (23) reported that the use of an amino acid mixture lacking cysteine, tyrosine and glutamic acid produced acute papulopustular acne in three male patients on intravenous nutrition for 2–4 weeks.

Hitherto there have been no investigations of the specific effects of aspartic acid, glycine and serine on the utilization of an intravenous amino acid mixture. They may however be used as a source of non-specific nitrogen (table 2).

The essential amino acid requirements have been investigated in various respects. Previously, research workers usually adopted the recommendations made by ROSE (24). According to ROSE the minimum daily requirements for the adult male are 0.7 g isoleucine, 1.1 g leucine, 0.8 g lysine, 1.1 g methionine, 1.1 g phenylalanine, 0.5 g threonine, 0.25 g tryptophan and 0.8 g valine. Tyrosine can replace up to 50 percent of the phenylalanine (25) and cystine or cysteine, up to 30 percent of the methionine (26). More recently a number of other studies have been carried out to determine the requirements at various ages and under various conditions. The results reported by ROSE (24) have been confirmed by INOUE et al (27) for young Japanese, and by HEGSTED (28) for young women. WATTS et al (29) and TUTTLE et al (30) found that elderly persons need about twice the amount of methionine and lysine required by younger individuals. MUNRO (31) summarized the results obtained by various investigators for the individual essential amino acid requirements.

An amino acid mixture for intravenous nutrition involves two components: the essential amino acids and the nonessential amino acids or nitrogen for synthesis of the former. The proportion of essential amino acids (E) to total nitrogen (T) is important from a nutritional point of view. This proportion, the *E: T ratio*, is usually expressed as grams of essential amino acids per gram of total nitrogen (32). The proteins of high nutritive value have an E:T ratio of about 3 and those of the lowest nutritive value, about 2 or less.

A reference pattern for the essential amino acids is given by the *FAO/WHO Expert Group* (32) in terms of the relationship between each essential amino acid (A) and the *total essential amino acids* (E), which is termed the A/E ratio. The *FAO/WHO Expert Group* concluded in 1965 that all new data justified adoption of the essential amino acid pattern of either *egg or human milk protein for reference* instead of other earlier patterns, including the provisional pattern suggested by the *FAO Committee on Protein Requirement* (33).

The optimum pattern for nonessential amino acids is not yet known. The amino acids appear to be interchangeable as nonspecific nitrogen sources. This could be expected from the rapidity of transamination reactions in the body. It seems therefore that within limits the body is indifferent to the composition of the nonessential nitrogen component but single amino acids may, if fed in excess, produce toxic effects. As nitrogen source for the synthesis of nonessential amino acids, nitrogen-containing substances, such as diammonium citrate, urea and biuret, have also been shown to be effective in oral feeding. However, the different nitrogen sources are not equally effective for synthesis of the nonessential amino acid part of body proteins. The most effective is a mixture of all the nonessential amino acids (34). This is followed, in order of decreasing effectiveness, by glutamic acid, alanine, aspartic acid, asparagine, proline, glutamine, glycine, serine and an excess of essential amino acids (35, 36, 37). The relatively low utilization of some amino acids in this respect depends partly on the fact that during the deamination of these amino acids, nitrogen is rapidly converted into urea, which is excreted by the urine, and cannot be readily utilized for the synthesis of amino acids by the body (38, 39).

The effect of amino acid solutions of various composition on nitrogen balance has been studied in both animals and man. In rats severe inanition has been caused by 'amino acid imbalance'. In man pronounced differences in utilization were observed for the different types of amino acid solution. The explanation may be that certain non-essential amino acids were missing in some of the solutions. The degree of utilization may also depend on variations in the ratio between the essential amino acids and the total amount of amino acids in the various solutions.

3. *Blood amino acid levels*

ZIMMERMAN and SCOTT (40) fed chickens with amino acid mixtures in which the amount of lysine was too low to produce growth of the birds. As the concentration of this 'limiting' amino acid in the food was increased, growth was proportional to the lysine content up to 0.8 percent. When more lysine was added no further increase in weight occurred, but the level of lysine in the serum then started to increase. In analogous experiments valine and arginine produced similar effects. YOUNG et al (41) investigated the effect of increasing amounts of tryptophan in young humans. They found that when more than 3 mg per kg body weight was added to the food, there was a sharp rise in the tryptophan content of the serum. More than 5 mg/kg caused an increase in the liver tryptophan pyrrolase activity, limiting the serum tryptophan to a constant level. These results are in good agreement with other investigations which show that about 3 mg tryptophan per kg body weight per day is optimal for man. Studies of serum amino acids have been used by YOUNG et al (41) to determine the requirement of amino acids.

The regulating power of the liver keeps the serum concentration of the amino acids at a constant level. If the level drops, amino acids from the liver are mobilized to meet the need. The amino acid concentration in serum is also regulated by hormones such as insulin, growth hormone and glucocorticoids (14).

4. Comparison of enteral and intravenous supply of amino acids

The alimentary tract and the liver may protect the organism against too high a concentration of amino acids from food. Consequently, it is most likely that the composition of amino acid solutions for parenteral use may differ from the aminogram of the dietary proteins. The discovery by MILLER (15) that branched amino acids pass through the liver with only a slight breakdown may indicate that they have to be enriched in parenteral solutions in comparison with the other five essential amino acids.

On the other hand, quite extensive experience has demonstrated the expected effects of parenteral nutrition in spite of the theoretical questions about the composition of the solutions. In a series of studies, PEASTON (42) observed the same positive nitrogen balance during intravenous and oral feeding with identical amino acid mixtures. JOHNSTON and SPIVEY (43) reported investigations which indicated that the intravenous route was as effective as the alimentary route in maintaining nitrogen balance. Investigations by FÜRST et al (44) of nitrogen balance also showed that the need for total nitrogen as well as essential amino acids is the same, whether they are given by mouth or intravenously. The most likely explanation of the evident success of parenteral nutrition seems to be that the infusion is given so slowly that the liver and other organs are able to metabolize the amino acids – and other nutrients – in approximately the normal way. Because the liver receives a substantial part of the total blood circulation, all the infused amino acids will very soon reach the liver. In this respect it may be of interest to mention that HALLBERG and SODA (45) have shown a

significant increase in the blood flow through the portal vein and
hepatic artery in dogs during constant infusion of an amino acid
mixture containing fructose into a peripheral vein (Vamin, table 3b).
No effects on the systemic blood pressure were observed. The possibility
of a specific effect of amino acids on hepatic circulation was indicated.

5. *Optimum amino acid composition and requirement*

The relationship between the various essential amino acids in commercially available amino acid mixtures for intravenous nutrition
(tables 3a and b) follows more or less the amino acid pattern found in
egg protein as well as the relationship between the essential amino acid
requirements found by Rose (24) in nitrogen balance investigations
in man.

Many investigations have shown a good utilization of amino acid
mixtures in the synthesis of body protein when the essential amino acid
requirement was met and the amino acid mixtures were well-balanced.
The best results in man have been obtained when the preparations
were complete and contained all essential and ten to twelve non-
essential amino acids (46, 47, 48). Studies on dogs also showed a better
utilization, and a more positive nitrogen balance, with a complete
crystalline amino acid mixture containing the essential and ten non-
essential amino acids, in comparison with incomplete mixtures containing essential amino acids, arginine, histidine and a high concentration of glycine.

In healthy adults it seems possible to maintain positive nitrogen
balance for a short period of time on an amino acid mixture with a
lower essential amino acid content (44, 18, 27). Here it is only a
question of covering the endogenous loss of essential amino acids. This
loss has been estimated to be 6.35 g per day (24) or about 80 mg per kg
body weight (28, 27). The nitrogen requirement for a healthy adult
may be 4–5 g, corresponding to 30–38 g amino acids per day. This implies that an essential amino acid content of about 20 percent might be
sufficient. In patients on intravenous nutrition it is usually desirable
to promote synthesis of body protein for growth in infants, and to
replace lost body protein. It would thus seem rational in intravenous
nutrition to always use amino acid mixtures with an essential amino
acid content corresponding to the content found in body proteins or
other proteins with high biological value. It is also important that the

Table 3a. *Amino acid content of egg protein and some commercial amino acid preparations. The amino acid values are given in grams per 16 g Total Nitrogen (T) of the protein or amino acid mixtures.*

L-AMINO ACIDS	Amount of amino acid in 16 gm total nitrogen				
	Egg protein	Aminosol[1]	Aminofusin L-Reihe[2]	Aminonorm[3]	Aminoplasmal L 5[3]
Isoleucine	6.6	6.5	3.3	2.6	5.1
Leucine	8.8	11.4	4.6	4.5	8.9
Lysine	6.4	10.1	4.2	7.2	5.6
Aromatic amino acids	10.0	7.5	4.6	4.7	6.4
Phenylalanine	5.8	6.4	4.6	4.2	5.1
Tyrosine	4.2	1.1	—	0.3	1.3
Sulphur-containing amino acids	5.5	5.5	4.4	4.5	4.3
Methionine	3.1	3.7	4.4	4.4	3.8
Cysteine-cystine	2.4	1.8	—	0.1	0.5
Threonine	5.1	5.0	2.1	4.1	4.1
Tryptophan	1.6	1.3	1.0	2.4	1.8
Valine	7.3	8.7	3.2	5.9	4.8
E = total amount of Essential Amino Acids per 16 gN	51.3	56.0	27.4	35.8	41.0
Alanine	7.4	4.1	12.6	9.4	13.7
Arginine	6.1	4.3	8.4	5.0	9.2
Asparagine	–	–	–	2.6	3.3
Aspartic acid	9.0	8.6	–	0.8	1.3
Glutamic acid	16.0	27.6	19.0	4.3	4.6
Glutamine	–	–	–	19.6	–
Glycine	3.6	2.4	21.1	4.9	7.9
Histidine	2.4	3.2	2.1	4.4	5.2
Ornithine	–	–	–	2.4	3.2
Proline	8.1	13.4	14.7	5.2	8.9
Serine	8.5	5.6	–	2.0	2.4
E/T ratio	3.2	3.5	1.7	2.24	2.6
E in per cent of total amino acids	46	45	26	37	41

1. VITRUM, Stockholm, Sweden   2. J. PFRIMMER, Erlangen, Germany   3. B. BRAUN, Melsungen, Germany

Table 3b. *Amino acid content of some commercial amino acid preparations. The amino values are given in grams per 16 g Total Nitrogen (T) of the protein or amino acid mixtures.*

L-AMINO ACIDS	FreAmine[1]	Intramin[2]	Intramin novum[2]	Trophysan[3]	Sohamin[4]	Vamin[5]
			Amount of amino acid in 16 gm total nitrogen			
Isoleucine	7.6	2.5	4.0	1.6	8.1	6.6
Leucine	9.9	4.0	6.2	2.6	12.2	9.0
Lysine	7.9	2.9	4.5	5.8	18.7	6.6
Aromatic amino acids	6.1	4.0	6.2	2.2	11.7	10.2
Phenylalanine	6.0	4.0	6.2	2.2	–	9.4
Tyrosine	–	–	–	–		0.8
Sulphur-containing amino acids	6.0	4.0	6.2	2.6	8.3	5.6
Methionine	5.8	4.0	6.2	2.6	–	3.2
Cysteine-cystine	0.2	–	–	–		2.4
Threonine	4.4	1.8	2.8	1.6	8.6	5.1
Tryptophan	1.7	0.9	1.4	1.0	3.7	1.7
Valine	7.2	2.9	4.5	2.2	7.8	7.3
E = total amount of Essential Amino Acids per 16 gN	50.8	23.0	35.8	19.6	79.1	52.1
Alanine	7.7	–	–	–	–	5.1
Arginine	4.0	4.0	6.2	1.8	11.0	5.6
Asparagine	–	–	–	–	–	–
Aspartic acid	–	–	–	–	–	7.0
Glutamic acid	–	–	–	–	–	15.3
Glutamine	–	–	–	–	–	–
Glycine	23.0	61.7	48.1	59.8	7.3	3.6
Histidine	3.1	2.0	3.1	–	4.2	4.1
Ornithine	–	–	–	–	–	–
Proline	12.2	–	–	–	–	13.8
Serine	6.4	–	–	–	–	12.8
E/T ratio	3.2	1.44	2.2	1.23	4.9	3.2
E in percent of total amino acids	47	25	38	24	78	44

1. McGaw Laboratories, Glendale, Calif., USA   2. Astra, Södertälje, Sweden   3. Egic, Montargis, France
4. Tanabe, Seiiaku Co., Osaka, Japan   5. Vitrum, Stockholm, Sweden

preparations contain tyrosine and cystine or cysteine. Only Aminosol, Aminonorm, Aminoplasmal and Vamin contain tyrosine (tables 3a and b). The concentration of cystine/cysteine in Aminonorm, Aminoplasmal, Aminosol, FreAmine and Vamin is shown in Tables 3a and b. The other amino acid products do not contain tyrosine and cystine/cysteine.

The results from various studies on the utilization of amino acid mixtures indicate that an optimum amino acid preparation for intravenous nutrition should contain both the essential and the nonessential amino acids in the L-configuration, and in the same proportions as found on the aminogram of body proteins or other proteins of high biological value (5). The essential amino acids should amount to about 45–50 percent of the total amino acids. A high glycine content should be avoided as it has been shown to produce ammonia intoxication.

The amino acid requirements can be calculated from known nitrogen losses and also from investigations of the nitrogen balance in patients. Considering the results and calculations from various investigations, a daily basal amino acid allowance of not less than 95 mg N or 0.7 g amino acids/kg is recommended for adults or 6–6.5 g N or 50 g amino acids for individuals weighing 70 kg (5). This quantity exceeds somewhat the protein supplied (calculated as protein with an NPU value of 70–80) by the average Swedish diet with an energy supply of 1,500–2,000 kcal/day.

About 330 mg nitrogen or 2.5 g amino acid mixture/kg/day is recommended for neonates and infants on total intravenous nutrition (5).

6. *Nutritional effects of amino acids supplied intravenously*

The utilization by the body of amino acid mixtures supplied intravenously has been confirmed by the effect on nitrogen balance and body weight.

The nitrogen balance technique has been used to show that the amino acids are utilized. It has also been used to determine the biological value of an amino acid mixture (49). In several investigations it has been shown that it is possible to maintain a positive nitrogen balance and weight increase for several months in adults. For infants on intravenous nutrition a positive nitrogen balance with body growth has been reported (50, 51, 52, 8, 53, 54). In one case, BERGSTRÖM et al

(55) reported that the average daily nitrogen balance was positive during total intravenous nutrition lasting 7 months and 13 days. DUDRICK *et al* (8) obtained positive nitrogen balance in adults on total intravenous nutrition for 7 to 210 days. Many other investigators have also obtained a positive nitrogen balance in adults (56, 57, 20, 42).

Many studies have shown that postoperatively complete intravenous nutrition with amino acid mixtures reduces nitrogen loss (50, 59, 60).

The amino acids and energy-supplying nutrients must be given simultaneously in order to obtain an optimum nutritional effect. The general tendency is, and will continue to be, to meet the energy requirement with the infusion of a carbohydrate solution and fat emulsions. A minimum of 100 g per day, or 20 energy percent carbohydrates, should always be supplied in order to avoid undesirable metabolic effects. An exogenous supply of energy in the form of carbohydrates or fat also produces a greater reduction in protein breakdown in a patient than in a healthy person.

The optimum utilization of an amino acid mixture occurs when the ratio of kilocalories to gram nitrogen in the amino acids is between 150:1, as recommended by MOORE (61) and applied by LAWSON (62), and 200:1 as used by JOHNSTON *et al* (63). In order to have the best possible utilization of amino acids, it is important to ensure an adequate supply of all other nutrients. Physical activity will favour anabolism, and will increase the retention of amino acids and the synthesis of body proteins (64). Anabolic steroids may stimulate the synthesis of body proteins and reduce the nitrogen loss provided adequate amounts of proteins and energy are supplied (65).

The factors required to ensure the best possible utilization of the proteins or amino acids given are summarized in table 4. Continuous application of these factors – day by day – also makes it possible to

Table 4. *Factors for obtaining optimum nutritional effects of intravenous alimentation*

1. Adequate amounts of amino acids; for adults: minimum 0.7 g/kg/day for infants: 2.5 g/kg/day
2. Adequate energy supply
3. At least 20 cal. percent carbohydrates
4. Simultaneous supply of amino acids and energy
5. Adequate supply of other nutrients
6. Mobilization; physical activity

maintain or replace the labile body protein, which is the best indication that the patient is in a good nutritional state.

D. CARBOHYDRATES

A minimal requirement for carbohydrates is difficult to define. For individuals living on an ordinary average diet, 100 g carbohydrates/day or 20 cal percent seems to be enough to avoid ketosis, increased protein catabolism and other undesirable metabolic effects (66, 67, 41). The human brain needs 100–150 g glucose per day which has to be added to avoid uneconomical 'gluconeogenesis' from amino acids. Of the carbohydrates, glucose and fructose are used for intravenous feeding. In order to follow normal oral nutrition, up to 100 g fructose might be given daily to an adult. In addition to this, glucose should be supplied in the amounts required to fulfill the need for carbohydrates.

There is a tendency to regard glucose as the chosen carbohydrate for intravenous nutrition of patients who are not in a stress situation. Future investigations will show whether there is a good glucose substitute which is metabolized independently of insulin. Such a substitute might be fructose, which is more rapidly metabolized than glucose. The rapid disappearance of fructose from the blood stream depends on a quick distribution in the total body fluid (68), the transformation of fructose into glucose and rapid conversion into glycogen. A manifestation of the rapid turnover of fructose is an increase in the concentrations of pyruvic and lactic acid. It has been stated that the loss of fructose in the urine is smaller than that of glucose. The tolerance for fructose, locally in the infused veins, is higher than that for the same concentration of glucose (69, 70). The uptake in the liver and in adipose tissue is independent of insulin. That fraction of fructose which is converted into glucose requires however for its further metabolism the presence of insulin (71). The rapid metabolism of fructose produces an increase in the lactic acid level in the liver (72). It has also been shown that infusions of fructose (20 percent solution) in a dosage of 0.5–3.5 g/kg/hour to healthy individuals and diabetics produce an increase of 0.9–8 mEq blood lactate/l(73). These investigations thus show that rapid infusions of fructose produce a lactic acid acidosis. In a dehydrated child with metabolic acidosis, a 20 percent fructose solution was infused at the

15

rate of 3 g fructose/kg/hour for 7 hours (74). The child died and it was assumed that death was caused by an acidosis during the fructose infusion. In another dehydrated child with acidosis, similar large and rapid fructose infusions produced a severe reaction with increased acidosis (74). In part the explanation for the reaction might also be the infusion of hypertonic fructose solutions. The results indicate however that rapid and large infusions of concentrated fructose are contraindicated in cases of dehydration and acidosis. Fructose infusions at a rate of less than 0.5 g/kg/hour seem to cause only small or insignificant changes in the lactate concentration in the blood.

The sugar alcohols, sorbitol and xylitol, have been used instead of carbohydrates in intravenous nutrition. There does not seem to be any convincing advantage from a nutritional point of view in using these substitutes for carbohydrate.

E. FAT IN THE INTRAVENOUS FEEDING PROGRAMME

1. *Intravenous fat emulsions*

Intravenous fat emulsions – in combination with not less than 20 cal percent carbohydrate – can easily supply the required amount of energy. The advantage of fat emulsions is that a large amount of energy can be given in a small volume of isotonic fluid. Because of their isotonicity, fat emulsions may be administered via the peripheral veins in contrast with the concentrated glucose solutions which have to be given through catheters in a central vein. Thrombophlebitis occurs seldom with an isotonic fat emulsion. The infusions do not cause diuresis and furthermore no losses are observed either in the urine or faeces. Fat emulsions also supply the body with essential fatty acids (75) and triglycerides, which are part of ordinary food. In this way the normal lipid composition of the body may be maintained.

The four commercial fat emulsions now available are *Intralipid, Lipiphysan, Lipofundin* and *Lipofundin S* (table 5). The most widely used fat emulsion is Intralipid.

SCHOEFL (76) as well as FRASER and HÅKANSSON (77) has carried out a series of electron microscopic studies of chylomicrons and Intralipid. These studies and other investigations have shown very pronounced physical and chemical similarities between natural chylomicrons and the fat particles in the egg yolk phospholipid-soybean oil emulsion, Intralipid.

Table 5. *Composition of commercial fat emulsions.*

	Intralipid[1]	Lipiphysan[2]	Lipofundin[3]	Lipofundin S[3]
Soybean oil	100 or 200 g			100 or 200 g
Cottonseed oil		10 g	100 g	
Egg yolk phospholipids	12 g			
Soybean lecithine		20 g		
Soybean phospholipids			7.5 g	7.5 or 15 g
Glycerol	25 g			
Sorbitol		50 g	50 g	
Xylitol				50 g
DL-α-tocopherol	4 g	0.5 g	0.585 g	
Distilled water to a volume of	1000 ml	1000 ml	1000 ml	1000 ml

1. Vitrum, Box 12 170, 102 24 Stockholm 12, Sweden
2. Egic, Loiret, France
3. Braun, Melsungen, Germany
4. 100 mg tocopherol are supplied by the soybean oil. About 25 percent of this amount is biologically active as vitamin E.

Many investigations have demonstrated that fat emulsions are utilized in more or less the same way as fat from ordinary food. Great biological differences have been found to exist between the various fat emulsions. Some of these have been summarized by WRETLIND (5).

2. *Tolerance and physiological effects of fat emulsions*

The *chronic toxicity* of fat emulsions in dogs has been studied in many laboratories. The egg yolk phospholipid-soybean oil emulsion Intralipid seems to be the least toxic. In some long-term tolerance tests of intravenous fat emulsions, the planned infusion period was 4 weeks (78). The daily infusions were given over a period of about 4 hours at a rate of 9 g fat/kg/day, which represents the total energy requirement of the dog (about 80 kcal/kg/day). All 28 dogs who received the egg yolk phospholipid-soybean oil emulsion (Intralipid) survived the 4-week experimental period, and were in good condition and showed no abnormal reactions throughout. All the other emulsions tested caused severe toxic reactions in the dogs, all of whom died before the end of the test period.

The effect of induced serum lipoprotein lipase on different fat emulsions has been investigated by BOBERG and CARLSON (99). They found that the artificial fat emulsion Intralipid and chylomicrons had very similar effects, whereas other substrates or fat emulsions had quite different properties in this respect.

After an infusion of fat emulsion, temporary hyperlipaemia invariably occurs. The kinetic principles of elimination from the blood stream are similar for both chylomicrons and the fat emulsion Intralipid in dog and man (80, 81). This principle is as follows: At high concentrations of the infused lipids in the blood stream, the elimination process is maximal and proceeds at a constant rate down to a so called 'critical concentration'. Below this 'critical concentration', the rate of elimination is dependent on the concentration and is therefore a fractional removal rate.

From studies in man on the rate of elimination of infused Intralipid from the blood, HALLBERG (80, 81) found in control adult subjects fasting overnight that 3.8 g fat per kg body weight per 24 hours was eliminated. This amount corresponds to 35 kcal/kg/24 hours. After fasting for 38 hours the elimination capacity increased to 52 kcal/kg/24 hours. In the postoperative period, after fasting for about two days, the elimination capacity was equivalent to 100 kcal per kg per 24 hours. WILMORE et al (82) showed that fat clearance curves also demonstrated an accelerated disappearance of the emulsion (Intralipid) from plasma in acutely burned patients.

SCHOLLER (83) found that the fat from some fat emulsions is accumulated in the reticuloendothelial cells. After a single infusion of Intralipid no accumulation of the fat particles in the Kupffer cells was observed (84, 83). Moreover, no significant reduction in the formation of antibodies was found in guinea pigs after administration of Intralipid.

Thrombophlebitis is very seldom observed when the infusions of fat emulsions are administered via a peripheral vein. This is in good agreement with the findings of DUCKERT and HARTMANN (85) and CRONBERG and NILSSON (86), who showed that infusion of Intralipid has no effect on either the coagulation or the fibrinolytic system.

The pulmonary diffusion capacity determined by the [133]Xenon perfusion-diffusion and the carbon monoxide rebreathing techniques was found to be normal after the infusion of Intralipid (82). Blood gas levels did not change following infusion of single or multiple units of the fat emulsion.

Because of the pronounced differences in tolerance and toxicity between the various fat emulsions it is incorrect to speak of fat emulsions for intravenous nutrition in general terms. The name of the product and its composition should always be stated.

A pigment – 'intravenous fat pigment' – is found in the liver and spleen of both man and animals after long-term fat infusions. Numerous liver function tests were performed in an attempt to assess the potential hazards which might be associated with large doses of emulsion (87). It was not possible to demonstrate that large doses of emulsion produced any impairment of liver function, either during the course of infusion or subsequently.

3. *Fat emulsions as a supply of energy*

Using the soybean oil – egg yolk phospholipid emulsion, Intralipid, PEASTON (88, 42) and STELL (89) gave 200 g fat (about 3 g/kg) per day which was equivalent to 60–80 percent of the total energy supply. BERGSTRÖM *et al* (55) supplied about 40 percent of the energy in the form of fat, equivalent to about 2 g fat/kg. Fat emulsion was administered, along with other caloric support, by WILMORE *et al* (82) to 10 critically injured individuals. The fat appeared to be utilized without complication, and the fat emulsion contributed 38 percent of the total caloric intake in this group of patients.

In view of the experience gained with the intravenous supply of fat, a quantity of 2 g fat/kg is recommended to fulfil the requirements of energy and fat in adults. This quantity has been recommended previously by HALLBERG *et al* (90), STEINBEREITHNER (91), LEE (92) and others.

To neonates and infants on intravenous nutrition, RICKHAM (93) gave 2.5–3 g fat/kg body weight/day in the form of Intralipid. BØRRESEN and KNUTRUD (50), BØRRESEN *et al* (94, 95) as well as GROTTE (54) have given 3–4 g fat (Intralipid)/kg/day to neonates and infants with good results. On the basis of these investigations, an amount of up to 4 g fat, for instance Intralipid, per kg per day may be recommended for neonates and infants.

Fat will be a part of the intravenous supply of energy in the future. The fat to be preferred seems to be the soybean oil – egg yolk phospholipid emulsion.

4. *Fat emulsions as a supply of essential fatty acids*

A certain quantity of fat is necessary to provide the body with the required amount of essential fatty acids. COLLINS *et al* (75) observed linoleic acid deficiency, in the form of dermatitis, in an adult on total parenteral feeding for more than three months. With intravenous infusions of Intralipid, the symptoms of insufficiency disappeared. The authors found 0.1 g linoleic acid/kg/day to be the required dose. This quantity can be obtained from 15 g soybean oil, which is the main constituent of the fat emulsion Intralipid. This fact also indicates that the future trend in intravenous feeding for adults will be the use of a fat emulsion.

Many other investigators have observed symptoms of linoleic acid deficiency in children on intravenous feeding without fat. Infants should have a supply of linoleic acid corresponding to 3–4 percent of the total energy intake. This amounts to about 0.4 g linoleic acid/kg body weight/day.

F. RATIO BETWEEN AMINO ACIDS, CARBOHYDRATES AND FAT

It is important, from a nutritional point of view, to balance the diet – oral or parenteral – correctly. The ratio between protein, carbohydrates and fat in the ordinary diet varies. The ordinary diet in Sweden and in most other developed countries contains about 10–13 energy percent protein, about 50 energy percent carbohydrates and about 40 energy percent fat.

The biological value of protein in the normal diet is about 70 percent when whole hen's egg is used as the standard and is defined as 100 percent. Furthermore some loss occurs due to inadequate absorption. An intravenous amino acid preparation with a correct composition has a biological value of more than 90. In view of this and the nitrogen content of protein and amino acids, respectively, the weight ratio between an intravenous amino acid mixture, carbohydrates and fat should be 1:5:1.8, if one wishes to simulate the conditions of an ordinary diet. The trend seems to be to keep the balance between the energy sources in intravenous nutrition about the same as in the normal oral diet. This trend will undoubtedly continue.

To achieve an adequate energy supply of not less than 30 kcal/kg, or 0.13 MJ/kg, about 2 g carbohydrates in the form of carbohydrates with a simultaneous supply of 2 g fat and 0.7 g amino acids per kg body weight per day are the quantities that have been recommended for intravenous nutrition for adults by various authors (90, 92, 91, 5).

Neonates and infants on complete intravenous nutrition should receive 90–120 kcal/kg, or 0.38–0.50 MJ/kg, in the form of 2.5 g amino acids (330 mg nitrogen), 12–18 g carbohydrates (glucose and fructose) and up to 4 g fat (Intralipid) per kg per day (5).

G. PARENTERAL SUPPLY OF VITAMINS

As mentioned previously, there are good reasons for including all of the necessary nutrients in an intravenous feeding programme (table 6).

Table 6. *Tentatively recommended daily allowances of energy and nutrients for patients on complete intravenous nutrition. The allowances cover resting metabolism, moderate physical activity of a patient and specific dynamic action, but not the increase in need caused by trauma, burns, etc.*

	ADULT Allowance per kg body weight per day	NEONATE and INFANTS Allowance per kg body weight per day
Water	30 ml	120–150 ml
Energy	30 kcal = 0.13 MJ	90–120 kcal = 0.38–0.50 MJ
Amino acid nitrogen	90 mg (0.7 g amino acids)	330 mg (2.5 g amino acids)
Glucose or fructose	2 g	12–18 g
Fat	2 g	4 g
Sodium	1–1.4 mmol	1–2.5 mmol
Potassium	0.7–0.9 mmol	2 mmol
Calcium	0.11 mmol	0.5–1 mmol
Magnesium	0.04 mmol	0.15 mmol
Iron	1 μmol	2 μmol
Manganese	0.6 μmol	1 μmol
Zinc	0.3 μmol	0.6 μmol
Copper	0.07 μmol	0.3 μmol
Chlorine	1.3–1.9 mmol	1.8–4.3 mmol
Phosphorus	0.15 mmol	0.4–0.8 mmol
Fluorine	0.7 μmol	3 μmol
Iodine	0.015 μmol	0.04 μmol
Thiamine	0.02 mg	0.05 mg
Riboflavin	0.03 mg	0.1 mg
Nicotinamide	0.2 mg	1 mg
Pyridoxine	0.03 mg	0.1 mg
Folic acid	3 μg	20 μg
Cyanocobalamin	0.03 μg	0.2 μg
Pantothenic acid	0.2 mg	1 mg
Biotin	5 μg	30 μg
Ascorbic acid	0.5 mg	3 mg
Retinol	10 μg	0.1 mg
Ergocalciferol or cholecalciferol	0.04 μg	2.5 μg
Phytylmenaquinone	2 μg	50 μg
α-Tocopherol	1.5 mg	3 mg

All of the vitamins are important in both oral and parenteral feeding.

There is a special reason for considering the need for vitamin K in parenteral nutrition. Vitamin K is formed in healthy adults by certain bacteria in the intestine, probably in sufficient quantity to meet the requirements. In a patient treated with antibiotics and on intravenous nutrition without vitamin K, signs of vitamin K deficiency were observed within 9 days (96). This is one example that antibiotics may cause a change in the intestinal flora and a decreased intestinal vitamin K production, causing vitamin K deficiency with severe or fatal bleeding. Consequently vitamin K_1, as well as other vitamins, should always be given daily to every patient on intravenous alimentation.

H. ELECTROLYTES IN INTRAVENOUS NUTRITION

As early as 1832, LATTA (97) reported on the infusion of salts in patients with cholera. Since that time, infusions containing sodium, potassium, magnesium, calcium and chloride solutions have been used and investigated in connection with intravenous feeding. It is obvious that the other essential minerals or electrolytes must also be included in complete intravenous nutrition. Of these minerals, phosphorus and zinc are of special interest for patients on intravenous nutrition.

Phosphorus has long been known to be one of the main constituents of bone tissue. In the twenties the discovery of phosphorylation in sugar metabolism, followed by that of adenosinetriphosphate (ATP), placed phosphorus in the centre of energy metabolism. A decade ago, cyclic adenosine monophosphate was shown to be a transmitter of hormonal effects in the cells. Finally it has been found that 2, 3-diphosphoglycerate is important for the affinity of haemoglobin for oxygen. Within seven to ten days on total intravenous nutrition with solutions lacking phosphate, adult patients were found to be significantly hypophosphataemic (98). The reduced amount of 2, 3-diphosphoglycerate and adenosine triphosphate in the erythrocytes was accompanied by an increase in the affinity of the red cells for oxygen, causing a reduced oxygen tension in the cells of the body tissues. In the future, phosphates should be included in the solutions for intravenous nutrition.

Zinc is present in several enzymes, such as carbonic anhydrase, carboxypeptidases, lactic acid dehydrogenase and other dehydrogenases. A zinc deficiency causes anaemia, splenomegaly, a small body, hypogonadism and geophagy. The quantity of zinc included in the daily diet is about 200 μmol or 10–15 mg, which is considered sufficient to prevent symptoms of zinc deficiency. Several groups of scientists have claimed that zinc intake accelerates the rate of wound healing. Tissue repairs make substantial demands on the body reserves of zinc (99, 100, 101, 102, 103, 104).

I. NUTRIENT REQUIREMENTS FOR PATIENTS ON INTRAVENOUS NUTRITION

Table 6 summarizes the tentative recommendations for the amounts of energy and nutrients to be supplied to patients during complete parenteral nutrition (5). The recommended intravenous supply is in agreement with the recommendations for ordinary food, when the biological values of normal food protein are taken into account as well as the inadequate absorption of some nutrients such as calcium, magnesium, iron, zinc, manganese, copper and phosphorus.

A practical guide for the preparation of infusion solutions, as used in Stockholm, is given in table 7. The amounts of energy and nutrients supplied in this way are listed in table 8.

Table 7. *Examples of infusion solutions and supplements for an adult on complete intravenous nutrition.*

Solution 1	
a. *Solution of crystalline amino acids (7%) and carbohydrates (10%) (Vamin[1])* Supplemented with	1000 ml
b. *Electrolyte solution*	10 ml
containing 5 mmol Ca, 1.5 mmol Mg, 50 μmol Fe, 20 μmol Zn, 40 μmol Mn, 5 μmol Cu, 50 μmol F, 1 μmol J and 13.3 mmol Cl^-	
Solution 2	
a. *Fat emulsion* (20%) (Intralipid 20%[2]) supplemented with	500 ml
b. *Emulsion of Fat-Soluble Vitamins*	10 ml
containing 0.75 mg retinol, 3 μg calciferol and 0.15 mg vitamin K_1	
Solution 3	
a. *10% Glucose solution* for intravenous infusion supplemented with	1000 ml
b. *Solution of Lyophilized Water-Soluble Vitamin Mixture*	10 ml
containing 1.2 mg thiamine, 1.8 mg riboflavine, 10 mg nicotinamide, 2 mg pyridoxine, 0.2 mg folic acid, 2 μg vitamin B_{12}, 10 mg pantothenic acid, 0.3 mg biotin and 30 mg ascorbic acid as well as	
c. Potassium phosphate solution	15 ml
containing 30 mmol K, 4 mmol P and 12 mmol lactate	

1. Table 3 b
2. Table 5

Table 8. *Complete intravenous nutrition for an adult using the solutions given in table 7.*

Energy and nutrients	Amount per day							
	Solution 1 in Table 7 1010 ml		Solution 2 in Table 7 510 ml		Solution 3 in Table 7 1025 ml		Total	
Water	0.94	l	0.38	l	0.98	l	2.3	l
Energy	650	kcal	1000	kcal	410	kcal	2.060	kcal
Amino acids	70	g	—		—		70	g
Glucose or fructose	100	g	12.5	g[1]	100	g	213	g
Fat	—		106	g[2]	—		106	g
Sodium	50	mmol	—		—		50	mmol
Potassium	20	mmol	—		30	mmol	50	mmol
Calcium	7.5	mmol	—		—		7.5	mmol
Magnesium	3.0	mmol	—		—		3.0	mmol
Iron	50	μmol	—		—		50	μmol
Zinc	20	μmol	—		—		20	μmol
Manganese	40	μmol	—		—		40	μmol
Copper	5	μmol	—		—		5	μmol
Chlorine	68.3	mmol	—		—		68.3	mmol
Phosphorus	—		7.5	mmol	6	mmol	13.5	mmol
Fluorine	50	μmol	—		—		50	μmol
Iodine	1	μmol	—		—		1	μmol
Thiamine	—		—		1.2	mg	1.2	mg
Riboflavine	—		—		1.8	mg	1.8	mg
Niacin	—		—		10	mg	10	mg
Vitamin B_6	—		—		2	mg	2	mg
Folic acid	—		—		0.2	mg	0.2	mg
Vitamin B_{12}	—		—		2	μg	2	μg
Pantothenic acid	—		—		10	mg	10	mg
Biotin	—		—		0.3	mg	0.3	mg
Ascorbic acid	—		—		30	mg	30	mg
Vitamin A	—		0.75	mg	—		0.75	mg
Vitamin D	—		3	μg	—		3	μg
Vitamin K_1	—		0.15	mg	—		0.15	mg
Tocopherol	—		100	mg	—		100	mg

1. Glycerol
2. 6 gm phospholipids

When the quantities of nutrients indicated in table 6 are supplied and the energy intake is adjusted to maintain weight in adults and growth in infants, the nutritive requirements of the patient should be completely satisfied.

In many clinical conditions there is an increased need for nutrients. After prolonged starvation, extra nutrients have to be added to replenish the patient and to increase the body weight. Infection, trauma, surgery and especially burns demand a considerable increase in all nutrients of up to 200–300 percent of the basal or normal requirement. The amounts of energy and nutrients required under these conditions will be further investigated in the future. This will be one of the most important activities of the scientists in the field of intravenous nutrition.

J. COMPLETE INTRAVENOUS NUTRITION

A large number of investigations have shown that it is possible to supply all essential nutrients in adequate amounts intravenously.

Studies of complete intravenous alimentation in dogs by means of the available fat emulsion have been successfully carried out in our Nutrition Unit during experimental periods lasting up to 12 weeks. In order to reduce the volume of the infusions, as much as 87 percent of the energy requirement was given as fat. One dog was maintained on complete or total intravenous nutrition, with 40 percent of the total energy supplied by fat (Intralipid[R]), during the whole period of gestation. After 61 days on complete or total intravenous nutrition, the dog gave birth to six puppies without anatomical abnormalities. This study indicated that complete intravenous nutrition with fat emulsions does not produce any teratogenic effects. It also demonstrates that our knowledge of the nutrients required for satisfactory nutrition during the gestation period and rapid fetal growth is fairly reliable (5).

That long-term complete intravenous nutrition can be achieved in man, by using a fat emulsion as part of the energy supply, has been illustrated in a large number of cases. In one case reported by JACOBSON and WRETLIND (47), and subsequently by BERGSTRÖM et al (55), complete intravenous nutrition was maintained for 7 months and 13 days. JACOBSON (105) has successfully used complete intravenous nutrition in a 70-year-old male patient after a massive resection of the small intestine and the ascending colon for 69 days after the operation. HALLBERG et al (59) reported complete intravenous nutrition for more than 5 months in a patient suffering from Crohn's disease.

Investigations which indicated that the intravenous route was as effective as the alimentary route in maintaining nitrogen balance have been published by JOHNSTON and SPIVEY (43).

The above-mentioned investigations as well as a large number of other investigations in adult patients, which were reviewed by WRET-

LIND (5), have demonstrated that complete intravenous nutrition which includes fat emulsions enables patients to maintain, or obtain, a good nutritional state.

Complete intravenous nutrition in neonates and infants has been studied in detail by BØRRESEN and KNUTRUD (50), BØRRESEN et al (94, 95) and GROTTE (54). These authors have also recommended complete intravenous nutrition via a peripheral vein. By using 3–4 gm fat/kg body weight, it was possible to reduce the hypertonicity of the carbohydrate solution.

K. DEVELOPMENT OF INFUSION TECHNIQUE

The infusion technique varies widely. The tendency in parenteral nutrition will be to find an easy and convenient way to give intravenous infusions without severe or serious complications.

In short-term intravenous feedings which include a fat emulsion, a cannula can be inserted in a peripheral vein. When peripheral vein infusions are performed there are several rules to be followed. The cannula should not be left in the vein for more than 8–12 hours. HALLBERG et al (59) have reported a comprehensive investigation of 2,781 infusions of fat emulsions in man. The very low incidence (1 case) of thrombophlebitis is impressive.

For long-term intravenous infusions a central vein catheter is used. This method is also necessary when the energy is supplied by glucose without fat. The elaborate techniques for this type of intravenous nutrition were developed by DUDRICK et al (7, 8). A large number of complications associated with central vein catheters have been reported (106, 107, 108, 109). Among these are thrombosis, embolism and infections. A summary of the potential complications with this technique has been given by DUDRICK and RUBERG (110).

SOLASSOL et al (111) and JOYEUX (112) have given infusions via a catheter implanted in the vena subclavia or vena epigastrica for long periods without any recorded complications.

The infusions have also been given via an arteriovenous shunt (113), or by a cannula in a subcutaneous arteriovenous fistula (114, 115). WIRBATZ et al (116) have used the vena umbilicalis for intravenous infusion; the same approach has been applied by FROHM (117) for neonates.

L. INTRAVENOUS NUTRITION AND FUTURE BALANCE STUDIES

Parenteral nutrition is being used with increasing frequency in exact metabolic studies. The supply of nutrients may be determined exactly. There will be no complications due to variations in absorption, which always occur when nutrients are given orally or by tube. The endogenous loss via faeces can easily be determined. In a number of investigations, the balances of nitrogen and minerals have been determined. In this way it will be possible to learn more about the essentiality of trace elements. Studies of the requirements of energy and nutrients for various ages and conditions may also be carried out.

SUMMARY

The trend in the development of intravenous nutrition is to supply all nutrients in the proportions known to exist when they enter the general circulation after well-balanced oral food intake.

With our present knowledge of intravenous nutrition it is possible to eliminate, or greatly reduce, the incidence of malnutrition as a complication of various medical and surgical conditions in modern hospitals. This is and will be a result of the tendency to include supplementary and total intravenous nutrition in the feeding programme of the hospital to ensure that patients in any condition receive an adequate daily amount of nutrients.

Various mixtures of amino acids have been used in complete intravenous nutrition. All studies in this field indicate a trend toward those amino acids mixtures which contain the essential and the nonessential L-amino acids in the proportions found on the aminogram of proteins with high biological value.

There is a trend to include fat in the form of a fat emulsion (soybean oil-eggy olk phospholipid emulsion) for intravenous nutrition in an amount corresponding to about 40 energy percent, as the source of both energy and essential fatty acids for the body.

To make intravenous nutrition as complete as possible, all essential minerals should be included. Phosphorus is of special interest here as it aids in the prevention of hypophosphataemia and tissue anoxia caused by deficiency of diphosphoglycerate in the erythrocytes. Zinc seems to be important for wound healing.

There is also a tendency to include all thirteen necessary vitamins in an intravenous feeding programme. In this respect vitamin K_1 is of special importance. If patients on intravenous nutrition are treated with antibiotics, this may result in a change in the intestinal flora and a reduced intestinal vitamin K production, causing vitamin K deficiency with severe or fatal bleeding. Consequently, vitamin K_1 should be given daily to every patient on intravenous alimentation.

The future trend in the field of parenteral nutrition will be to use this method for exact nutrition balance. In this way it may be possible to determine the endogenous loss via faeces, as well as to study the requirements of nutrients under different conditions.

REFERENCES

1. Thorén, L., (1969) *Vätskebalans*. Almquist & Wiksell, Uppsala, Sweden.
2. Wilkinson, A. W., (1969) *Body fluids in surgery*. 3rd ed. E. & X. Livingstone Ltd., Edinburgh and London.
3. Reissigl, H., (1965) *Praxis der Flüssigkeitstherapie*. Urban & Schwarzenberg, München and Berlin.
4. Allen, P. C. and Lee, H. A., (1969) P. C. Allen and H. A. Lee, (eds.), *A clinical guide to intravenous nutrition*. Blackwell, Oxford.
5. Wretlind, A., (1972) Complete intravenous nutrition. Theoretical and experimental background. *Nutr. Metabol.*, 14, Suppl. p. 1.
6. Elman, R., (1937) Urinary output of nitrogen as influenced by intravenous injection of a mixture of amino acids. *Proc. Soc. exp. Biol. Med.*, 37, 610.
7. Dudrick, S. J., Wilmore, D. W., Vars, H. M. and Rhoads, J. E., (1968) Long-term total parenteral nutrition with growth, development and positive nitrogen balance. *Surgery*, 64, 134.
8. Dudrick, S. J., Wilmore, D. W., Vars, H. M. and Rhoads, J. E., (1969) Can intravenous feeding as the sole means of nutrition support growth in the child and restore weight loss in an adult? *Ann. Surg.*, 169, 974.
9. Elwyn, D., (1970) The role of the liver in regulation of amino acid and protein metabolism. In: H. N. Munro, (ed.), *Mammalian protein metabolism*. Vol. 4, p. 523. Academic Press, New York.
10. Harper, A. E., (1968) Diet and plasma amino acids. *Am. J. Clin. Nutr.*, 21, 358.
11. Fishman, B., Whitman, R. J. and Munro, H. N., (1969) Daily rhythms in hepatic polysome profiles and tyrosine transaminase: Role of dietary protein. *Proc. Nat. Acad. Sci.*, 64, 677.
12. Soliman, A. G. and Harper, A. E., (1971) Effect of protein content of diet on lysine oxidation by the rat. *Biochim. Biophys. Acta*, 244, 146.
13. Wurtman, R. J., (1970) Diurnal rhythms in mammalian protein metabolism. In: H. N. Munro, (ed.), *Mammalian protein metabolism*. Vol. 4, p. 445. Academic Press, New York and London.
14. Munro, H. N., (1970) A general survey of mechanisms regulating protein metabolism in mammals. In: H. N. Munro, (ed.), *Mammalian protein metabolism*. Vol. 4, p. 299. Academic Press, New York.
15. Miller, L. L., (1962) The role of the liver and the non-hepatic tissues in the

regulation of free amino acid levels in the blood. In: T. T. Holden, (ed.), *Amino acid pools* p. 708. Elsevier, Amsterdam.

16. STURMAN, J. A., GAULL, G. and RAIHA, N. C. P., (1970) Absence of cystathionase in human fetal liver. Is cystine essential? *Science*, 169, 74.

17. STEGINK, L. D. and DEN BESTEN, L., (1972) Synthesis of cystine from methionine in normal subjects: Effect of route of alimentation. *Science*, 178, 514.

18. HOLT, L. E. JR. and SNYDERMAN, S. E., (1961) The amino acid requirements of infants. *J. Am. Med. Ass.*, 175, 100.

19. BERGSTRÖM, J., FÜRST, P., JOSEPHSON, B. and NORÉE, L.-O., (1970). Improvement of nitrogen balance in a uremic patient by the addition of histidine to essential amino acid solutions given intravenously. *Life Sci.*, 9, 787.

20. JÜRGENS, P. and DOLIF, D., (1972) Experimental results of parenteral nutrition with amino acids. In: A. W. Wilkinson, (ed.), Parenteral nutrition p. 47. Churchill Livingstone, Edinburgh and London.

21. JÜRGENS, S. P. and DOLIF, D., (1968) Die Bedeutung nichtessentieller Aminosäuren für den Stickstoffhaushalt des Menschen unter parenteraler Ernährung. *Klin. Wschr.*, 46, 131.

22. DOLIF, D. and JÜRGENS, P., (1969) Die Bedeutung der nichtessentiellen Aminosäuren bei der parenteralen Ernährung. In: G. Berg, (ed.), Advances in parenteral nutrition. Symposium of the International Society of Parenteral Nutrition, Prague, p. 126. G. Thieme Verlag, Stuttgart.

23. SCHLAPPNER, O. L. A., SHELLEY, W.B., RUBERG, R. L. and DUDRICK, S. J., (1972) Acute papulopustular acne associated with prolonged intravenous hyperalimentation. *JAMA*, 219, 877.

24. ROSE, W. C., (1957) The amino acid requirements of adult man. *Nutr. Abstr. Rev.*, 27, 631.

25. ROSE, W. C., OESTERLING, M. J. and WOMACK, M., (1948) Comparative growth on diets containing ten and nineteen amino acids, with further observations upon the role of glutamic and aspartic acids. *J. Biol. Chem.*, 176, 753.

26. WOMACK, M. and ROSE, W. C., (1941) Partial replacement of dietary methionine by cystine for purposes of growth. *J. Biol. Chem.*, 141, 375.

27. INOUE, G., FUJITA, T. and NIIJAMA, Y., (1971) Unpublished data.

28. HEGSTED, D. M., (1963) Variation in requirements of nutrients. Amino acids. *Fed. Proc.* 22, 1424.

29. WATTS, J. H., MANN, A. N., BRADLEY, L. and THOMPSON, D. J., (1964) Nitrogen balances of men over 65 fed the FAO and milk patterns of essential amino acid. *J. Gerontol.*, 19, 370.

30. TUTTLE, S. G., BOSSET, S. H., GRIFFITH, W. H., MULCARE, D. B. and SWENSEID, M. E., (1968) Further observations on the amino acid requirements of older men. I. Effects of nonessential nitrogen supplements fed with different amounts of essential amino acids. *Amer. J. Clin.*, 16, 225.

31. MUNRO, H. N., (1972 a) Adaptation of mammalian protein metabolism to hyperalimentation. In: G. S. M. Cowan and W. L. Scheetz, (eds.), Intravenous hyperalimentation, p. 34. Lea & Febiger, Philadelphia.
   MUNRO, H. N., (1972 b) Amino acid requirements and metabolism and their relevance to parenteral nutrition. In: A. W. Wilkinson, (ed.), Parenteral nutrition, p. 34. Churchill Livingstone, Edinburgh and London.

32. FAO/WHO Expert Group, (1965) *Protein requirements*. FAO Nutr. Meet. Rep. Ser. No. 37.

33. FAO Committee, (1957) *Protein requirements*. FAO Nutritional Studies No. 16, Rome.

34. SWENSEID, M. E., FEELEY, R. J., HARRIS, C. L. and TUTTLE, S. G., (1959)

Egg protein as a source of the essential amino acids. Requirement for nitrogen balance in young adults studied at two levels of nitrogen intake. *J. Nutr.*, 68, 203.

35. FROST, D. V., (1959) Methods of measuring the nutritive value of proteins, protein hydrolysates, and amino acid mixtures. The repletion method. In: A. A. Albanese (ed.), *Protein and amino acid nutrition*, p. 225. Academic Press, New York and London.

36. FROST, D. V. and SANDY, H. R., (1949) Rat-repletion studies with amino acid solutions. Role of nonessential amino acids. *Fed. Proc.*, 8, 383.

37. REISSIGL, H., (1957) Blut oder Plasmaersatzstoffe? Eine kritische Betrachtung der Indikation in Hinblick auf den biologischen Wert und die Gefahren. *Med. Klinik*, 52, 1357.

38. CAMMARATA, P. S. and COHEN, P. P., (1950) Scope of transamination reaction in animal tissues. *J. Biol. Chem.*, 187, 439.

39. NAKADA, H. I. and WEINHOUSE, S., (1953) Studies of glycine oxidation in rat tissues. *Arch. Biochem.*, 42, 257.

40. ZIMMERMAN, R. A. and SCOTT, H. M., (1965) Interrelationships of plasma amino acid levels and weight gain in the chick as influenced by suboptimal and supraoptimal dietary concentrations of single amino acids. *J. Nutr.*, 8, 713.

41. YOUNG, V. R., HUSSEIN, E. M., MURRAY, E. and SCRIMSHAW, N. S., (1971) Plasma tryptophan curve and its relation to tryptophan requirements in young adult men. *J. Nutr.*, 101, 54.

42. PEASTON, M. J. T., (1967) Maintenance of metabolism during intensive patient care. *Postgrad. Med. J.*, 43, 31.

43. JOHNSTON, I. D. A. and SPIVEY, J., (1970) The use of longterm parenteral nutrients in alimentary failure. In: G. Berg (ed.), Advances in parenteral nutrition. Symposion of the International Society of Parenteral Nutrition. p. 82. G. Thieme Verlag, Stuttgart.

44. FÜRST, P., JOSEPHSON, B. and VINNARS, E., (1970) The effect on the nitrogen balance of the ratio essential/non-essential amino acids in intravenously infused solutions. *Scand. J. Clin. Lab. Invest.*, 26, 319.

45. HALLBERG, D. and SODA, M., (1973) Effect of different parenteral nutritional solutions on hepatic blood flow in dogs. To be published.

46. DECKNER, K., BRAND, K. and KOFRANY, E., (1970) Untersuchungen über die Verträglichkeit und biologische Wertigkeit von parenteral verabreichten Aminosäure-Mustern. *Klin. Wschr.*, 48, 795.

47. JACOBSON, S. and WRETLIND, A., (1970) The use of fat emulsions for complete intravenous nutrition. In: C. L. Fox Jr. and G. C. Nahas (eds.), Body fluid replacement in the surgical patient. p. 334. Grune & Stratton, New York.

48. MAYER, G., KNAUFF, H. C., MILLER, B., SCHMIDT, H. and STAIB, I., (1969) Beeinflussbarkeit der Stickstoffbilanz durch eine verschiedene Zusammensetzung parenteral verabreichter Aminosäurelösungen bei Frischoperierten. *Klin. Wschr.*, 47, 1275.

49. LIDSTRÖM, F. and WRETLIND, A., (1952) The effect of intravenous administration of a dialyzed, enzymatic casein hydrolysate (Aminosol) on the serum concentration and on the urinary excretion of amino acids. Peptides and nitrogen. *Scand. Lab. Clin. Invest.*, 4, 167.

50. BØRRESEN, H. C. and KNUTRUD, O., (1969) Parenteral feeding of neonates undergoing major surgery. *Acta Paediatr. Scand.*, 58, 420.

51. BØRRESEN, H. C. and KNUTRUD, O., (1972) The clinical use of complete parenteral feeding in the neonate. In: A. W. Wilkinson (ed.), *Parenteral nutrition*, p. 176, Churchill Livingstone, Edinburgh and London.

52. DAS, J. B., FILLER, R. M., RUBIN, V. G. and ERAKLIS, A. J., (1970) Intravenous dextrose-amino-acid feeding. The metabolic response in the surgical neonate. *J. Pediat. Surg.*, 5, 127.
53. FILLER, R. M., ERAKLIS, A. J., RUBIN, V. G. and DAS, J. B., (1969) Long-term total parenteral nutrition in infants. *N. Engl. J. Med.*, 281, 589.
54. GROTTE, G., (1971) Nutrition parentérale du nourrisson. In: G. G. Nahas et P. Viars, (eds.), Les solutés de substitution et rééquilibration métabolique. p. 509. Librairie Arnette, Paris.
55. BERGSTRÖM, K., BLOMSTRAND, R. and JACOBSON, S., (1972) Longterm complete intravenous nutrition in man. *Nutr. Metabol.*, 14, Suppl. p. 118.
56. HALMAGYI, M. and KILBINGER, G., (1972) Clinical experimental study on the relationship between energy supply and nitrogen balance. In: A. W. Wilkinson (ed.), Parenteral Nutrition. p. 283. Churchill Livingstone, Edinburgh and London.
57. JOSEPHSON, B., FÜRST, P. and VINNARS, E., (1972) Metabolic aspects on the use of amino acid mixtures. In: A. W. Wilkinson, (ed.), Parenteral nutrition. p. 68 Churchill Livingstone, Edinburgh and London.
58. ABBOTT, W. E. and ALBERTSEN, K., (1963) Intravenous protein alimentation. *Nutr. Diet.*, 5, 339.
59. HALLBERG, D., HOLM, I., OBEL, A.-L., SCHUBERTH, O. and WRETLIND, A., (1967) Fat emulsion for complete intravenous nutrition. *Postgrad. Med.*, 42, A-71, A-87, A-99, A-149.
60. LARSEN, V. and BRØCKNER, J., (1965) Nitrogen balance and operative stress. Effect of early postoperative nutrition on nitrogen balance following major surgery. *Acta Chir. Scand. Suppl.*, 343, 191.
61. MOORE, F. D., (1959) Metabolic care of the surgical patient. Saunders, Philadelphia and London.
62. LAWSON, L. J. (1965) Parenteral nutrition in surgery. *Brit. J. Surg.*, 52, 795.
63. JOHNSTON, I. D. A., TWEEDLE, D. E. F. and SPIVEY, J., (1972) Intravenous feeding after surgical operation. In: A. W. Wilkinson (ed.), *Parenteral nutrition* p. 189. Churchill Livingstone, Edinburgh and London.
64. JORDAL, K., (1965) Proteinzufuhr in der parenteralen Ernährung in der Chirurgie. *Internat. Zschr. Vitaminforsch.*, 35, 26.
65. SAARNE, A., BJERSTAF, L. and EKMAN, B., (1965) Studies on the nitrogen balance in the human during long-term treatment with different anabolic agents under strictly standardized conditions. *Acta Med. Scand.*, 177, 199.
66. GAMBLE, J. L., (1958) *Chemical anatomy. Physiology and pathology of extracellular fluid.* Harward University Press, Cambridge.
67. Recommended Dietary Allowances (1968). National Academy of Sciences. 7th ed. Publ. 1694. Washington, D. C.
68. WEICHSELBAUM, T. E. and ELMAN, R., (1951) The distribution of fructose and of glucose in total body water after i.v. injection. *J. Lab. Clin. Med.*, 38, 958.
69. JOB, C. and HUBER, O., (1961) Zur Permeabilität menschlicher Erythrocyten für Glucose und Fructose. *Arch. exp. Path. Pharmakol.*, 241, 53.
70. THORÉN, L., (1964) Parenteral nutrition with carbohydrate and alcohol. *Acta Chir. Scand.* 325, Suppl. p. 75.
71. FROESCH, E. R. and U. KELLER, (1972) Review of energy metabolism with particular reference to the metabolism of glucose, fructose, sorbitol and xylitol and of their therapeutic use in parenteral nutrition. In: A. W. Wilkinson (ed.), *Parenteral nutrition* p. 105. Churchill Livingstone, Edinburgh and London.
72. MENDELOFF, A. L. and WEICHSELBAUM, T. E., (1953) Role of the human liver in the assimilation of intravenously administered fructose. *Metabolism* 2, 450.

73. BERGSTRÖM, J., HULTMAN, E. and ROCH-NORLUND, A., (1969) Intravenös fruktostillförsel kan vara livsfarlif. *Läkartidningen*, 66, 2223.

74. ANDERSSON, G., BROHULT, J. and STERNER, G., (1969) Increasing metabolic acidosis following fructose infusion in two children. *Acta Paediat. Scand.*, 58, 301.

75. COLLINS, F. D., SINCLAIR, A. J., BOYLE, J. P., COATS, D. A., MAYNARD, A. T. and LEONARD, R. F., (1971) Plasma lipids in human linoleic acid deficiency *Nutr. Metabol.*, 13, 150.

76. SCHOEFL, G. I., (1968) The ultrastructure of chylomicrons and of the particles in an artificial fat emulsion. *Proc. Roy. Soc.* Ser. B., 169, 147.

77. FRASER, R. and HÅKANSSON, I., (1973) *A comparison of artificial fat emulsions with chylomicrons.* In press.

78. HÅKANSSON, I., (1968) Experience in long-termsstudies on nine intravenous fat emulsions in dogs. *Nutr. Dieta*, 10, 54.

79. BOBERG, J. and CARLSON, L. A., (1964) Determination of heparin-induced lipoprotein lipase activity in human plasma. *Clin. Chim. Acta*, 10, 420.

80. HALLBERG, D., (1965 a) Studies on the elimination of exogenous lipids from the blood stream. The kinetics for the elimination of a fat emulsion studied by single injection technique in man. *Acta Physiol. Scand.*, 64, 306.

81. HALLBERG, D., (1965 b) Elimination of exogenous lipids from the blood stream. An experimental, methodological and clinical study in dog and man. *Acta Physiol. Scand.* 65 Suppl. p. 254.

82. WILMORE, D. W., MOYLAN, J. A., HELMKAMP, G. M. and PRUITT, B. A., (1973) *Clinical evaluation of a 10% intravenous fat emulsion for parenteral nutrition in thermally injured patients.* Paper presented at the 1973 meeting of the American Surgical Association, April 27, Los Angeles, California. In press.

83. SCRIBNER, B. H., COLE, J. J., CHRISTOPHER, T. G., VIZZO, J. E., ATKINS, R. C. and BLAGG, C. R., (1970) Long-term parenteral nutrition. *JAMA*, 212, 457.

84. LEMPERLE, G., REICHELT, M. and DENK, S., (1970) *The evaluation of phagocytic activity in men by means of a lipid-clearing-test.* Abstract from 6th International Meeting of the Reticuloendothelial Society, p. 83.

85. DUCKERT, F. and HARTMANN, G., (1966) Intravenöse Fettinfusion und Blutgerinnung. *Schweiz. Med. Wschr.*, 96, 1205.

86. CRONBERG, S. and NILSSON, I.-M., (1967) Coagulation studies after administration of a fat emulsion Intralipid. *Thromb. Diath. Haemorrh.*, 18, 364.

87. THOMPSON, S. W., JONES, L. D., FERRELL, J. F., HUNT, R. D., MENG, H. C., KUYAHA, T., SASAKI, H., SCHAFFNER, F., SINGLETON, W. S. and COHN, J., (1965) Testing of fat emulsions and emulsion components. *Am. J. Clin. Nutr.*, 16, 43.

88. PEASTON, M. J. T., (1966) Design of an intravenous diet of amino acids and fat suitable for intensive patient-care. *Brit. Med. J.*, 2, 388.

89. STELL, P. M., (1970) Esophageal replacement by transposed stomach. *Arch. Otolaryng.* 91, 166.

90. HALLBERG, D., SCHUBERTH, O. and WRETLIND, A., (1966) Experimental and clinical studies with fat emulsion for intravenous nutrition. *Nutr. Dieta*, 8, 245.

91. STEINBEREITHNER, K., (1966) Problems of artificial alimentation in an intensive therapy unit. (Possibilities and limitations,) In: F. T. Evans and T. Gray (eds.), *Modern trends in anaesthesia* Chapter 11, Butterworths, London.

92. LEE, H. A., (1969) Design of an intravenous diet and some practical observations. In: P. C. Allen and H. A. Lee, (eds), A clinical guide to intravenous nutrition. p. 141. Blackwell, Oxford.

93. RICKHAM, P. P., (1967) Massive small intestinal resection in newborn infants. Hungerian lecture delivered at the Royal College of Surgeons of England. *Ann. Roy. Coll. Surg.*, 41, 480.

94. BØRRESEN, H. C., CORAN, A. G. and KNUTRUD, O., (1970 a) Postoperative parenteral ernaering av nyfødte. *Nordisk Medicin*, 84, 1089.

95. BØRRESEN, H. C., CORAN, A. G. and KNUTRUD, O., (1970 b) Parenteral feeding of newborns undergoing major surgery. In: G. Berg (ed.), *Advances in parenteral nutrition*. Symposium of the International Society of Parenteral Nutrition, Prague, September 3-4, 1969. p. 93. Georg Thieme Verlag, Stuttgart.

96. BERTHOUD, M., BOUVIER, C. A. and KRÄHENBÜHL, B., (1966) Diagnostic différential d'une diathèse hémorragique aigue: hypothrombinémie au course d'une alimentation parénterale prolongée. *Schweiz. Med. Wschr.*, 96, 1522.

97. LATTA, T., (1832) Relative to the treatment of cholera by the copious injection of aqueous and saline fluids into the veins. *The Lancet*, II, 275.

98. TRAVIS, S., SUGERMAN, H. J., RUBERG, R. L., DUDRICK, S. J., DELIVORIA-PAPADOPOULOS, M., MILLER, L. D. and OSKI, F. A., (1971) Alterations of red-cell glycolytic intermediates and oxygen transport as a consequence of hypophosphatemia in patients receiving intravenous hyperalimentation. *New Engl. J. Med.*, 285, 763.

99. Editorial, (1973) *Zinc deficiency in man*. Lancet, I, 299.

100. GREAVES, M. W. and SKILLEN, A. W., (1970) Effects of long-continued ingestion of zinc sulphate in patients with venous leg ulceration. *The Lancet II*, 889.

101 HALLBÖÖK, T. and LANNER, E., (1972) Serum-zinc and healing of venous leg ulcers. *The Lancet*, II, 780.

102. HUSSEIN, S. L., (1969) Oral zinc sulphate in leg ulcers. *The Lancet*, I. 1069,

103. MILLS, C. F., (1972) Some aspects of trace element nutrition in man. *Nutrition* 26, 357.

104. PULLEN, F. W., PORIES, W. J. and STRAIN, W. H., (1971) Delayed healing: The rationale for zinc therapy. *Laryngoscope*, 81, 1638.

105. JACOBSON, S., (1972) Long-term parenteral nutrition following massive intestinal resection. *Nutr. Metabol.*, 14, Suppl. p. 150.

106. ABRAHAMSSON, J. DOMELLÖF, L. and NORRINDER, B., (1971) Intrapleural infusion som senklomplikation till central venkateter. *Nordisk Medicin*, 85, 241.

107. ADAR, R. and MOZES, M., (1970) Hydromediastinum. *JAMA*, 214, 272.

108. AULENBACHER, C. A., (1970) Hydrothorax from subclavian vein catheterization. *JAMA*, 214, 372.

109. BADEN, H., (1971) Kateter i sentrale vener. *Nordisk Medicin*, 86, 1306.

110. DUDRICK, S. J. and RUBERG, R. L., (1971) Principles and practice of parenteral nutrition. *Gastroenterology*, 61, 901.

111. SOLASSOL, C., JOYEUX, H., SERROU, B., CALLIS, A., PUJOL, H. and ROMIEU, C., (1972) Long-term parenteral hypernutrition in cancer patients. In: P. Arroyo, S. S. Basta, H. Bourges, A. Chávez, M. Coronado, M. Munoz and S. E. Zuiroz (eds.), *Abstracts of short communications. IX International Congress of Nutrition*. p. 15. Committee of the IX International Congress of Nutrition, México.

112. JOYEUX, H., (1972) *L'intestin artificiel. Etude clinique de la nutrition parentérale prolongée. Etude expérimentale de la nutrition par voie portale*. Montpellier, France.

113. SCHOLLER, K. L., (1968) Transport und Speicherung von Fettemulsionsteilchen. *Z. prakt. Anästhesie und Wiederbelebung* 3, 193.

114. ALVAREZ, J. J. P., VARGAS-ROSENDO, R., GUTIÉRREZ-BOSQUE, R., DIAZ-ORDAZ, M. M. and SANTOS-ATHERTON, D., (1970). A new type of subcutaneous arteriovenous fistula for chronic hemodialysis in children. *Ped. Surg.*, 67, 355.

115. BRESCIA, M. J., CIMINO, J. E., APPEL, K. and HURWICH, B. J., (1966) Chronic hemodialysis using venipuncture and a surgically created arteriovenous fistula. *N. Engl. J. Med.*, 275, 1089.

116. WIRBATZ, W., KIESSLING, J., BAUKE, G., MATEEV, B. and WITTBRODT, S., (1969) Langzeitkatheterismus der Vena portae. *Bruns' Beitr. Klin. Chir.* 217, 330.
117. FROHM, M. J. N., (1971) Cannulation of the umbilical vein. *Proc. Roy. Soc. Med.*, 64, 568.

PARENTERAL NUTRITION IN PAEDIATRIC SURGERY

U. G. STAUFFER, D. SHMERLING AND P. DANGEL*

Parenteral nutrition is always indicated when it is impossible to provide adequate oral nutrition (1). By definition parenteral nutrition is quite different from postoperative intravenous fluid therapy and infusions to combat shock. In the last few years, numerous authors have reported on their experience with intravenous infusions in children using amino acids, sugars in high concentration and fat emulsions. However in the majority of cases these infusions were only given for a few days. Exact information about the type and concentration of these solutions is often missing. There are relatively few papers in literature which deal with the problem of long-term parenteral nutrition (1–10).

In order to compare results from different centres, exact data concerning the solutions for parenteral nutrition, the dosages per kg body weight and the length of therapy are needed, as well as detailed reports on any complications.

Up to now there has been no general agreement on what constitutes total parenteral nutrition. We suggest that one should talk about total parenteral nutrition when at least 50% of the calory and protein requirements are supplied intravenously. This definition would exclude all those cases in which an insufficient amount of amino acids, carbohydrates or fat emulsions has been given. This definition does however allow inclusion of those cases in which repeated attempts have been made to feed the patient orally, as for instance in cases of extensive resection of the small intestine.

The expression 'long-term parenteral nutrition' has been used very differently by various authors. We suggest that parenteral nutrition which lasts for more than 4 weeks should be described as long-term. Parenteral nutrition lasting for less than 4 weeks should be described as short-term. Today the problem of short-term parenteral nutrition

* University Children's Hospital Zürich, Switzerland

in infants and children has more or less been solved. (1, 4, 5, 7, 9, 10, 11, 12, 13). Short-term parenteral nutrition can be given via either peripheral veins or central veins without much difficulty. All that is necessary is to administer adequate amounts of amino acids, sugar and electrolyte mixtures with or without fat emulsions. Severe deficiency diseases secondary to an insufficient supply of trace elements, vitamins, calcium, phosphorus, etc. are rarely seen.

Insufficient growth and weight gain are usually not of great importance.

The clinical indications for short-term parenteral nutrition are a subject of considerable debate. It has become fashionable to prescribe prophylactic intravenous amino acids and sugar mixtures, and even intravenous fat emulsions, for the first postoperative days. This has been done in cases of perforated appendicitis, severe trauma and even after correction of non-intestinal malformations. We should like to sound a note of warning about the uncritical use of intravenous parenteral nutrition. It is often unnecessary, it is expensive and it is not without danger to the patient. We believe that intravenous parenteral nutrition is only indicated if a child cannot be adequately fed orally for a period of more than four to five days. An exception to this rule are those children whom one can confidently predict will need parenteral nutrition for long periods, for instance cases with extensive resection of the small intestine. In these cases we start with parenteral nutrition on the second postoperative day.

A number of authors have suggested that parenteral nutrition is indicated for tetanus and in the post-traumatic period for cases with severe burns (1, 10, 20, 22, 23, 24). In our experience with 15 children suffering from tetanus, all of whom survived, and children treated during the fast few years for burns, including 50 children with burns over 40% of their body surface, parenteral nutrition has never been necessary. All of these children could be fed perfectly satisfactorily per os or by tube.

The problems of long-term parenteral nutrition are considerably greater than those of short-term intravenous feeding. We therefore want to report on our experience and our difficulties with long-term parenteral feeding in children.

Between 1966 and 1972 six children were given long-term parenteral feeding in our clinic (table 1).

Table 1. *Total long-term parenteral nutrition (Universitätsklinik Zürich, Dept. of Surg.).*

Case Year	Age	Diagnosis	Residual (cm) small intestine Jej.	Ileum	*Parenteral nutrition* Total Weeks	Partial	Outcome
1 A.C. 1966	2 days	Mesenteric cyst, necrosis of the small intestine	25	30 5	7		well
2 P.N. 1970	10 days premature 1920 g	Multiple atresias of the small bowel	3	23 20	7	11	well
3 S.R. 1970	9 11/12 y	Ulcerative colitis, toxic megacolon			12	13	improved 3–5 stools a day
4 K.D. 1970	9 years	Intestinal obstruction due to adhesions			14	17	well
5 R.J. 1971	9 weeks	Aganglionosis Colon + 50 cm ileum, ileorectal anastomosis			30	32	improved
6 P. MP 1971	2 days 1680 g	Multiple atresias of the small bowel and volvulus	19	21 2	68	–	died

1. The first child was a two-day-old neonate with a mesenteric cyst and extensive gangrene of the entire small intestine, with the exception of 25 cm of jejunum and 5 cm of ileum. The gangrenous gut was resected. The child was fed intravenously for seven weeks; he is now seven years old and perfectly well.

2. The second child, a premature infant weighing 1920 grams at birth with multiple intestinal atresias, was left with 23 cm of small intestine after resection. After seven weeks of total and four weeks of partial parenteral nutrition, it became possible to feed him orally. This child is now 3 years old and somewhat small, but otherwise healthy. The length of the remaining intestine, 23 cm, is perhaps close to being the lowest limit for survival. Only very few such cases have been described in literature.

3. The third case was a 10-year-old boy with ulcerative colitis and severe toxicity; he had to be fed parenterally for 13 weeks. A partial colectomy was performed and today he is much improved although he still has 3–5 defaecations containing a little blood each day.

4. Case 4 was a nine-year-old boy with chronic intestinal obstruction due to adhesions following a perforated appendix. He was admitted in a desperate state with several intestinal perforations. Total parenteral nutrition carried out over a period of several weeks improved the general condition to such an extent that it was possible to operate on him and close the perforations and fistulae. After 17 weeks of parenteral nutrition and more than 20 weeks in the hospital, we were able to discharge the boy in good health.

5. Case 5 indicates another reason for long-term parenteral nutrition. This was a 9-week-old girl with Hirschsprung's disease. The aganglionic segment included the entire colon and the distal 50 cm of the ileum. The aganglionic segment was resected and an ileorectal anastomosis was performed. This resulted in a malabsorption syndrome with severe diarrhoea. She needed total parenteral nutrition for 30 weeks. This child is now two years old, and has occasional slight attacks of diarrhoea alternating with mild obstruction.

6. The last patient was a premature infant weighing 1680 grams who received parenteral nutrition for a total period of 68 weeks; the parenteral feeding of this child is therefore one of the longest described in

literature. He suffered from multiple intestinal atresias and volvulus; when he was two days old, the entire small intestine with the exception of 21 cm of jejunum was resected. This segment of intestine proved to be too short for oral nutrition. The child finally died of intercurrent pneumonia. The management of this infant provided is considerable experience in parenteral nutrition.

These in brief are the clinical data of the patients who received long-term parenteral nutrition. We should now like to discuss the difficulties and complications we encountered.

The first major problem of long-term parenteral nutrition is the availability of veins for infusion. After several months of parenteral nutrition, this becomes problem no. 1. For the last three years we have preferred to use the subclavian vein which is entered percutaneously below the clavicle (14, 15, 16). This procedure is carried out under general anaesthesia. The patient is placed in Trendelenburg's position to increase the pressure in the subclavian vein. This will also prevent any danger of air emboli. The operation is carried out under strict aseptic conditions. We use a siliconized PVC-catheter made by Intra-cat. We agree with other authors (9, 17, 18, 19) that only very thin catheters should be used. The tip of the catheter lies correctly in the right atrium if one can aspirate blood, and if the pressure measured by a manometer is that of normal venous pressure. The correct position of each catheter is checked by radiography. The catheter is fixed to the skin with two silk stitches. Using this technique, the distance between the puncture wound in the skin and the vessel is relatively short. There is therefore a relatively greater risk of infection. More recently we have followed the advice of COLVIN (18) and have placed the catheter sub-cutaneously at a distance of 10 to 12 cm from the puncture wound, either up towards the skull or down towards the flank. This modification has two advantages. Firstly it diminishes the risk of infection, and secondly it prevents dislodgement of the catheter by movements of the patient, which is especially important in children who should be nursed without any restrictions whatsoever. Introduction of a catheter into the subclavian vein is not without danger and demands consider-able experience. Out of 350 cases in which we inserted subclavian catheters we had five complications. A pneumothorax occurred twice and had to be drained. Haemathorax was encountered 3 times. In one of these patients the haemorrhage was so massive that a thoracotomy had to be performed. The haemathorax was caused by puncture of an intercostal artery. All 5 patients survived their complications without any permanent damage. It should be added that in all of these cases, the physician was relatively inexperienced; with adequate experience and good technique, these complications should be avoidable.

We believe that complications are least common if the subclavian vein is used. Today we only use other veins if it is not possible to use the subclavian. The peripheral veins in the antecubital fossa are very useful for the introduction of central catheters, but can only be used for a few days as phlebitis invariably occurs. The internal jugular vein can be punctured relatively easily, but it is often difficult to advance the catheter into the thorax. Puncture of the femoral vein in infants is also feasible technically but our experience is that the danger of thrombosis and emboli is higher with femoral catheters than with subclavian catheters. Scalp vein infusions will only last for a few days. It is impossible to give high concentrations of carbohydrate solutions through a scalp vein infusion. We only use scalp veins to tide the patient over, especially when he is suffering from an infectious complication.

BELIN (21) reported on a trial with a subcutaneously placed Pudenz-Heyer-valve draining via the internal jugular vein into the right atrium. The valve can be punctured again and again with a needle at an angle of 90°. BELIN used this method successfully in a patient for a period of 22 months. We have not been successful as the Pudenz-valve started to leak after a few days. We have therefore developed a special reservoir but have had as yet insufficient experience with it.

Table 2 shows the veins used in our 6 patients on long-term parenteral nutrition. The average time a catheter could be left in place is given. The 39 subclavian catheters remained in situ for an average of 22 days. Catheters inserted into the internal and external jugular veins lasted for about the same time, but the catheters in the femoral vein lasted for an average of only 9 days; peripherally placed catheters only lasted for an average of four days. We were forced to change the catheters three times because of thrombosis, but the main complica-

Table 2. *Intravenous catheters in 6 patients with long-term parenteral nutrition.*

| | Number | Time (days) catheters were in place | | |
		Mean	Minimum	Maximum
V. subclavia	39	22	5	45
V. femoralis	10	9	2	15
V. jug.int + ext	4	22	4	38

tion was infection. This cannot always be prevented even with the most careful nursing. In three of our patients we saw 19 cases of infection. All these infections could finally be cured, but this is only possible if they are recognized early. It is therefore important to examine each patient every day for early signs of infection. The skin puncture should be inspected daily and redressed. Inexplicable fever, deterioration in the peripheral circulation, hepatomegaly, thrombocytopenia and the appearance of fat vacuoles in the leucocytes indicating a diminished fat clearance are all danger signals. If infection is confirmed or strongly suspected, the catheter must be removed and antibiotics have to be given. Prophylactic antibiotics are in our experience quite useless. They do not prevent infection and only stimulate the growth of resistant pathogens. In recent years we have placed a bacterial filter immediately proximal to the implanted catheter. This filter has perforations 0.22 μ in diameter. The filter must be changed every day. Unfortunately it is impossible to give fat emulsions through the filter. In our experience the use of a filter has unfortunately not greatly reduced the incidence of infection.

A problem which is relatively easily solved is the maintenance of a continuous infusion rate. If hypertonic solutions with a high sugar content are infused, a hyperglycaemia is produced causing diuresis and therefore marked fluid loss via the kidneys. On occasion oligaemic shock has even been observed. In addition large amounts of glucose are lost to the body. On the other hand if the patient is adapted to the infusion of large amounts of sugar, a slow infusion rate may produce hypoglycaemia. If amino acids are infused too rapidly, a hyperaminoacidaemia is produced. It is not certain to date whether this can cause damage to the central nervous system in young infants.

These dangers can be prevented by using an infusion pump. The pump ensures a uniform rate of flow throughout each 24 hour period. In cases where less than 500 ml are given over 24 hours, i.e. in newborn and small infants, the use of such a pump is absolutely vital.

Having described these practical problems, we should now like to discuss the infusions used. Table 3 shows the amounts per kg of body weight of fluid, calories, amino acids and fat that we generally like to use for infants and older children. For every gram of protein, the patient receives about 35 calories in the form of carbohydrates and fat. The carbohydrates were given as 10–50% glucose solutions. The amino acids were pure L-amino acids (Vamin,). In these solutions

Table 3. *Total long-term parenteral nutrition volume/kg of body weight/day*

Volume	ml	Infants 100–140	Toddlers 40–80
Calories	k cal	100–140	40–80
Protein (L-amino acids)	g	2–3	1–2
Carbohydrates (Glucose)	g	10–20	5–15
Lipids	g	1–4	1–2

the percentages of methionine and phenylalanine are rather high, especially for infants. Most of these solutions are in addition rather sour with a pH of 5.2; furthermore they contain fructose or sorbitol or both. These amino acid solutions lead to an acidosis and in our experience this tendency toward acidosis is further increased by the administration of fructose. The relatively high methionine and phenylalanine contents are also not suitable for infants. Finally it is possible in patients with fructose intolerance that solutions containing fructose will produce a catastrophe. For all of these reasons, we have used a new preparation during the last year which is not yet commercially available. It contains a mixture of L-amino acids with low methionine and phenylalanine contents, without fructose and sorbitol and with a pH between 7.2 and 7.4 as well as a titrable acidity of 0. In order to provide enough calories, glucose is added to the solution just before it is used.

All 6 patients received fat emulsions intravenously, usually 10 or 20% Intralipid. Fat emulsion infusions were usually given for 10 days without interruption, followed by a 3-day pause. If a thrombopenia or an inclusion of fat in thrombocytes or leukocytes was noticed, the fat infusions were interrupted. Some of these children received fat emulsions for several months without ever having serious complications. The need for electrolytes was covered by a special glucose-electrolyte mixture. Calcium was given separately as 10% calcium gluconate in a dosage of 1–4 ml per day. The need for trace elements was satisfied by giving 10–15 ml per kg body weight of fresh plasma once a week. 0.2 ml vitamin mixture (Pancebrin Lilly), 0.5 ml Becozym and 20 mg vit. C were also given each day. In addition, once a week we gave 1 mg of vit. K, vit. B 12 and folic acid intravenously.

Long-term parenteral nutrition requires very careful control. This is summarized in tables 4 and 5. Only by this careful clinical and

Table 4. *Clinical Controls in long-term parenteral nutrition*

Daily	Weight, oedema
Weekly	Head circumference (infants), size of liver, spleen, skin folds
Monthly	Length, psychomot. development, general development, 3-monthly radiogram of hand.

Table 5. *Laboratory investigations in long-term parenteral nutrition*

URINE

Daily	Volume ⎫	
	Glucose ⎪ after 2 weeks	
	Acetone ⎬ twice a week	
	pH ⎭	
Weekly	microscopy, protein, glucose, acetone, osmolarity	

HEMATOLOGY

2 times/week	Hb, Hkrit, leucocyte count, thrombocyte cell count
If needed	White, red blood count (incl. MCHC, reticulocytes)

BLOOD CHEMISTRY

Daily	Na, Cl, K ⎫ after 2 weeks Glucose ⎬ 2–3 times/week Astrup ⎭
Weekly	Ca, P, alc. phosphatase, total protein, electrophoresis, urea, SGOT, SGPT, osmolarity
Every 2 weeks	magnesium, ammonia

laboratory supervision will it be possible to recognize mistakes in parenteral nutrition at an early stage.

RESULTS

In our 6 patients on long-term parenteral nutrition we were able to achieve a weight gain between 15 and 475 grams per month. Growth was markedly retarded in all patients. This retardation of growth could not be completely explained. The protein intake in the form of amino acid mixtures in dosages of 2–3 grams per kg of body weight per day should assure normal growth. Some of our patients showed transient hypokalaemia and hypophosphataemia. Potassium and phosphorus are essential for the metabolism of proteins. It is possible that the rather limited administration of these two elements in former years may have been the cause of the retarded growth. Table 6 shows

Table 6. *Six patients with long-term parenteral nutrition, metabolic complications*

Metabolic acidosis	6
Hypoproteinaemia (slight)	4
Hypophosphataemia	2
Hepatomegaly	1*
Rickets	1*
Vit. B 12 and folic acid deficiency	1*
Deficiency of antibodies	1*

* same patient, 68 weeks long-term parenteral nutrition.

the main metabolic complications. All 6 children had a moderate metabolic acidosis with a base deficit between —4 and —8 mEq/l. This was corrected by daily administration of sodium bicarbonate solutions. This acidosis was less marked in children who had received an amino acid solution without fructose and sorbitol. In four children there was a mild hypoproteinaemia, secondary to diarrhoea, and in two a hypophosphataemia. The cause of the hypophosphataemia was most likely an insufficient phosphorus intake. Children need much more phosphorus for their protein and bone metabolism than adults. The infant who was fed parenterally for 68 weeks developed a hepatomegaly, rickets and vitamin B 12 and folic acid deficiencies. There was also a hypoproteinaemia and an antibody deficiency probably caused by the repeated infections. The rickets could be cured by vitamin D and the signs of pernicious anaemia were cured by folic acid and vitamin B 12. As a result of our experience with this patient, we now give higher dosages of vitamins to all patients on long-term parenteral nutrition.

CONCLUSIONS

Today it is possible to give long-term parenteral nutrition and to insure a good food intake in infants for a period of several months. The possibility of feeding infants parenterally for several months raises many ethical problems in the case of children with subtotal resection of the small intestine. Some of the infants as well as some older patients could only be helped by intestinal transplantation. Transplantation of irreversibly damaged organs necessary to life has, during the last few years, become one of the main problems of experimental surgery. Up till now only renal transplantation has become a clinically acceptable method. On the other hand intestinal transplantation is still very much in its infancy and has only been studied in a few centres. One of the great problems in transplantation of the small intestine is the early recognition of rejection. We have been performing experiments in intestinal transplantation for the last $1\frac{1}{2}$ years. After numerous preparatory experiments we transplanted the small intestine in forty 4 to 6-week-old minipigs weighing between $2\frac{1}{2}$ and 6 kgs. 20–60 cm long jejunum allografts were prepared from the donors (fig. 1). The recipient had a right nephrectomy and the intestinal vessels were anastomosed end-to-end to the renal vessels. The two ends of the intestine were implanted in the abdominal wall as enterostomies. Daily biopsies were then taken from the transplanted loop of intestine to examine the histology.

These experiments are not yet completed. We hope that this work will later enable us to recognize rejection crises early so that we will be able to control them by the administration of drugs, or if necessary to remove the segment of intestine without danger to the patient. We believe that transplantation of the small intestine in infants and children has thus become at least technically feasible. I therefore close my lecture by quoting FIKRI ALICAN who carried out one of the seven intestinal transplants which has been performed so far in man: 'It appears that when clinical intestinal transplantation is advanced to a level comparable to that of kidney transplantation, the improved methods of total intravenous nutrition will represent as useful an adjunct as the artificial kidney is to renal transplantation.'

SUMMARY

Parenteral nutrition is only indicated when it is impossible to feed the children orally for a prolonged period, i.e. a minimum of about 4–5 days. In order to be able to compare the results from different centres, it is absolutely essential to have precise information about the nature of the intravenous infusions used, the quantity given per kilogram of body weight, the length of treatment and any complications encountered.

We suggest that the term complete parenteral nutrition should be used only when at least 50% of the calories and proteins are given intravenously. Long-term parenteral nutrition must also be defined. We suggest that total parenteral nutrition of more than four weeks' duration should be described as long-term. The practical problems of long-term parenteral nutrition are still very great.

Between 1966 and 1972 we used total long-term parenteral nutrition for periods of 6½ to 68 weeks in 6 children; two premature infants, one neonate, one infant and two older children.

The infusions used were synthetic L-amino acid mixtures, fat emulsions, carbohydrates, electrolytes and vitamins. The children were given 80 to 140 ml infusion fluid, 80 to 140 ca'ories, 2–3 grams amino acids and 1–4 grams fat per kg of body weight per day. The infusion was administered via a central vein with a bacterial filter and an infusion pump. In most cases the intravenous catheter was placed percutaneously through the subclavian vein into the superior vena cava. Of the complications encountered infection was by far the most common. Hepatomegaly, hypophosphataemia, metabolic acidosis, rickets and vitamin B 12, folic acid and iron deficiencies were all encountered. In all patients there was a weight gain between 15 and 500 grams per month. Growth was retarded in all patients.

The possibility of total parenteral nutrition carried out successfully for many months causes great ethical problems in the case of subtotal resection of the small intestine. Some of the children and possibly also some adults could only be helped by transplantation of the small intestine. The preliminary results achieved in our laboratory with small intestinal transplantations in young minipigs are discussed briefly.

REFERENCES

1. WRETLIND, A., (1972) Ernährungsphysiologische und pharmakologische Gesichtspunkte in der kompletten parenteralen Ernährung. *Parenterale Ernährung, Internationale Zeitschrift für Vitamin- und Ernährungsforschung*, Beiheft 12. Verlag H. Huber, Bern, Stuttgart, Wien.
2. DUDRICK, S. I., WILMORE, D. W., VARS, H. M. und RHOADS, J. E., (1969) Can intravenous feeding as the solum means of nutrition support growth in the child and restore weight loss in adults. An affirmative answer. *Annals of Surgery*, 169, 974.
3. WILMORE, D. W., GROFF, D. B., BISHOP, H. C. und DUDRICK, S. I., (1969) Total parenteral nutrition in infants with catastrophic gastrointestinal anomalies. *Journal of Paediatric Surgery*, 4, 181.
4. BÖRRESEN, H. C., CORAN, A. G. und KNUTRUD, O., (1970) Metabolic results of parenteral feeding in neonatal surgery. *Annals of Surgery*, 17, 2291–2301.
5. BÖRRESEN, H. C. und KNUTRUD, O., (1969) Parenteral feeding of neonates undergoing major surgery. *Acta Paediatrica Scandinavica*, 58, 420.
6. HARRIS, J. T., (1971) Intravenous feeding in infants. *Archives of Diseases of Childhood*, 46, 855–863.
7. FILLER, R. M., ERAKLIS, A. J., RUBIN, V. G. and DAS, J. B., (1969) Long-term parenteral nutrition in infants. *New England Journal of Medicine*, 281, 589–594.

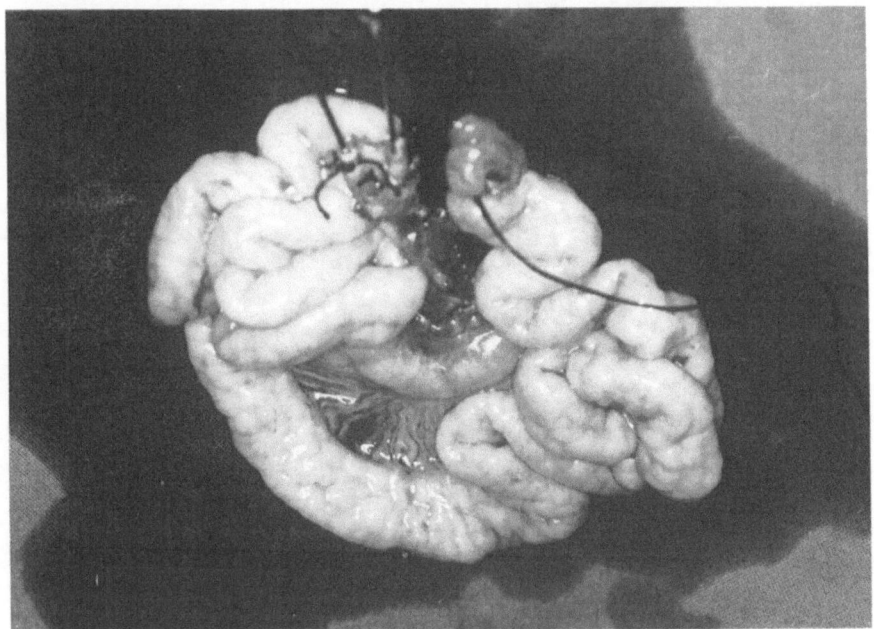

Fig. 1. Small intestinal transplant for heterotopic transplantation in a four-week-old minipig.

8. LLOYD-STILL, J. D., SHWACHMAN, H. and FILLER, R. M., (1972) Intravenous hyperalimentation in pediatrics. *American Journal of Digestive Diseases*, 17, 1043.
9. RICOUR, C., NIHOUL-FÉKÉTÉ, CL., VERTIN, P., ROYER, P. and PELLERIN, D., (1971) Alimentation parentérale continue par cathéter intracave chez l'enfant. *Annales de Chirurgie Infantile*, 13, 7–16.
10. BERGER, H., (1972) Grundsätzliches über die parenterale Ernährung beim Kind. *Parenterale Ernährung, Internationale Zeitschrift für Vitamin- und Ernährungsforschung*, 1284. Verlag Hans Huber, Bern, Stuttgart, Wien.
11. RICKHAM, P. P., (1968) Ausgedehnte Dünndarmresektion beim Neugeborenen. *Zeitschrift für Kinderchirurgie*, Supplement zu Band 5, 2.
12. KIM, S. H. und RICKHAM, P. P., (1972) Parenteral lipids and amino acids in surgical neonates. *Zeitschrift für Kinderchirurgie*, 11, 277.
13. SHMERLING, D. H. und DANGEL, P., (1972) *Praktische Erfahrungen mit vollständiger langfristiger parenteraler Ernährung in der Paediatrie*. Symposium Homburg/Saar, Dezember 1972.
14. WRBITZKY, R. und VOGEL, W., (1967) Zur Technik der infraklaviculären Punktion der V. subclavia und Indikation des Cavakatheters. *Zeitschrift für praktische Anästhesie*, 2, 120–128.
15. DANGEL, P., (1968) Blutentnahme und intravenöse Infusion beim Kleinkind. *Therapeutische Umschau*, 25, 679.
16. DANGEL, P., (1973) *Die Technik der langfristigen parenteralen Ernährung in der Pädiatrie und in der Kinderchirurgie*. Symposium Obergurge, Februar 1973.
17. BOLSANY, B. L., MARTIN, C. E. und CONKLE, D. M., (1971) Careful technique with plastic intravenous catheters. *Surgery, Gynecology and Obstetrics*, 132, 1030–1032.
18. COLVIN, M. P., BLOGG, C. E., SAVEGE, T. M., JARVIS, J. D. and STRUNIN, L., (1972) A safe long-term infusion technique? *Lancet* 2, 317–320.
19. LIEBERT, P. S., (1971) Central venous catheters in children – their placement and care. *Clinical Pediatrics*, 10, 218–222.
20. CUTHBERTSON, D. P., G. S. FELL, C. M. SMITH and W. J. TILSTONE, (1972) Nutrition in the Post-traumatic Period. *Nutrition and Metabolism*, 141, Supplement, 92–109.
21. BELIN, R. P., KOSTER, J. K., BRYANT, L. J. and GRIFFEN, W. O., (1972) Implantable subcutaneous feeding chamber for non-continuous central nervous alimentation. *Surgery*, 134, 491.
22. BIRKE, G., LILJEDAHL, S. O. und NYLEN, B., (1970) Behandling av mycket utbredda brännskador. *Läkartidningen*, 67, 3760.
23. LILJEDAHL, S. O., (1972) Behandlungen von Verbrennungen am Karolinischen Krankenhaus. *Parenterale Ernährung, Internationale Zeitschrift für Vitamin- und Ernährungsforschung*, Verlag Hans Huber, Bern, Stuttgart, Wien.
24. FEISCHL, P. und HIOTAKIS, K., (1969) Vollständige parenterale Ernährung bei schwerem Tetanus. *Wochenschrift für Klinik und Praxis*, 64, 2296.

PARENTERAL NUTRITION IN LOW
BIRTH WEIGHT BABIES

J. C. L. SHAW*

INTRODUCTION

From the moment of birth the low birthweight infant faces a period of malnutrition that may last several weeks. It is most severe in those infants who are the most premature, and calculations based on their estimated energy reserves and rate of energy expenditure show that the smallest of these infants will die in four days of starvation unless adequate nutrition is provided (1). In addition to these immediate hazards there is accumulating evidence that malnutrition early in development may permanently affect the developing brain by reducing it in size and cell number, a situation that cannot be reversed by a period of liberal feeding later on (2). It is considerations such as these that have led paediatricians to apply modern techniques of intravenous feeding to low birthweight infants, in order to bridge the gap between placental and effective gastrointestinal nutrition.

REFERENCE STANDARD FOR THE NUTRITION OF LOW BIRTH-WEIGHT INFANTS

The ideal nutrition of the low birthweight infant should be such that his postnatal growth is both qualitatively and quantitatively similar to that that would have occurred had he remained *in utero*, and so by studying intrauterine growth it is possible to obtain information on the nutritional requirements of these infants, and to show that they differ in some respects from those of full-term infants. Figure 1 compares two intrauterine growth curves obtained from the mean values for birthweight of infants born at different periods of gestation. The data of KLOOSTERMAN (3) were from infants born at sea level whereas those of LUBCHENKO et al (4) were from infants born one mile above sea

* Department of Paediatrics, University College Hospital, London, U.K.

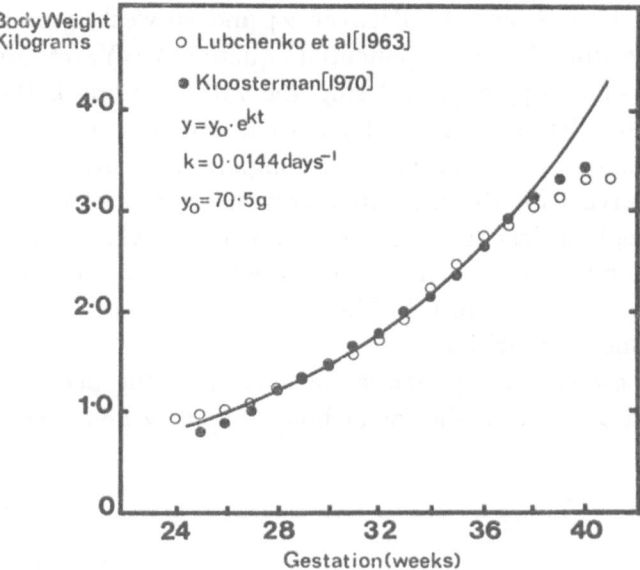

Fig. 1. Comparison of two intrauterine growth curves for infants born at sea level (KLOOSTERMAN 1970) and those born at 6000 feet (LUBCHENKO et al 1963), weight gain between 24 and 36 weeks is exponential.

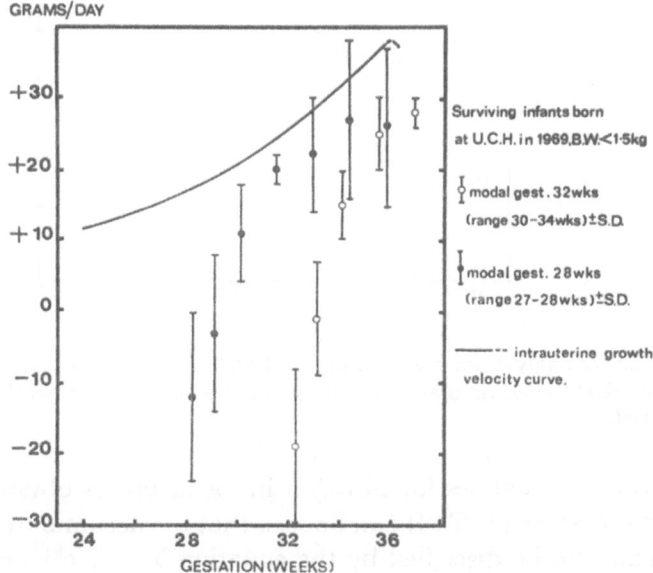

Fig. 2. Comparison of calculated intrauterine growth velocity curve, with the measured growth velocity of two groups of infants of less than 1.5 kg birthweight who did not receive parenteral nutrition.

level in Denver, Colorado. Between 24 and 36 weeks growth *in utero* can be described by the exponential equation $Y = Y_0 . e^{kt}$ and occurs at a rate of 0.0144 days^{-1}. Using the rate constant k the growth velocity at different periods of gestation can be calculated and an incremental curve plotted. Figure 2 compares the intrauterine growth velocity curve with the measured growth velocity of two groups of infants weighing less than 1.5 kg at birth and who were not given parenteral nutrition. Their rate of growth was mostly substantially below the calculated intrauterine growth rate, and this represents quite serious malnutrition.

Just as growth is exponential *in utero* so is the accumulation of different substances in the foetal body. Figure 3 gives the results of

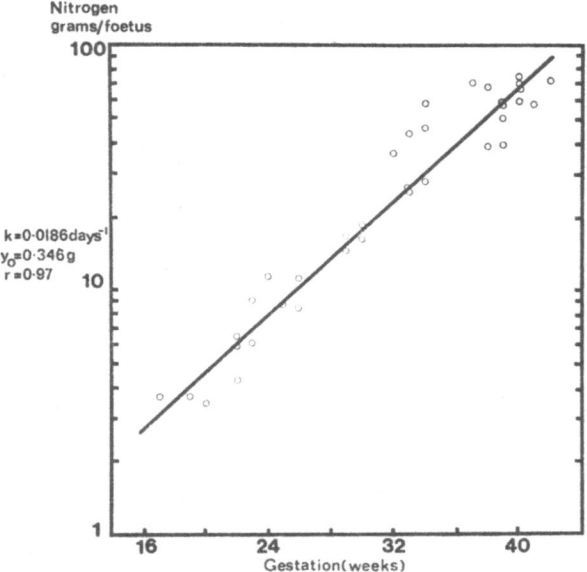

Fig. 3. Results of analyses for nitrogen in foetal bodies at different periods of gestation showing that the accumulation of nitrogen between 16 and 40 weeks gestation is exponential.

all the available analyses for nitrogen in foetal bodies obtained from the world literature (5, 6). It can be seen that the accumulation of this element can also be discribed by the equation $Y = Y_0 . e^{kt}$ and occurs at a rate of 0.0186 days^{-1}. Using this rate constant the rate of acculation of nitrogen at different periods of gestation can be calculated and an incremental curve plotted. Figure 4 gives the results of such calculations for all the substances that have been measured in foetal bodies (5, 6). These data provide a reference standard which I think will prove useful in the evaluation and design of solutions used for parenteral feeding. I would like now to turn to the more practical aspects of parenteral nutrition, but I will have occasion to refer to these data from time to time.

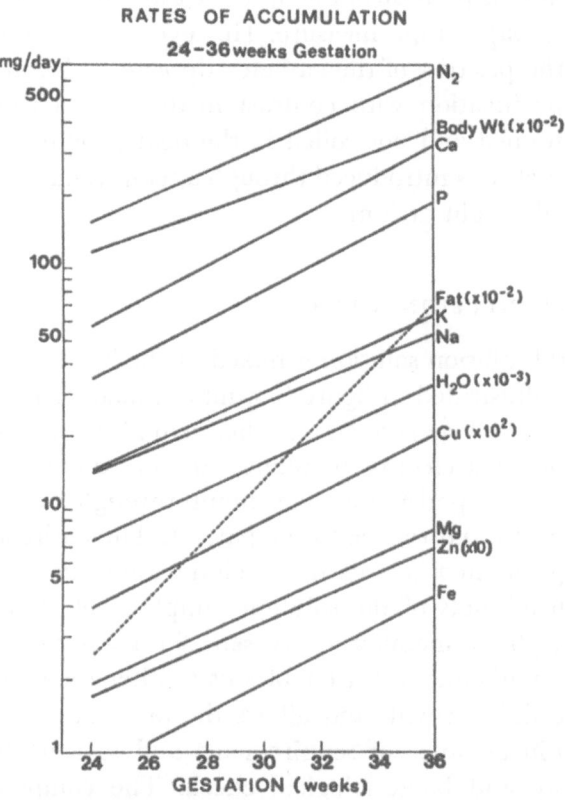

Fig. 4. Incremental curves giving the rate of accumulation of different substances by the human foetus *in utero* between 24 weeks and 30 weeks of gestation.

TECHNIQUE OF INTRAVENOUS FEEDING

The technique used in the Neonatal Intensive Care Unit at University College Hospital, London, is based on the methods of WILMORE & DUDRICK (7). It consists of the continuous infusion of a fat-free hyperosmolar solution of glucose, amino acids, minerals and vitamins into the

right atrium of the heart. In order to achieve this we have developed a
technique of introducing a very fine silicone rubber catheter of 0.6 mm
o.d. (A) through a 19 guage scalp vein needle (B) into a peripheral
vein, and threading it into the right atrium of the heart (8). Scalp
veins are to be preferred but veins in the wrist or antecubital fossa,
and the long saphenous veins have all been successfully used. Certain
precautions must be observed. The catheters are exactly 50 cm long
and this enables the position of the tip to be estimated during insertion,
using a sterile paper tape measure. However, before the infusion is
commenced the position of the catheter tip *must* be located radiologi-
cally after opacification with contrast medium, to ensure that it is
correctly positioned and not coiled in the heart. Figure 5 shows such
a catheter, which was introduced through a scalp vein, and is correctly
positioned in the right atrium.

PARENTERAL INFUSION SOLUTION

The parenteral infusion solution is mixed at the bed side in the closed
circuit system illustrated in figure 6. 5 ml of molar K_2HPO_4 is added
to the Aminosol (C) by syringe and then, equal volumes of Aminosol
glucose and Dextrose electrolyte solution are mixed in the beurette (D)
and are driven by a peristaltic finger pump through a 0.22 μ pore size
bacterial filter (F) and thence to the patient. The entire system up to
and including the filter is discarded each day, and the infusion bottles
together with aliquots of the solution sampled before and after the
filter, and the filter membrane are sent for bacterial culture. This
system has two advantages; it enables us to alter the glucose concentration of the fluid at will, and allows the pharmacy to prepare the
solutions well in advance of requirements and to issue them after a
chemical assay and bacteriological check. The composition of the
solutions used and the approximate daily intake of the different
nutrients are shown in tables 1, 2 and 3. The Dextrose electrolyte
solution is available in three concentrations of glucose, which when
mixed with the Aminosol will give a final concentration of 10%, 15%
or 20%. Very low birthweight infants are given initially 10% glucose
which corresponds to a rate of 0.63 g/kg/hr. While keeping a close
watch on the urine for glycosuria, the glucose concentration can be
increased stepwise until the intake reaches maximum values corresponding to a rate of 1.25 g/kg/hr. We selected glucose as the principle

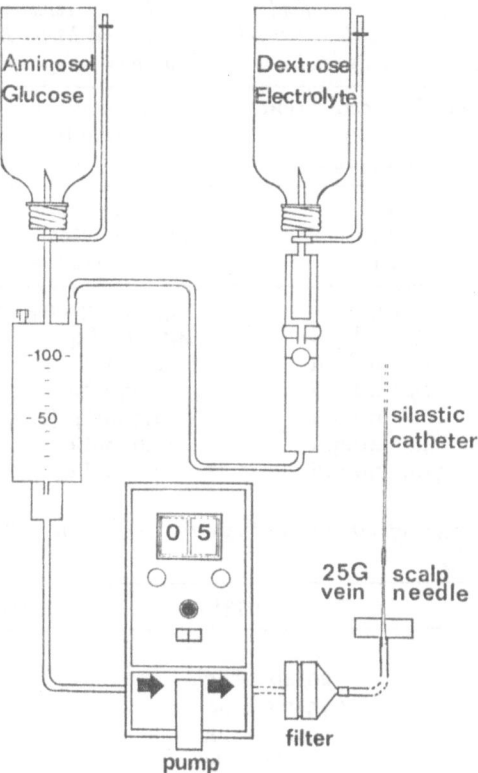

Fig. 6. Diagram showing the arrangement for mixing the parenteral infusion solution at the bedside.

Table 1.

A. *Dextrose Electrolyte Solution*

Potassium	15	mEq./l
Calcium (as gluconate)	30	mEq./l
Magnesium	8	mEq./l
Chloride	23	mEq./l

Dextrose: 15%, 25% or 35%

B. *Aminosol Glucose (Vitrum) Solution*

Amino acids	3.3	g%
Sodium	54	mEq./l
Potassium	0.15	mEq./l
Dextrose	5	%

C. *Phosphate Solutions:* (5 ml ampules)*

M K$_2$HPO$_4$ 2 mEq. of Cation and 30 mg Phosphorus/ml
M Na$_2$HPO$_4$

* either salt can be used depending on the plasma electrolyte results

Table 2. *Composition of intravenous fluid made up of equal volumes of aminosol glucose (Vitrum) and dextrose electrolyte solution + 0.5 ml Molar K_2HPO_4, per 100 ml of infusate, and the daily intakes when administered at 150 ml/kg day.*

	Final concentration in infusate	Daily intake per Kilogram body weight	Rate per kg per hour
Dextrose 15%	10%	15.0 g (68 cals)	0.63 g
25%	15%	22.5 g (98 cals)	0.93 g
35%	20%	30.0 g (128 cals)	1,25 g
Amino Acids	1.7 g%	2.5 g (320mg N_2)	
Sodium	27 mEq./l	4.0 m Eq.	
Potassium	17.5 mEq./l	2.6 mEq.	
Calcium	15.0 mEq./l	2.25 mEq. (45 mg)	
Phosphate	10.0 mEq./l	1.5 mEq. (22.5 mg)	
Magnesium	4.0 mEq./l	0.6 mEq.	
Chloride	31.5 mEq./l	4.5 mEq.	

Table 3. *Daily allowances of vitamins and essential fatty acids. All values per kg body weight and day.*

	Shaw (1973)		Wretlind (1972) (16)	
Fat soluble viatmins				
Retinol	20–40	μg	100	μg
Cholecalciferol	1.75–3.5	μg	2.5	μg
Phytylmenaqinone	35	μg	50	μg
αtocopherol	0.25	mg	3.0	mg
Water soluble vitamins				
Thiamin	1.0	mg	0.05	mg
Riboflavine	0.05	mg	0.1	mg
Nicotinamide	2.0	mg	1.0	mg
Pyridoxine	0.5	mg	0.1	mg
Folic acid	0.07	mg	0.02	mg
Cyanocobalamine	15.0	μg	0.2	μg
Ascorbic acid	15.0	mg	3.0	mg
Pantothenic acid	–		1.0	mg
Biotin	–		30.0	μg
Essential fatty acids				
Ethyl linoleate	300 mg/kg/day orally			
or Intralipid	2.5 ml/kg/day I.V.			

energy source because the foetus is thought to derive most of its energy from glucose, and because fat is not thought to be a major energy substrate for the foetus. However the recent report by GUSTAF-SON et al (9) suggests that low birthweight preterm infants can meta-bolise infused soy fat emulsions quite readily.

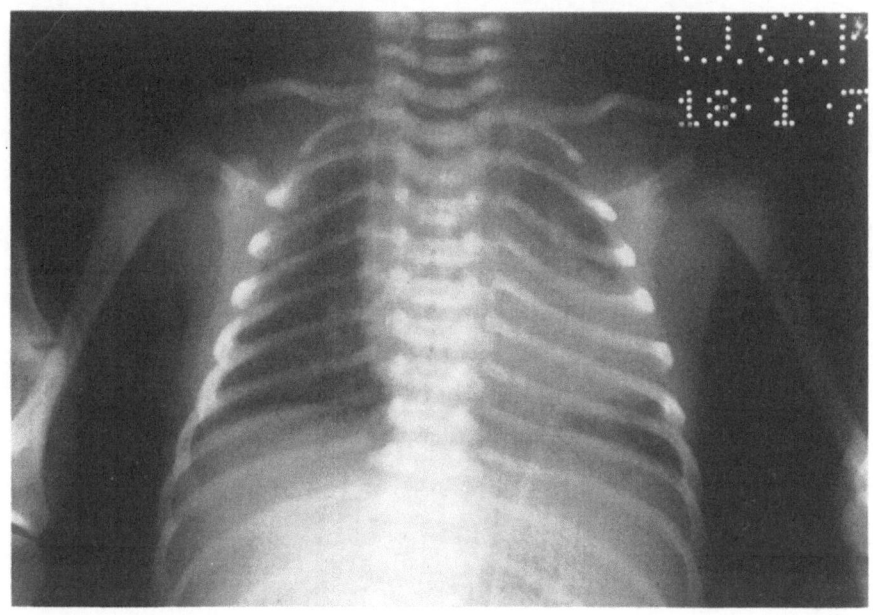

Fig. 5. X-ray showing a fine silicone rubber catheter, 0.6 mm o.d., and opacified with contrast medium, correctly positioned in the right atrium, the tip being located just below the lower border of the 5th rib.

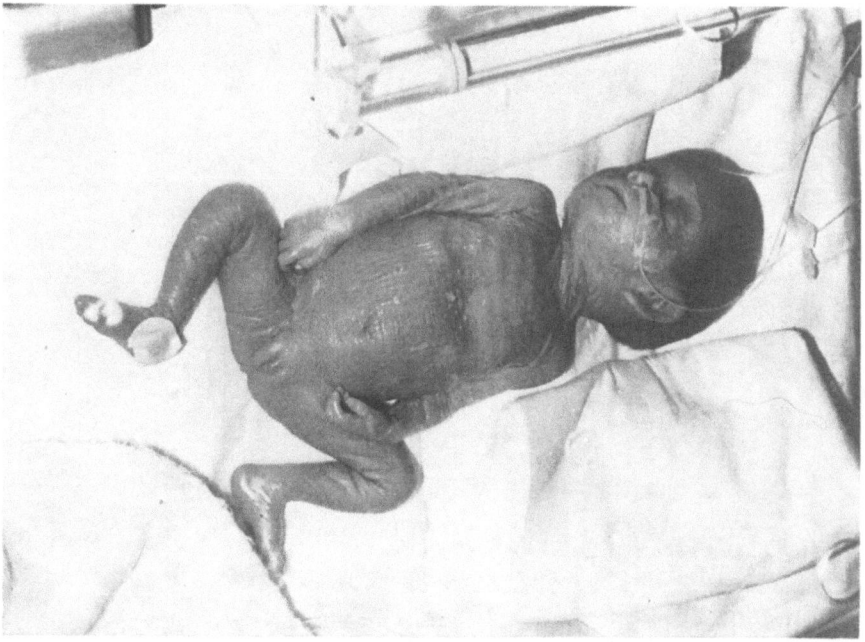

Fig. 8. Exfoliative skin condition occurring in a 765 gram infant of 25 weeks gestation who received virtually no dietary fat for the first 39 days of life.

Table 4. *Comparison of daily allowances of various substances, with their rate of accumultation by the human foetus in utero.*

	I.V. allowance per kg day		Rate of intrauterine accumulation per kg day
Nitrogen	320	mg	319–350 mg
Sodium	4.0	mEq.	1.0– 1.3 mEq.
Potassium	2.6	mEq.	0.75 mEq.
Calcium	2.25	mEq.	5.9–7.5 mEq.
Phosphorus	22.5	mg	70–86 mg
Magnesium	0.6	mEq.	0.32 mEq.

Table 4 compares the daily allowances of various substances with the rate of accumulation in utero. Two striking facts emerge; first that the infusion solution contains scarcely sufficient nitrogen, and also quite inadequate amounts of calcium and phosphorus. In practice, because these infants will tolerate fluid intakes of up to 200 ml/kg/day we find it possible to provide an adequate nitrogen intake by increasing the rate of infusion. However, since serious hyperammonaemia has been reported in infants given both protein hydrolysates and l-amino acid mixtures (10,11), we prefer at present to administer rather modest amounts of nitrogen. Because the period of parenteral feeding in these infants is usually relatively short we do not attempt to provide the amount of calcium and phosphorus required for normal skeletal mineralisation *in utero*, but provide an amount that is sufficient to maintain normal serum calcium. The infusion of much larger amounts of calcium and phosphorus, by binding basic ions in the bone mineral, would release substantial amounts of hydrogen ions in the E.C.F. and this might be undesirable in sick low birthweight infants whose acid base homeostasis is often already compromised (12).

For the provision of trace minerals we have relied upon plasma and blood transfusions. Table 5 shows that when the amounts of trace metals recommended by various authors are compared with the rate they accumulate *in utero*, there is a considerable discrepancy, and it seems likely from this data that we should be providing much more of these substances than we are at present.

RESULTS

We have now maintained thirty six infants on parenteral feeding for a mean period of 11 days (range 1–34 days). Of these cases 28 were of

Table 5. *A comparison of the suggested I.V. allowance of some trace elements with the daily rate of accumulation in utero. Values in mg/kg/day.*

	Wilmore et al (1969) (13)	Plasma at 40 ml/kg/wk* (14)	Daily increments in utero
Iron	0.020	0.008	1.6 –2.0
Copper	0.022	0.006	0.078–0.092
Zinc	0.040	0.007	0.272–0.337
Manganese	0.040	0.0006	?
Cobalt	0.014	0.002	?
Iodine	0.015	0.0004	?

* Calculated from values in Geigy Scientific Tables 1970 (15)

less than 2.5 kg birthweight. The mean birthweight of these 28 infants was 1223 grams (range 765 g–2270 g) and the mean gestation 29 weeks (range 25–33 weeks). They were fed intravenously because it was judged that their survival was seriously jeopardised by their inability to tolerate oral feeding. The principle indications were – oesophageal atresia, intestinal obstruction, severe hyaline membrane disease, apnoea of prematurity or very low birthweight (< 1.0 kg). Because they were all seriously ill the mortality was high in these infants (43%). There were no deaths in infants of more than 2.5 kg birthweight. The immediate cause of death in all cases was unrelated to intravenous feeding but in one case dehydration due to glycosuria and in two cases thrombosis associated with badly positioned catheters may have been a contributory cause of death.

Figure 7 gives as an example the growth chart of a 765 gram infant of 25 weeks gestation who was maintained on intravenous feeding for 34 days, because of severe recurrent neonatal apnoea. After the initial weight loss she gained weight at a mean rate of 11.0 grams per day, a rate comparable to orally fed infants of similar gestation but rather less than the calculated intrauterine rate of weight gain over an equivalent period. From the thirty fifth to the thirty ninth day of life this infant developed an exfoliative skin condition shown in figure 8. Because of its resemblance to reported cases (17) we think it is probably due to essential fatty acid deficiency, and the skin lesions recovered rapidly when a breast milk diet was introduced. Since an infant of this birthweight has only 5 grams of body fat to subsidise her future growth it is not surprising that such a deficiency state should arise on a fat free diet.

Because we have not conducted a controlled trial it is difficult to

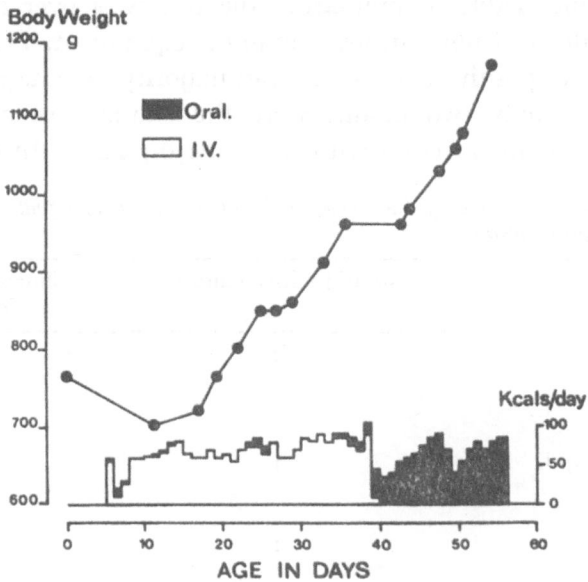

Fig. 7. Growth curve of a 765 gram infant of 25 weeks gestation who was maintained on total parenteral nutrition for a period of 34 days. After an initial weight loss she gained weight at a rate of about 11 grams per day.

establish beyond doubt that parenteral feeding has benefitted all the patients, some would undoubtedly have died without it but in other cases the benefit is not so easily evaluated. Analyses of our data for infants of less than 1.5 kg birthweight and fed intravenously shows that the mean weight gain over the first ten days of life was $+3$ g/day (± 6.0 g S.D.) whereas it was -6.8 g/day ($\pm$ 8.5 g S.D.) for all the infants of birthweight less than 1.5 kg surviving on our Unit in 1969 before the introduction of parenteral nutrition.

INFECTION

Finally, I would like to deal briefly with the question of infection, which is the commonest reported complication in parenteral nutrition. The prognosis for septicaemia in these infants is so bad that it is very important to be able to prevent it by knowing where the organisms are introduced. Sometimes there is pre-existing sepsis, and in other cases organisms are thought to track down the catheter, and in yet other instances it has been shown that the infusate has been infected

at some point. Table 6 summarises the results of over a thousand
bacterial cultures from various sites in the equipment. From a total
of seventy three positive cultures the vast majority were staphylococcus
albus, but in only two infants were the cultures associated with
clinically apparent infection with the same organism. In one case a

Table 6. *Summary of results of bacteriological investigations in 36 infants maintained on parenteral nutrition.*

Organism	No. of positive cultures	Clinically apparent infection
Staphylococcus Albus	61	1
Streptococcus haemolyticus Gp.D	1	0
Streptococcus Viridans	1	0
Escherichia Coli	1	0
Alkaligenes Species	1	0
Bacillus Species	4	0
Aspergillus Fumigatus	2	0
Candida Albicans	2	1

Frequency of positive culture by site

	Total	No. of positive cultures	Percentage positive cultures
Dextrose	305	12	3.9%
Aminosol	282	15	5.3%
Prefilter sample	193	15	7.7%
Filter membrane	76	7	9.2%
Post filter sample	151	17	11.3%
Catheter tip	23	4	17.0%
Skin swab before removal of catheter	12	2	16.0%

connector on the patient's side of the bacterial filter had split, and the infusion became infected with staphylococcus albus. Though this made the patient very ill, he recovered when the catheter was removed and penicillin given. The other case was a child who died on artificial ventilation from a candida albicans septicaemia. In this instance we are fairly certain that the catheter was infected from the patient because she had candida albicans in her lungs and blood culture at a time when all cultures from the infusion equipment were sterile. Since the skin swab at the point of entry of the catheter was also sterile, it seems improbable that the intravenous feeding was responsible for the septicaemia. Thus our overall infection rate attributable to the procedure is at present 2.7% and is zero for the low birthweight infants. The majority of the positive cultures were sporadic, and probably represent contamination from the outside of the apparatus during sampling. Examining the frequency of positive cultures by site probably indicates therefore the relative risk of introducing organisms at different places on the equipment. The highest risk would seem to be at the junction on the patient's side of the filter assembly which is usually in the incubator close to the infant, and which is broken each day when the apparatus is changed. Because of this we have placed this filter outside the incubator and at present we are studying different ways of protecting this junction from contamination. The high incidence of positive cultures from the catheter tips is worrying. Two were associated with proven infection described above and the other two were due to staphylococcus albus and occurred in otherwise healthy infants who had negative blood cultures. Since the skin swab at the time of removal were sterile these positive cultures probably represent colonisation of the catheter tip.

SUMMARY

Because of their poor energy reserves and rapid rate of growth, low birthweight infants are likely to be particularly vulnerable to malnutrition. Judging from the rate at which elements accumulate in the foetus *in utero* their requirements for nitrogen, calcium and some trace minerals are likely to be greater per kg body weight than those of a full-term infant. A simple technique of long-term intravenous infusion into the right atrium of the heart using fine silicone rubber catheters has been developed which is suitable and safe for low birthweight infants. Our experience with the first 36 cases managed in this way shows that low birthweight infants can grow when fed entirely intravenously, and also that it is a useful adjunct to oral feeding. The risk of infection is great but can be reduced to acceptable levels by sufficient attention to detail.

MATHEMATICAL METHODS

The regression lines were fitted to the data using the method of least squares and the equation $l_nY = l_nY_0 + kt$ (t = gestational age in days, Y_0 is taken for convenience as the value for Y when t = 0, k = a rate constant. The growth velocity or rate of accumulation of a substance at any moment $\left(\dfrac{dy}{dt}\right)$ is equal to k x Y_t).

APPENDIX
Equipment referenced by letter in text

A. Silastic Medical Grade Tubing. Dow Corning Corporation, Products Division, Midland (Mich.) U.S.A. 48640.
B. 19 guage Scalp Vein needle. Abbott Laboratories, North Chicago (Ill.) U.S.A.
C. Aminosol Glucose Vitrum. Stockholm, Sweden.
D. Drip Sets. AKCO 135, & AKC 2045. Baxter Laboratories Ltd., Thetford, Norfolk, England.
E. Ivac 500 Infusion Pump. Tekmar Medical Ltd., Harrow-on-the-Hill, Mddx., England.
F. Filter Millex T.M. disposable filter unit. SLGS. 0250S–0.22 μ. Millepore Corporation, Bedford (Mass.) 01730 U.S.A.

REFERENCES

1. HEIRD, W. C., DRISCOLL, J. M., JR., SCHULLINGER, J. N., GREBIN, B. and WINTERS, R. W., (1972) Intravenous alimentation in pediatric patients. *Journal of Pediatrics*, 80, 351.
2. Lipids, Malnutrition and the Developing Brain. *Ciba Foundation Symposium.* Associated Scientific Publishers. Amsterdam, London, New York. (1972).
3. KLOOSTERMAN, G. J., (1970) On intrauterine growth. *International Journal of Gynaecology and Obstetrics*, 8, 895.
4. LUBCHENKO, L. O., HANSMAN, C., DRESSLER, M. and BOYD, E., (1963) In-

trauterine growth as estimated from liveborn birthweight data at 24 to 42 weeks of gestation. *Pediatrics*, 32, 793.

5. WIDDOWSON, E. M. and DICKERSON, J. W. T., (1961) In: Comar, C. L. and Bronner, F. (eds.), *Mineral Metabolism*. Vol. II, Part A. Academic Press. New York and London.

6. KELLY, H. J., SLOAN, R. E., HOFFMAN, W. and SAUNDERS, C., (1950) Accumulation of nitrogen and six minerals in the human foetus during gestation. *Human Biology*, 2, 61.

7. WILMORE, D. W. and DUDRICK, S. J., (1968) Growth and development of an infant receiving all nutrients exclusively by vein. *Journal of the American Medical Association*, 203, 860.

8. SHAW, J. C. L., (1973) Parenteral nutrition in sick low birthweight infants. *Pediatric Clinics of North America*, 20, 333.

9. GUSTAFSON, A., KJELLMER, I., OLEGARD, R. and VICTORIN, L., (1972) Nutrition in low birthweight infants. 1. Intravenous injection of fat emulsion. *Acta Paediatrica Scandinavica*, 61, 149.

10. HEIRD, W. C., NICHOLSON, J. F., DRISCOLL, J. M., JR., SCHULLINGER, J. N. and WINTERS, R. W., (1972) Hyperammonaemia resulting from intravenous alimentation using a mixture of synthetic 1-amino acids: A preliminary report. *Journal of Pediatrics* 81, 162.

11. JOHNSON, J. D., ALBRITTON, W. L. and SUNSHINE, P., (1972) Hyperammonaemia accompanying parenteral nutrition in newborn infants. *Journal of Pediatrics* 81, 154.

12. KILDEBERG, P., ENGEL, K. and WINTERS, R. W., (1969) Balance of net acid in growing infants. Endogenous and Transintestinal Aspects. *Acta Paediatrica Scandinavica*, 58, 321.

13. WILMORE, D. W., GROFF, D. B., BISHOP, H. C. and DUDRICK, S. J., (1969) Total parenteral nutrition in infants with catastrophic gastrointestinal anomalies. *Journal of Pediatric Surgery*, 4, 181.

14. FILLER, R. M., ERAKLIS, A. J., RUBIN, V. G. and DAS, J. B., (1969) Long-term total parenteral nutrition in infants. *New England Journal of Medicine*, 281, 589.

15. Documenta Geigy – Scientific Tables, (1970) Ed: Diem, K.

16. WRETLIND, A. (1972). Complete intravenous nutrition theoretical and experimental background. *Nutrition and Metabolism 14* Suppl: 1.

17. HANSEN, A. E., WIESE, H. F., BOELSCHE, A. N., HAGGARD, M. E., ADAM, D. J. D. and DAVIS, H., (1963) Role of linoleic acid in infant nutrition. *Pediatrics*, 31, 171.

PARENTERAL NUTRITION IN LOW-BIRTH WEIGHT INFANTS

H. K. A. VISSER*, W. BLOM**, J. F. VAN GILS* AND T. ZURCHER*

INTRODUCTION

For a long time there has been a difference of opinion among pediatricians as to the timing of the first feeding as well as the type of food for the low-birth weight infant.

During the twenties and thirties early feeding of the premature baby was recommended on the assumption that these small infants do not tolerate starvation (1) (2) (3) (4). During the forties and fifties it was strongly advocated that feeding should be delayed until several days after birth to prevent vomiting and aspiration; it was thought that many premature infants were overhydrated at birth (5) (6) (7). This concept was challenged by YLPPÖ in 1954. Noting that fasting caused acidosis and disturbances of the renal function, he recommended that premature babies be given fluids and food as early as possible (8).

Since the early 1960's increasing evidence has shown that early feeding of low-birth weight infants is highly beneficial to their metabolic homeostasis. Numerous studies have indicated that an early intake of fluid and calories will reduce the hazards of thirst and fasting in these babies: depletion of glycogen stores and hypoglycaemia; metabolic acidosis; dehydration with increases in serum osmolality, and urea, potassium and sodium concentrations; hyperbilirubinaemia; protein catabolism (9) (10) (11) (12) (13) (14) (15).

Although comparative studies have not been carried out and are now ethically impossible, there is considerable evidence that the influence of early feeding on metabolic homeostasis will lower the risk of permanent brain damage (16).

* Departments of Pediatrics* and Clinical Chemistry**, Erasmus University and Academic Hospital/Sophia Children's Hospital and Neonatal Unit, Rotterdam, The Netherlands.

The rate of growth in length, weight and head circumference is very high during the last trimester of pregnancy. It is important to avoid nutritional restrictions during the period in which the brain grows the fastest (17) (18) (19) (20).

In this paper we will discuss our experience with early intake of fluid and calories (humanized milk and 10% glucose intravenously) in low-birth weight infants, and its effect on growth during the first weeks of life. We would also like to present the data of a pilot study on some metabolic effects of intravenous alimentation with amino acids and fats in 4 low-birth weight infants. We will not discuss the management of low-birth weight infants who have undergone neonatal surgery.

EARLY INTAKE OF FLUID AND CALORIES (HUMANIZED MILK AND I.V. GLUCOSE): ITS EFFECT ON GROWTH DURING THE FIRST WEEKS OF LIFE

Since 1968 it has been our practice to give all low-birth weight infants (birth weight < 2500 grams) 10% or 15% glucose and water intravenously (via the umbilical vein but preferably via a scalp or peripheral vein) as soon as possible after birth. Milk feeding is started 2–4 hours after birth. We have used humanized milk feedings (Almiron-A and Almiron-M₂; Nutricia) exclusively and the milk is given continuously by gastric drip. An indwelling plastic feeding catheter is inserted through a nostril into the stomach. To administer small amounts of milk accurately and continuously we use an i.v. drip system (infant-model). Great care is taken to control the ambient temperature of the infants.

During the first 24 hours 60 ml/kg combined parenteral and oral feeding is given; this is increased each day to 80, 100, 120, 140, 160 and 180 ml/kg, respectively. The total quantity of milk feeding is 20–40 ml/kg on the first day and is increased up to 200 ml/kg on the 8th day of life. Average caloric intake is 60–80 kcal/kg/d during the first week, and 130–140 kcal/kg/d during the second and following weeks of life. Length, head circumference and skin folds are measured every 1–2 weeks. Weight is recorded each day. After discharge (weight about 3000 grams) the infants are seen at regular intervals at a special outpatient clinic. More than 200 infants and children are now included in this long-term study of the postnatal growth and development in low-birth weight infants. Full details of this study will be presented in a thesis by J. F. VAN GILS.

Figures 1–9 and 10–16 present weight, length and head circumference data for a small number of low-birth weight infants during the first weeks of life. These infants are a representative sample of the above-mentioned group.

In premature infants (without respiratory distress syndrome) initial weight loss during the first week of life is limited (usually less than 5 percent of birth weight) and in many premature infants (including twins) there is an increase in weight (up to 5 percent) after one week. This is illustrated in figures 10, 13 and 14. When compared with the intra-uterine growth curves (from USHER and McLEAN, *J. Pediat.* 74, 901, 1969) growth in length, weight and head circumference lags for one or two weeks after birth, but from then on it is normal for the gestational age (figures 1, 2 and 3). In some cases catch-up-growth can be demonstrated.

In small-for-date babies there is usually an immediate increase in weight, length and head circumference. In small-for-date babies with a gestational age of less than 36 weeks, growth rates lag for one or two weeks. Further growth rates are either normal for the gestational age or demonstrate catch-up-growth, particularly in head circumference (21). This is illustrated in figures 1, 2, 3, 11 and 12.

In premature infants with respiratory distress syndrome initial weight loss may be 5–10 percent of birth weight. Although caloric intake is not different, growth rates during the first two weeks are usually less than those of infants without RDS (figures 7, 8, 9, 15 and 16).

Some low-birth weight infants, particularly very small premature infants and infants with respiratory distress syndrome, do not tolerate a rapid increase in the volume of oral intake during the first week of life and demonstrate symptoms of abdominal distension and regurgitation. To avoid the risks of aspiration the rate of increase of oral feeding is reduced and parenteral fluid is continued for a longer period of time. In such infants it is difficult to meet the nutritional needs over a period of several weeks after birth. In an attempt to provide these infants with adequate nutrition at a critical time of maturation, total or partial intravenous alimentation with amino acid solutions and/or fat emulsions has been used. A limited number of studies have been reported and most authors remain cautious (22) (23) (24) (25). More experience has been gained from the use of intravenous alimenta-

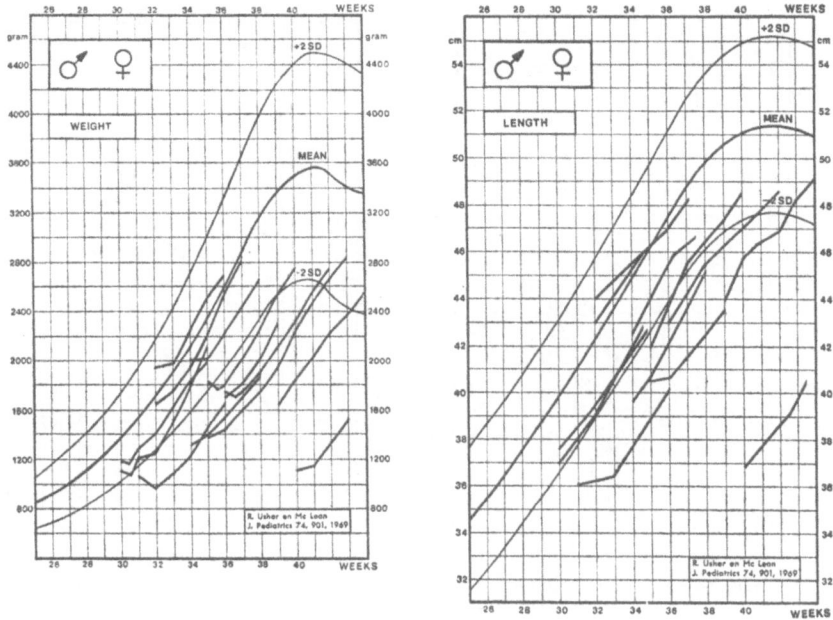

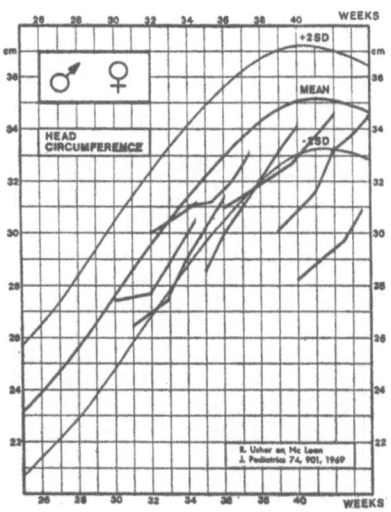

Figures 1, 2 and 3. Weight, length and head circumference data for a small number of low-birth weight infants during the first weeks of life. See text. (Standard growth curves are from USHER and McLEAN, *J. Pediat.* 74, 901, 1969).

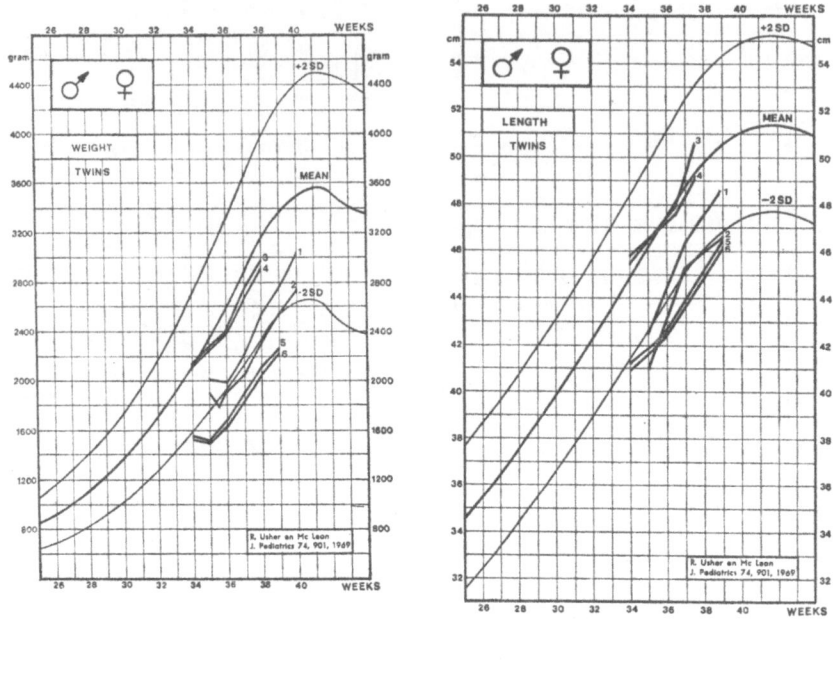

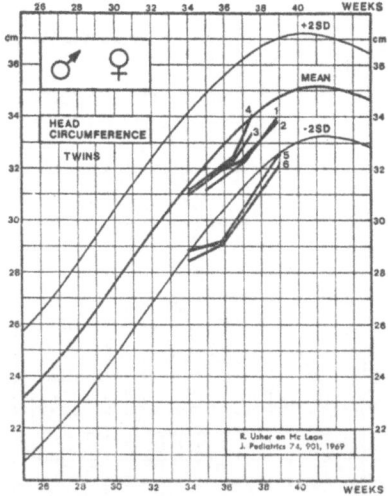

Figures 4, 5 and 6. Weight, length and head circumference data for 3 pairs of twins with low birth weight during the first weeks of life. See text. (Standard growth curves are from USHER and McLEAN, *J. Pediat.* 74, 901, 1969).

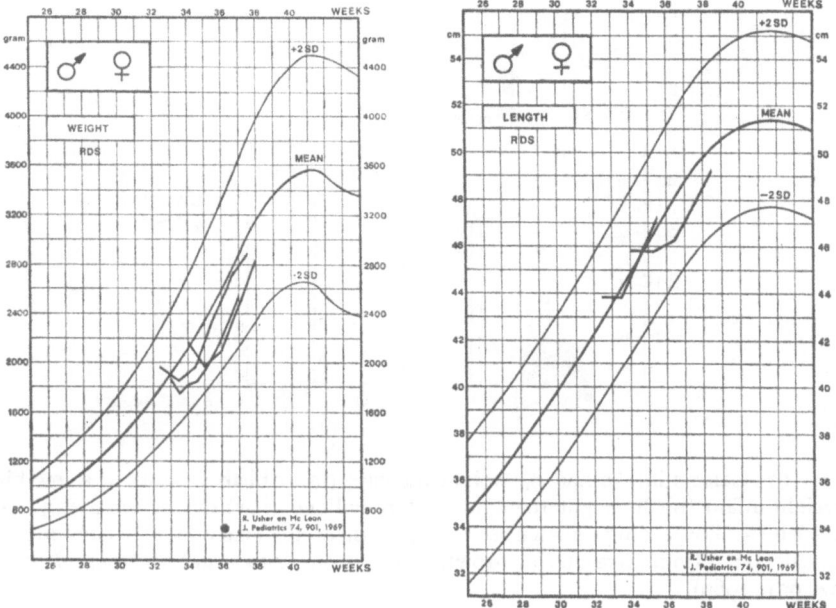

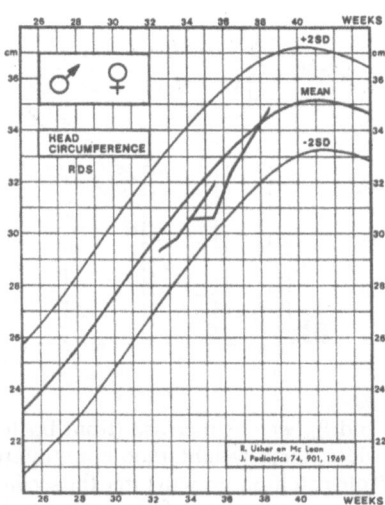

Figures 7, 8 and 9. Weight, length and head circumference data for a few low-birth weight infants with severe respiratory distress syndrome. See text. (Standard growth curves are from USHER and McLEAN, *J. Pediat.* 74, 901, 1969)

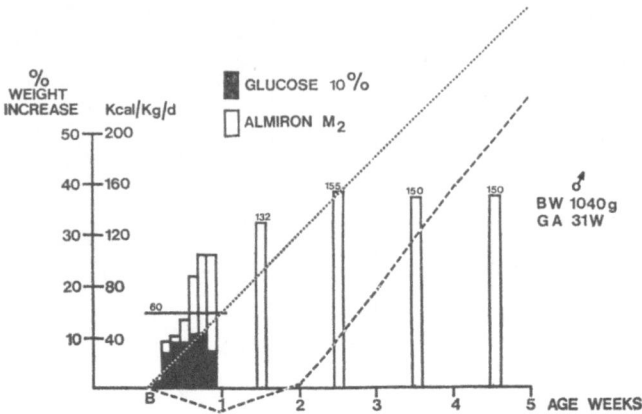

Fig. 10. Caloric intake and % weight increase (from birth weight) in a low-birth weight infant (birth weight 1040 gm, gestational age 31 w) during the first 5 weeks after birth. For feeding regimen see text. (. . . theoretical curve of % weight increase as calculated from intra-uterine growth curves from USHER and McLEAN, *J. Pediat.* 74, 901, 1969).

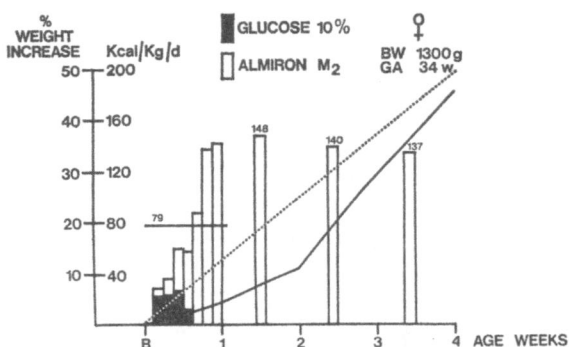

Fig. 11. Caloric intake and % weight increase (from birth weight) in a low-birth weight infant (small-for-date, birth weight 1300 gm, gestational age 34 w) during the first 4 weeks of life. Note catch-up-growth after the second week. (. . . theoretical curve of % weight increase as calculated from intra-uterine growth curves from USHER and McLEAN, *J. Pediat.* 74, 901, 1969).

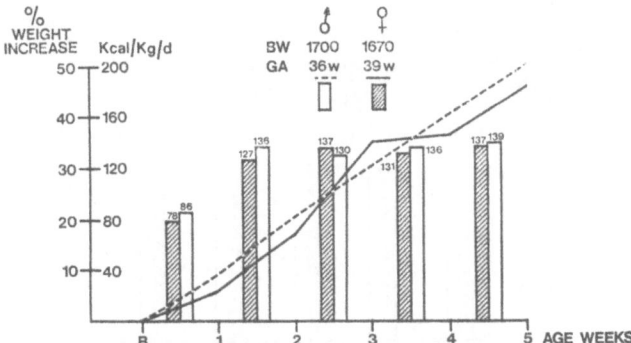

Fig. 12. Caloric intake and % weight increase (from birth weight) in two low-birth weight infants (small-for-date) during the first 5 weeks after birth. Theoretical curve (as calculated from intra-uterine growth curves) for 36–40 weeks of gestational age is the same as observed curve for infant GA 36 w. (. . .).

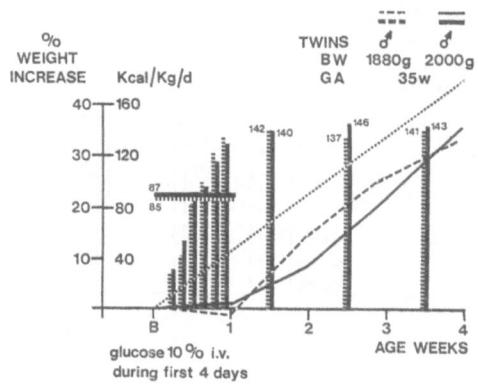

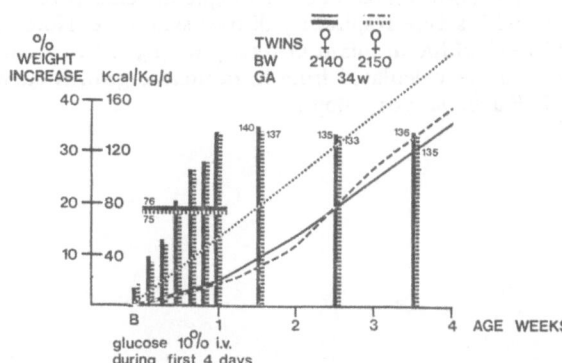

Figures 13 and 14. Caloric intake and % weight increase (from birth weight) in two pairs of twins with low birth weight. (. . . theoretical curve of % weight increase as calculated from intra-uterine growth curves from USHER and MCLEAN, *J. Pediat.* 74, 901, 1969).

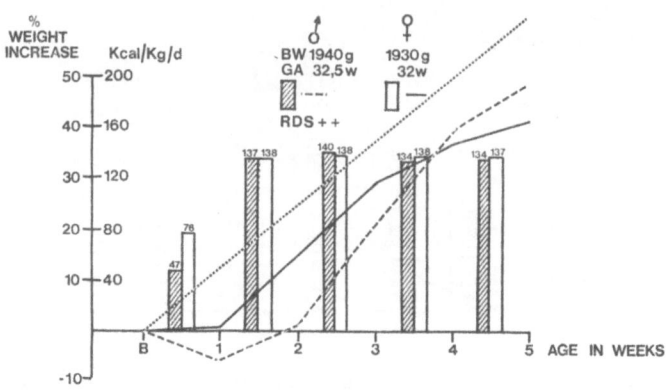

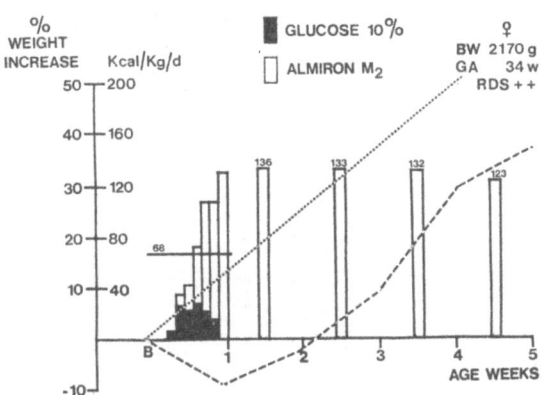

Figures 15 and 16. Caloric intake and % weight increase (from birth weight) in two LBW infants with severe respiratory distress syndrome. Note catch-up-growth after the second week of life in infant GA 32, 5 w. (fig. 15). (... theoretical curve of % weight increase as calculated from intra-uterine growth curves from USHER and McLEAN, *J. Pediat.* 74, 901, 1969).

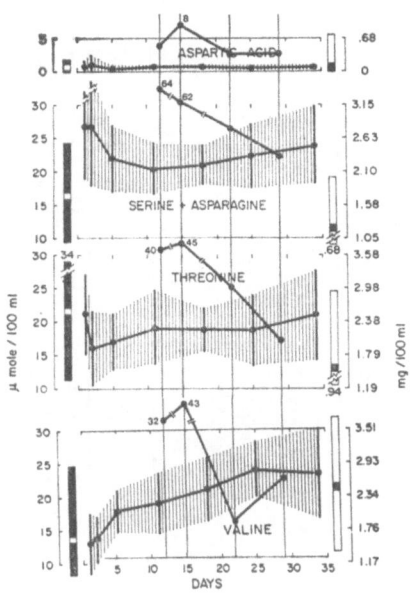

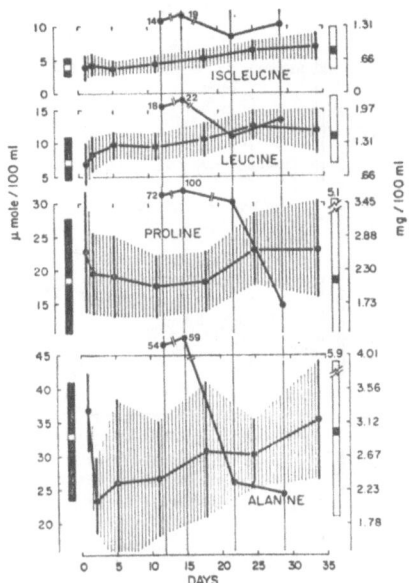

Fig. 17a, b, c, d. Plasma amino concentrations in patient 1. (See table 8). Data are plotted against the data for normal LBW infants from DICKINSON et al. (42), reproduced with permission of authors and publisher.

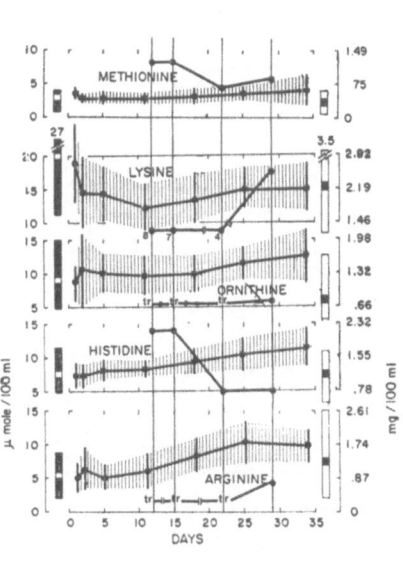

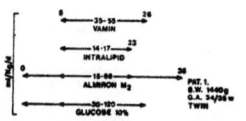

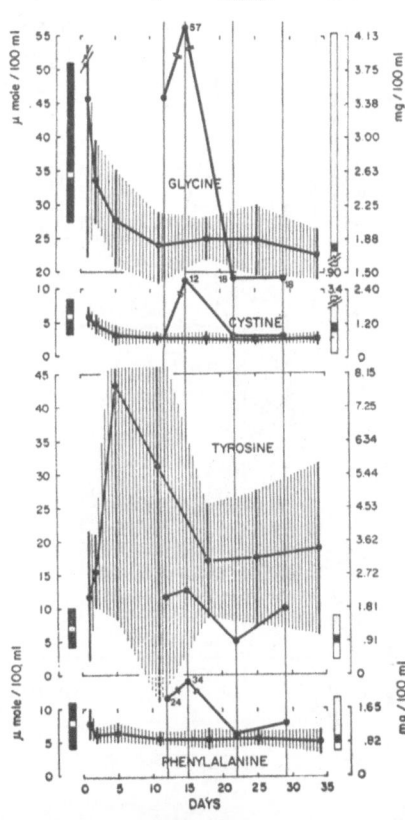

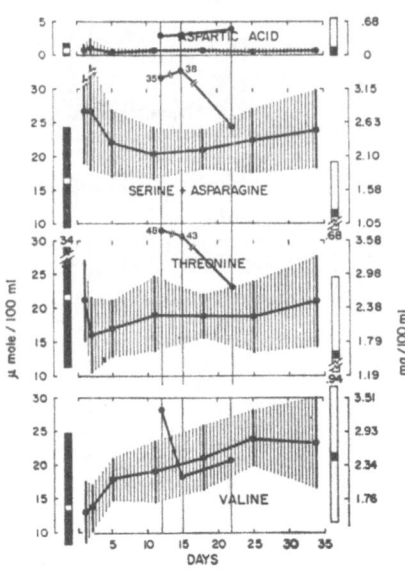

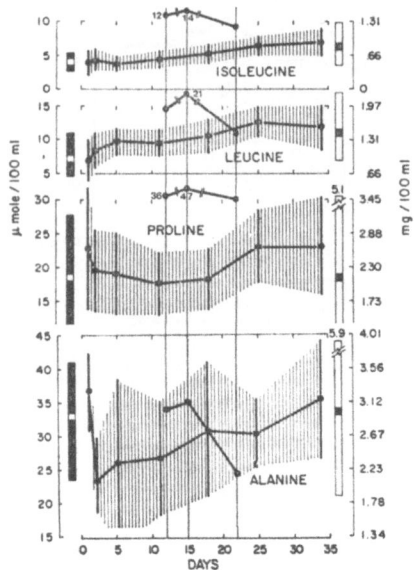

Fig. 18a, b, c, d. Plasma amino acid concentrations in patient 2 (See table 9). Data are plotted against the data for normal LBW infants from DICKINSON et al. (42), reproduced with permission of authors and publisher.

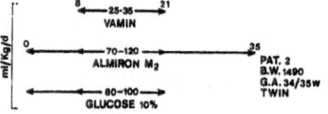

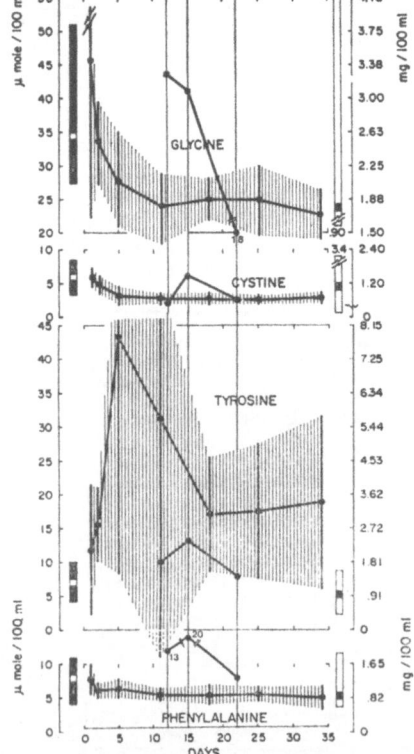

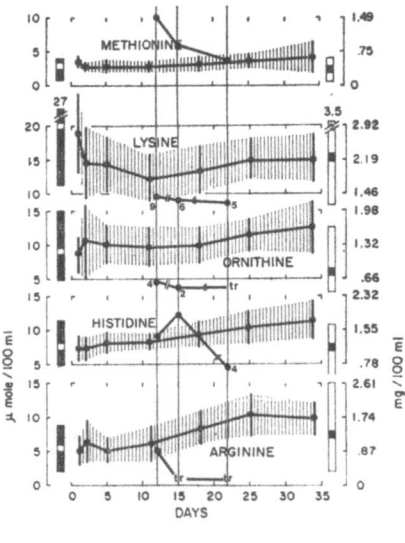

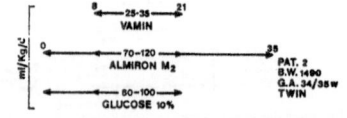

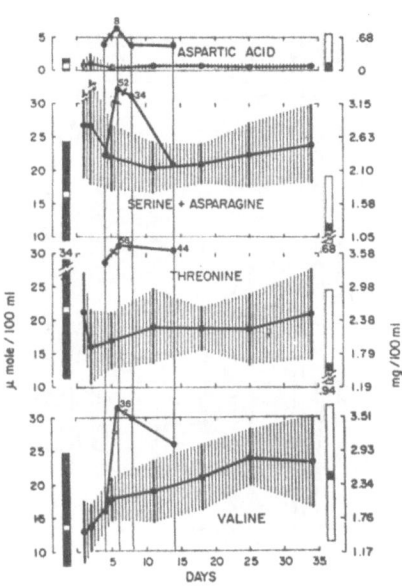

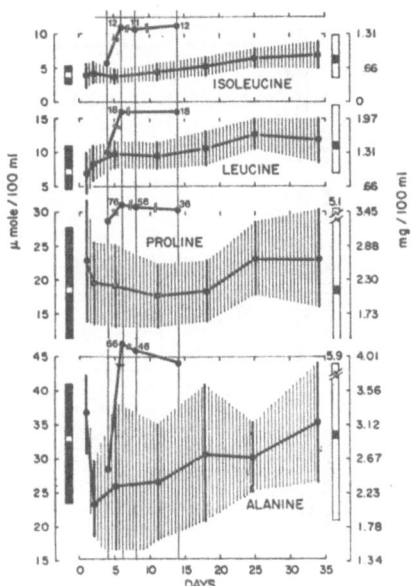

Fig. 19a, b, c, d. Plasma amino acid concentrations in patient 3 (See table 10). Data are plotted against the data for normal LBW infants from DICKINSON et al. (42), reproduced with permission of authors and publisher.

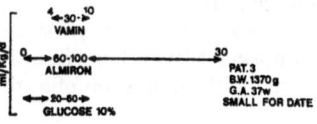

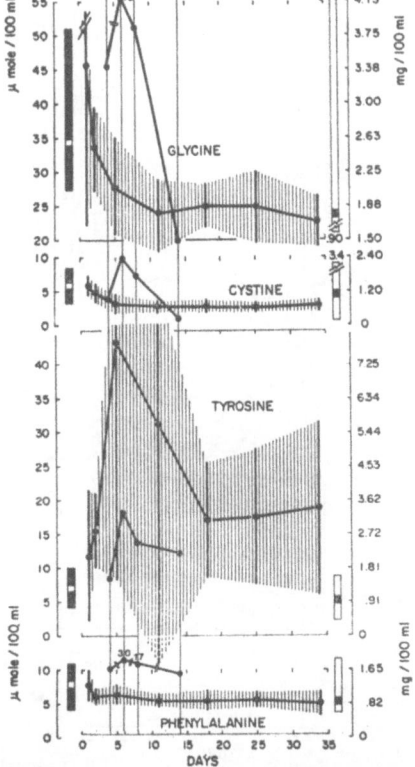

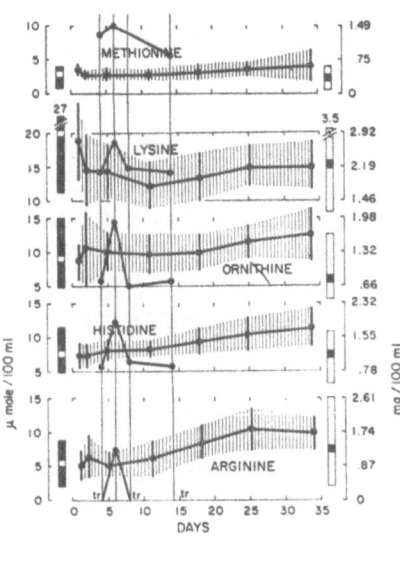

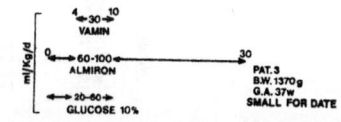

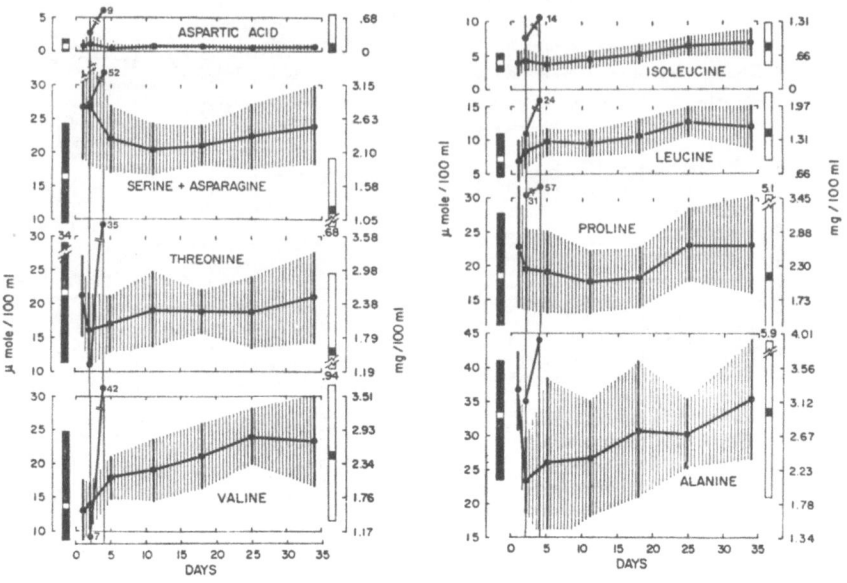

Fig. 20a, b, c, d. Plasma amino acid concentrations in patient 4 (See table 11). Data are plotted against the data for normal LBW infants from DICKINSON et al. (42), reproduced with permission of authors and publisher.

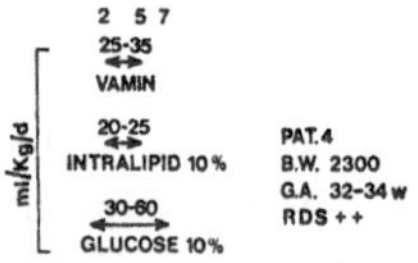

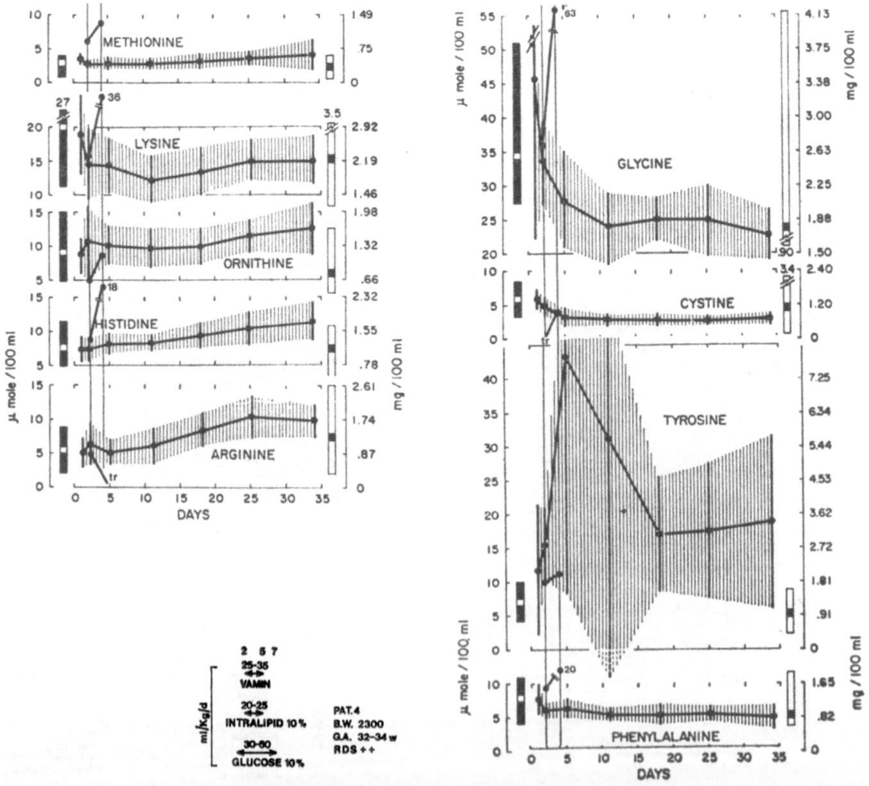

tion after neonatal surgery (26) (27) and in the treatment of protracted diarrhoea (28). Such feedings are administered via either a
central venous or a peripheral catheter (29). Apart from technical
and other problems, such as septicaemia and phlebitis, metabolic
problems such as hyperammonaemia (30) (31), imbalance of plasma
amino acids (32) and metabolic acidosis (33) have been reported.

SOME METABOLIC EFFECTS OF INTRAVENOUS ALIMENTATION IN 4 LOW-BIRTH WEIGHT INFANTS: A PILOT STUDY

In a pilot study some metabolic effects of intravenous alimentation in
4 low-birth weight infants were studied.
Two premature babies (patients 1 and 2; twins; birth weight 1440 and
1490 grams; gestational age 34–35 weeks) were given humanized milk
(Almiron-M$_2$: Nutricia) by gastric drip and 10% glucose (intravenously) for the first 21 and 26 days of life, respectively. An amino
acid solution (7% Vamin, Vitrum) was administered to one infant
(patient 2) between the 8th and 21st days; the other infant (patient 1)
received Vamin (8th–26th day) and a fat emulsion (10% Intralipid,
Vitrum) from the 8th to the 23rd day (tables 1 and 2). Both infants

Tables 1–4. *Feeding regimen in 4 low-birth weight infants. Combined parenteral and oral
feeding in patients 1, 2 and 3. Parenteral feeding in patient 4. For further
explanation see text.*

Table 1

Patient 1 Days after birth	BW 1440 g 8	GA 34–35 w	(twin) 23 26
Vamin ml/kg/d protein g/kg/d	– –	35–55 2.1–3.3	– –
10% Intralipid ml/kg/d fat g/kg/d	– –	14–17 1.4–1.7	– –
Almiron M$_2$ ml/kg/d protein g/kg/d	10–80 0.15–1.2	15–80 0.25–1.2	185–200 2.8–3.0
10% Glucose ml/kg/d	45–80	30–120	–
Calories Kcal/kg/d	25–80	65–120 (average 104)	125–140

Table 2.

Patient 2	BW 1490 gm	GA 34–35 w	(twin)
Days after birth	8		21
Vamin			
ml/kg/d	–	25–35	–
protein g/kg/d	–	1.5–2.1	–
Almiron M₂			
ml/kg/d	10–100	70–120	185–200
protein g/kg/d	0.15–1.5	1.1–1.8	2.8–3.0
10% Glucose			
ml/kg/d	35–50	80–100	–
Calories			
Kcal/kg/d	25–85 (av. 56)	70–120 (av. 108)	125–140

Table 3.

Patient 3	BW 1370 gm	GA 37 w	(small-for-date)
Days after birth	4	10	
Vamin			
ml/kg/d	–	30	–
protein g/kg/d	–	1.8	–
Almiron M₂			
ml/kg/d	5–50	60–100	200
protein g/kg/d	0.075–0.75	0.9–1.5	3
10% Glucose			
ml/kg/d	25–60	20–60	–
Calories			
Kcal/kg/d	10–60	75–125	140

Table 4.

Patient 4	BW 2300 gm	GA 32–34 w	RDS++
Days after birth	2	5	7†
Vamin			
ml/kg/d	25–35		
protein gm/kg/d	1.5–2.1		
10% Intralipid			
ml/kg/d	20–25		
fat g/kg/d	2.0–2.5		
10% Glucose			
ml/kg/d	30–60		
Calories			
Kcal/kg/d	20–75		

Table 5. *Total daily intake of protein, carbohydrates, fat and minerals (per kg body weight) on a combined feeding regimen of Almiron-M₂ 10% glucose, Vamin and Intralipid.*

	Volume ml	kcal.	Protein	Carbohydrates g	Fat	Na	K	Cl	P	Ca	Mg
								meq.			
Human milk	200	138	2.4	13.0	8.5	0.9	2.0	1.7	1.2	3.0	0.6
Almiron-M₂	200	138	3.0	15.0	7.0	1.3	2.4	1.4	3.2	5.0	0.8
Vamin	30	20	1.8	3.0 (fructose)	—	1.5	0.6	1.5	—	0.2	0.1
Almiron-M₂	80	55	1.2	6.0	2.8	0.5	1.0	0.6	1.3	2.0	0.3
10% Glucose	90	36	—	9.0	—	—	—	—	—	—	—
I.Total feeding i.v. + oral	200	110	3.0	18.0	2.8	2.0	1.6	2.1	1.3	2.2	0.4
10% Intralipid	20	22	—	—	2.0	—	—	—	—	—	—
II. Total feeding i.v. + oral	220	132	3.0	18.0	4.8	2.0	1.6	2.1	1.3	2.2	0.4

were healthy and gave no specific problems, but they did not tolerate large volumes of oral intake during the first weeks of life.

One small-for-date infant (patient 3; birth weight 1370 gram; gestational age 37 weeks) was given Almiron-M_2 and 10% glucose for the first 10 days of life; Vamin was added from the 4th to 10th day (table 3). In this otherwise healthy infant the low birth weight was the result of placental insufficiency with toxaemia of the mother.

One premature infant with severe respiratory distress syndrome (patient 4; birth weight 2300 gram; gestational age 32–34 weeks) received 10% glucose, Vamin and Intralipid during the first 6 days of life. This infant died on the 7th day.

7% Vamin was given continuously at a rate of 25–55 ml/kg/d (total protein 1.5–3.3 g/kg/d). Total daily protein intake (oral and parenteral feeding) was not more than 3.5 g/kg.

10% Intralipid was administered continuously at a rate of 14–25 ml/kg/d (total fat 1.4–2.5 g/kg/d).

10% Glucose was given at a rate of 25–120 ml/kg/d. Maximum fluid intake was 220 ml/kg/d. I. v. fluids were given via peripheral vein, using a constant infusion pump. Total caloric intake varied between 25–125 kcal/kg/d.

The total daily intake of protein, carbohydrates, fat and minerals on a combined feeding regimen of Almiron-M_2, Vamin and Intralipid is shown in table 5. This table also gives the total daily intake of nutrients from human milk and Almiron-M_2 (200 ml/kg/d).

The amino acid composition of two commercially available amino acid solutions (Aminosol, Vitrum; Vamin, Vitrum) is compared with that of egg protein, human milk and Almiron-M_2 in table 6. Vamin has a relatively high content of a number of amino acids: phenylalanine, proline, serine, glycine, alanine and arginine. The content of tyrosine is low.

Table 7 shows the daily intake of individual amino acids (mmol/ kg/d) when a low-birth weight infant is fed on human milk or Almiron-M_2 (200 ml/kg/d) or Vamin (intravenously; 50 ml/kg/d), or a combined oral (Almiron-M_2, 80 ml/kg/d) and parenteral feeding (Vamin, 30 ml/kg/d). On this combined feeding total protein intake is 3.0 g/kg/d. It is evident that when Vamin is given at a rate of 30–50 ml/kg/d, the daily intake of serine, proline, alanine, glycine, phenylalanine and arginine is relatively high. On the other hand the daily intake of tyrosine is low.

Table 6. *Amino acid composition of two commercially available amino acid solutions (Aminosol and Vamin, Vitrum) as compared with egg protein, human milk and Almiron-M₂ (Nutricia). E/T ratio is total amount of essential amino acids per 100 g protein or 16 g nitrogen.*

	Egg protein (1)	Human milk(2)	Almiron-M₂* (Nutricia)	Aminosol* (Vitrum)	Vamin* (Vitrum)
Isoleucine	5.8	5.6	5.7	7.3	6.6
Leucine	9.0	9.4	11.0	11.4	9.0
Lysine	6.7	6.2	9.0	7.4	6.6
Phenylalanine	5.3	4.0	3.8	} 6.9	9.4
Tyrosine	4.3	4.8	3.4		0.8
Methionine	3.0	2.1	2.4	} 4.5	3.2
Cysteine/cystine	2.1	2.0	1.6		2.4
Threonine	5.3	4.5	5.4	4.4	5.1
Tryptophan	1.8	1.6	1.3	1.1	1.7
Valine	7.2	6.2	6.8	5.2	7.3
E = tot. essential amino acids	50.5	46.4	50.4	48.2	52.1
Alanine	–	3.8	3.9	2.9	5.1
Arginine	6.4	3.4	2.6	2.9	5.6
Asparagine	–	–	–	–	–
Aspartic acid	10.7	9.3	9.0	6.0	7.0
Glutamic acid	12.3	19.8	19.2	22.7	15.3
Glycine	3.8	2.2	1.7	2.2	3.6
Histidine	2.6	2.2	2.1	2.6	4.1
Ornithine	–	–	–	–	–
Proline	4.3	8.6	6.8	9.4	13.8
Serine	7.7	4.8	4.8	7.5	12.8
E/T ratio	3.2	2.9	3.2	3.0	3.2

References 1 and 2: R. A. Mc Cance and E. M. Widdowson, (1960) *The composition of foods*, Medical Res. Council, Special report Series no.: 297, Her Majesty's Stationery Office, London, p. 253.

* Amino acid composition as given by the manufacturer.

Table 7. *Amino acid composition (mmol/l) of human milk, Almiron-M₂ (Nutricia) and Vamin (Vitrum). Calculated daily intake of individual amino acids (human milk and Almiron-M₂ 200 ml/kg/d; Vamin 50 ml/kg/d; Vamin 30 ml/kg/d and Almiron-M₂ 80 ml/kg/d in combination with Almiron-M₂ 80 ml/kg/d).*

| | Human milk mmol/l [2] | Vamin (Vitrum) mmol/l [1] | Human milk mmol/200 ml/kg/d | Vamin mmol/50 ml/kg/d | Minimum requirement infants [4] mmol/kg/d | Almiron-M₂ (Nutricia) mmol/l [1] | Almiron-M₂ mmol/200 ml/kg/d | Combined oral and parenteral feeding | | |
								Vamin mmol/30 ml/kg/d	Almiron-M₂ mmol/80 ml/kg/d	Total mmol/kg/d
Aspartic acid	—	30.80	—	1.54		9.74	1.95	0.92	0.78	1.70
Threonine	5.04	25.18	1.01	1.26	0.48	6.53	1.31	0.75	0.52	1.27
Serine	6.37	71.36	1.27	3.57		6.57	1.31	2.14	0.52	2.66
Asparagine	8.55	—	1.71	—		—	—	—	—	—
Glutamic acid	15.15	61.18	3.03	3.05		18.80	3.76	1.84	1.50	3.34
Proline	6.78	70.37	1.36	3.52		8.50	1.70	2.11	0.68	2.79
Glycine	3.13 [3]	27.96	0.63	1.40		3.26	0.65	0.83	0.26	1.09
Alanine	3.81	33.67	0.76	1.68		6.31	1.26	1.01	0.50	1.51
Valine	7.43	36.70	1.48	1.83	0.84	8.35	1.67	1.10	0.67	1.77
Cystine	1.16	5.82	0.23	0.29		0.96	0.19	0.17	0.07	0.24
Methionine	1.47	12.73	0.29	0.64	0.30	2.32	0.46	0.38	0.18	0.56
Isoleucine	6.33	29.72	1.26	1.49	0.91	6.26	1.25	0.89	0.50	1.39
Leucine	11.89	40.39	2.38	2.02	1.14	12.07	2.41	1.21	0.96	2.17
Tyrosine	3.31	2.76	0.66	0.14		2.70	0.54	0.08	0.22	0.30
Phenylalanine	3.75	33.29	0.75	1.66	0.54	3.31	0.66	0.99	0.26	1.25
Lysine	5.27	26.67	1.05	1.33	0.70	8.86	1.77	0.80	0.71	1.51
Histidine	1.42	15.46	0.28	0.77	0.22	1.95	0.39	0.46	0.16	0.62
Arginine	2.87	18.94	0.57	0.95		2.15	0.43	0.57	0.17	0.74
Tryptophan	1.03	4.90	0.20	0.25	0.11	0.92	0.18	0.15	0.07	0.22
Total protein g/kg/d	2.4			3.0		3.0		1.8	1.2	3.0

1. Aminoacid composition as given by the manufacturer
2. From I. G. MACY and H. J. KELLY, (1961) In: S. K. KON and A. T. COWIE (eds.), *Milk: the mammary gland and its secretion*, Academic Press, New York and London, p. 265.
3. Reference for glycine: R. A. McCANCE and E. M. WIDDOWSON, (1960) *The composition of foods*, Medical Res. Council, Special Report Series no.: 297; Her Majesty's Stationery Office, London, p. 253.
4. From L. E. HOLT JR. and S. E. SNYDERMAN, (1961) The aminoacid requirements of infants, *JAMA* 175, 100.

Blood samples were obtained from an umbilical artery or peripheral vein for the following determinations: P_H, PCO_2, total bicarbonate (Radiometer); osmolality (freezing point depression, Advanced Instruments); sodium, potassium (flame photometer, BECKMAN 105); chloride (Marius chlor-o-counter); calcium (Marius calcium-titrator); phosphorus (34); glucose (oxidase method); ammonia-nitrogen (35); urea (36); creatinine (37); individual amino acids (ion-exchange method, Technicon TSM1); triglycerides (38) and cholesterol (39). For technical and practical reasons it was not possible to carry out all determinations and only a few determinations of triglycerides and cholesterol were done.

Urine was collected for 24 hours on several days and the following were determined: volume, creatinine, sodium, potassium, chloride, osmolality, urea, glucose (Labstix, Ames), individual amino acids, total nitrogen (Kjeldahl method), total free α-amino-nitrogen (40) and total hydroxyproline (41).

Plasma and urinary amino acid concentrations in these 4 infants (before, during and after Vamin given intravenously) are listed in tables 8–11 and figures 17–20. In figures 17–20 plasma amino acid concentrations in our patients are compared with the normal data for LBW infants of DICKINSON et al. (42) As can be seen in these figures plasma amino acid concentrations during administration of Vamin generally reflect the amino acid composition of this solution. High plasma concentrations of phenylalanine, alanine, proline, serine and glycine were observed. Tyrosine concentrations were low. Concentrations of threonine, valine, isoleucine, leucine and methionine were slightly increased. Concentrations of aspartic acid, cystine, lysine, ornithinine, histidine and arginine were within normal limits for this age.

In patients 1, 2 and 3 plasma amino acid concentrations decreased during continuous administration of Vamin, which may indicate the induction of adaptive processes. This is supported by the fact that there is only a small increase in urinary excretion of amino acids during administration of Vamin.

Total urinary excretion of amino acids per 24 hours was less then 2 percent of the total daily intake of l-amino acids in Vamin (except on day 2 in patient 4).

Total urinary free α-amino-N per 24 hours was less than 5 percent of total daily intake of α-amino-N in Vamin (except on day 2 in patient 4).

Tables 8–11. *Plasma and urinary amino acid concentrations; urinary excretion of total free α-amino-nitrogen and total nitrogen in patients 1, 2, 3 and 4. See tables 1–4, figures 17–20 and text.*

Table 8

PATIENT 1 (concentrations in μmol/ml)

days after birth	URINE — INTRALIPID ▼23 / VAMIN						PLASMA — INTRALIPID ▼23 / VAMIN					
	▼8	12	14	21	▼26	29	▼8	12	15	22	▼26	29
Aspartic acid	−	.14	.06	.08	−	−	.04	.08	.03	.03	.03	.03
Threonine	.06	.21	.36	.48	.56	.60	.40	.45	.62	.21	.25	.27
Serine	.48	.56	.48	.60	−	−	.62	.62	1.00	.26	.26	.16
Asparagine	−	tr	.11	.16	−	−	.02	tr	.02	.06	.06	.06
Glutamic acid	.08	.06	.06	.04	−	−	.30	.28	.28	.26	.26	.27
Proline	−	.69	.50	.22	−	−	.72	1.00	.30	.30	.15	.15
Glycine	.93	1.39	1.53	1.02	−	−	.46	.57	.18	.18	.18	.18
Alanine	.16	.24	.46	.34	−	−	.54	.59	.26	.26	.24	.24
Valine	tr	tr	tr	.03	−	−	.32	.43	.16	.16	.22	.22
Cystine	.01	.02	.09	.11	−	−	tr	.12	.03	.03	.03	.03
Cystathionine	.02	.07	−	−	−	−	−	−	.04	.04	.06	.06
Methionine	.02	−	.09	−	−	−	.08	.19	.08	.08	.10	.10
Isoleucine	.02	.02	.03	.03	−	−	.14	.22	.11	.11	.13	.13
Leucine	tr	.02	.06	.07	−	−	.18	.13	.05	.05	.10	.10
Tyrosine	tr	.03	.04	.06	−	−	.12	.34	.06	.06	.08	.08
Phenylalanine	.02	.03	.02	.33	−	−	.24	.34	.06	.06	.08	.08
α-aminoisobut. acid	−	−	−	−	−	−	tr	tr	tr	tr	.06	.06
Ornithine	−	tr	−	.03	−	−	tr	.07	.04	.04	.17	.17
Lysine	.02	.03	.08	.32	−	−	.08	.14	.05	.05	.05	.05
Histidine	.09	.16	.33	.26	−	−	.14	.14	−	−	−	−
1-Me-His	tr	tr	tr	tr	−	−	tr	−	−	−	−	−
3-Me-His	tr	tr	−	.04	−	−	−	−	−	−	−	−
Carnosine	−	−	−	−	−	−	−	−	−	−	−	−
Arginine	−	−	−	−	−	−	tr	−	−	−	−	.04
Creatinine (mmol/L)	.62	.53	1.76	1.22								
Volume (ml/24 h)	160	145	60	82								
Total urinary excretion aminoacids (mmol/24 h)	.32	.52	.27	.35								
as % of Vamin intake	1.2	1.6	.82	−								
Total urinary free α-amino-N (mmol/24 h)	1.10	.93	.56	.67								
as % of Vamin intake	4.1	3.0	1.7	−								
Total urinary N (mg/24 h)	130	−	−	123								
as % of total N intake	20.5	−	−	14.2								
Total urinary free α-amino-N (mg N/24 h)	15.4	13.0	7.8	9.4								
as % of total urinary N excr.	11.8	−	−	7.6								
Total urinary excretion OH-proline (mg/24 h)	8.70	6.03	7.20	8.21								

Table 9

PATIENT 2 (concentrations in μmol/ml)

days after birth	URINE — VAMIN				PLASMA — VAMIN		
	▼8	12	14	▼18	12	15	22
Aspartic acid	.03	.03	−	.03	.03	.03	.04
Threonine	.08	.08	−	−	.48	.43	.23
Serine	.13	.13	−	−	.32	.38	.21
Asparagine	−	.03	−	−	.03	tr	.03
Glutamic acid	.03	.15	.15	.23	.27	.15	.24
Proline	.15	.70	.23	1.18	.36	.47	.30
Glycine	.70	.11	1.18	.22	.43	.41	.30
Alanine	.11	.34	.22	.22	.34	.35	.21
Valine	tr	.28	tr	tr	.28	.18	.21
Cystine	.05	.02	.12	.12	.06	.06	.03
Cystathionine	.08	.08	tr	.16	−	−	.03
Methionine	tr	tr	tr	.02	.10	.06	.04
Isoleucine	tr	.12	.02	.02	.12	.14	.09
Leucine	tr	.13	.13	.04	.13	.21	.11
Tyrosine	tr	.10	.04	.04	.10	.13	.08
Phenylalanine	tr	.13	.02	.02	.13	.20	.08
α-aminoisobut. acid	tr	tr	tr	−	−	−	−
Ornithine	tr	.04	tr	tr	.04	.02	−
Lysine	tr	.09	.06	.06	.09	.06	.05
Histidine	tr	.08	.15	.15	.08	.12	.04
1-Me-His	.16	.08	tr	tr	.08	−	−
3-Me-His	.12	.13	tr	tr	.13	−	−
Carnosine	−	−	−	tr	.05	−	−
Arginine	−	.05	tr	tr	−	−	−
Creatinine (mmol/L)	.57	.67					
Volume (ml/24 h)	135	100					
Total urinary excretion aminoacids (mmol/24 h)	.22	.24					
as % of Vamin-intake	.83	1.3					
Total urinary free α-amino-N (mmol/24 h)	.65	.50					
as % of Vamin intake	2.4	2.6					
Total urinary N (mg/24 h)	102	94					
as % of total N intake	13.8	15.5					
Total urinary free α-amino-N (mg N/24 h)	9.1	7.0					
as % of total urinary N excr.	8.9	7.4					
Total urinary excretion OH-proline (mg/24 h)	10.01	6.43					

Table 10

PATIENT 3

μmol/ml

days after birth	URINE VAMIN ↓4 ↓10							PLASMA VAMIN ↓4 ↓10			
	3	5	7	9	10	13	21	4	6	8	14
Aspartic acid	0.04	.09	—	.09	—	.02	.03	.04	.08	.04	.04
Threonine	.07	.14	.21	.18	.22	.32	.15	.28	.56	.32	.44
Serine	.16	.28	.33	.22	.02	.24	.20	.18	.50	.02	.13
Asparagine	.02	.03	.03	.02	.10	.02	.08	.04	.02	.02	.08
Glutamic acid	.02	.04	.04	.10	—	.16	.06	.22	.40	.32	.34
Proline	.07	.08	—	.08	.08	.22	.33	.28	.76	.56	.36
Glycine	.57	.89	.75	.77	.77	.86	.86	.46	.76	.52	.20
Alanine	.07	.09	.09	.15	.15	.27	.16	.28	.66	.46	.44
Valine	.01	.04	.02	.06	.06	.03	.02	.16	.36	.30	.26
Cystine	.01	.07	.09	.01	.01	.03	tr	.04	.10	.07	.01
Cystathionine	.06	.10	.09	.14	.14	.17	.08	—	—	—	—
Methionine	.04	.06	.05	.04	.04	.04	.02	.08	.10	—	.06
Isoleucine	.02	.02	.03	.05	.05	.04	.03	.06	.12	.11	.12
Leucine	.03	.05	.05	.06	.06	.08	.03	.10	.18	.07	.18
Tyrosine	.03	.03	.03	.03	.03	.03	.03	.08	.18	.13	.12
Phenylalanine	.02	.02	.03	.03	.03	.12	tr	.10	.30	.17	.09
β-aminoisobut. acid	.06	tr	tr	tr	tr	tr	—	—	—	—	—
Ornithine	.03	.01	tr	tr	tr	tr	tr	.06	.14	.05	.06
Lysine	tr	.05	.03	.12	.12	.19	.10	.14	.18	.15	.14
Histidine	.06	.09	.06	.10	.10	.13	.15	.06	.12	.07	.06
1-Me-His	tr	tr	tr	—	—	—	tr	—	—	—	—
3-Me-His	.04	.05	—	tr	tr	.03	tr	tr	—	—	—
Carnosine	—	—	—	—	—	.06	.08	.07	—	—	—
Arginine	—	—	—	tr	tr	tr	tr	tr	tr	tr	tr
Creatinine (mmol/L)	1.06	1.38	1.04		1.07	1.45	.60				
Volume (ml/24 h)	85	60	88		110	80	215				
Total urinary excretion amino acids (mmol/24 h)	.12	.13	.17		.25	.24	.52				
as % of Vamin intake	—	.63	.65		1.6	—	—				
Total urinary free α-amino-N (mmol/24 h)	.42	.37	.40		.58	.68	1.25				
as % of Vamin intake	—	1.8	1.5		3.7	—	—				
Total urinary N (mg/24 h)	84	76	104		134		216				
as % of total N intake	51.5	13.6	13.7		16.5		23.0				
Total urinary free α-amino-N (mg N/24 h)	5.9	5.2	5.6		8.1	9.5	17.5				
as % of total urinary N excr.	7.0	6.8	5.3		6.0	13.6	8.1				
Total urinary excretion OH-proline (mg/24 h)	4.25	3.57	5.72		7.04	13.6	23.1				

Table 11

PATIENT 4

μmol/ml

days after birth	URINE VAMIN ↓2 ↓5			PLASMA VAMIN ↓2 ↓5	
	1	2	4	2	4
Aspartic acid	.02	.02	.02	.03	.09
Threonine	.03	.07	.13	.11	.35
Serine	.11	.18	.31	.16	.43
Asparagine	.02	.03	.04	.05	.09
Glutamic acid	.01	.02	.01	.29	.45
Proline	.26	.56	.64	.31	.57
Glycine	.75	1.36	.46	.36	.63
Alanine	.08	.13	.12	.35	.44
Valine	.01	.02	.02	.07	.42
Cystine	.04	.07	.21	tr	.04
Cystathionine	.02	.03	.05	—	—
Methionine	.02	.01	.01	.06	.08
Isoleucine	.02	.02	.01	.07	.14
Leucine	.02	.05	.05	.11	.24
Tyrosine	tr	.02	.02	.10	.11
Phenylalanine	tr	tr	.02	.09	.20
β-aminoisobut. acid	—	—	—	—	—
Ornithine	.01	.01	.02	.05	.08
Lysine	.08	.23	.51	.16	.36
Histidine	.06	.15	.27	.08	.18
1-Me-His	tr	tr	tr	—	—
3-Me-His	.04	.08	.11	—	—
Carnosine	.06	.10	.06	—	—
Arginine	tr	—	tr	.05	tr
Creatinine (mmol/L)	1.14	1.16	1.04		
Volume (ml/24 h)	175	210	210		
Total urinary excretion amino acids (mmol/24 h)	.29	.66	.65		
as % of Vamin intake	—	12	1.5		
Total urinary free α-amino-N (mmol/24 h)	1.15	1.26	1.85		
as % of Vamin intake	—	22.5	4.3		
Total urinary N (mg/24 h)	350	555	730		
Total N-intake (mg/24 h)	—	95	740		
Total urinary free α-amino-N (mg N/24 h)	16.1	17.6	25.9		
as % of total urinary N excr.	4.6	3.2	3.5		
Total urinary excretion OH-proline (mg/24 h)	9.15	14.5	16.8		

Tables 12–15. *Further data in patients 1–4 as observed during pilot study. See tables 1–4 and text.*

Table 12

PATIENT 1	BLOOD							URINE				
	INTRALIPID ↓8 ——— ↓23							INTRALIPID ↓8 ——— ↓23				
	VAMIN ↓8 ——————— ↓26							VAMIN ↓8 ——————— ↓26				
days after birth	9	10	12	14	22	27	29	9	10	12	14	29
Na	131		135	133		137		5 (1.4)	3 (.6)	2 (.32)	2 (.29)	10 (.82)
K	5.0		4.6	3.8		5.3		3 (.84)	.5 (.10)	.6 (.96)	.4 (.06)	14 (1.2)
Cl (mmol/L)	102		98	102		106		3 (.84)	4 (.80)	2 (.32)	4 (.85)	16 (1.3)
Ca	2.44		2.54	2.39		2.13						
P			1.08				2.29					
Osm. (mosm/L)			274	281			278	60	51	61	61	117
pH	7.38	7.30	7.37	7.34		7.26						
Bic. (mmol/L)			21.0	16.0								
PCO₂ (mm Hg)			37.5	31.0								
glucose (mmol/L)	5.9	4.4	5.0	3.6		2.9		neg.	neg.	neg.	neg.	neg.
NH₃-N (µmol/L)	84		54	52	56		75					
urea (mmol/L)				2.5		3.2		17.2 (4.8)	15.0 (3.0)	11.6 (1.9)	15.7 (2.3)	32 (2.6)
triglycerides (mmol/L)			.86	.60	2.46	1.14						
			.89	.50	2.54	1.10						
cholesterol (mmol/L)				5.93		4.65						
total N (mgr/24 h)								223	137	130		123
α-amino-N (mg N/24 h)								20.7	15.7	15.4		9.4
volume (ml/24 h)								290	200	160	145	82
creatinine (mmol/L)								.80	.71	.62	.53	1.22
(mmol/24 h)								.23	.14	.10	.08	.10

Table 13

PATIENT 2	BLOOD				URINE		
	VAMIN ↓8 ——————— ↓21				VAMIN ↓8 ——————— ↓21		
days after birth	9	12	14	22	10	12	14
Na	132	132	134	139	8 (1.2)	4 (.5)	8 (.8)
K	4.8	5.1	4.9	6.0	3.2 (.48)	1.4 (.19)	3.9 (.39)
Cl (mmol/L)	103	99	103	100	7 (1.0)	3 (.4)	4 (.4)
Ca	2.40	2.40	2.33				
P		1.30	1.37	2.27			
Osm. (mosm/L)		266	276		64	48	61
pH		7.34	7.35	7.27			
Bic. (mmol/L)		22	20	18			
PCO₂ (mm Hg)		43	37.5	42			
glucose (mmol/L)	4.8	5.6	4.7	4.0	neg.	neg.	neg.
NH₃-N (µmol/L)	84	45	83	51			
urea (mmol/L)		1.9	2.2	2.5	19.4 (2.9)	13.3 (1.8)	20.3 (2.0)
triglycerides (mmol/L)		.55		1.16			
		.61		1.21			
total N (mgr/24 h)					132	102	94
α-amino-N (mg N/24 h)					13.9	9.1	7.0
volume (ml/24 h)					150	135	100
creatinine (mmol/L)					.71	.57	.67
(mmol/24 h)					.10	.07	.07

Table 14

PATIENT 3		BLOOD						URINE					
		VAMIN ↓4 ↓10						VAMIN ↓4 ↓10					
days after birth		3	4	5	7	9	13	3	5	7	9	13	21
Na		143		148	143		141	5 (.42)	2 (.12)	2 (.18)	12 (1.3)	4 (.32)	1 (.22)
K		3.8		4.0	3.5		5.9	4.3 (.36)	1.0 (.06)	9 (.80)	18 (.80)	22 (1.8)	9 (1.9)
Cl	(mmol/L)	107			99		101	1 (.09)	– –	4.7 (.41)	15.6 (1.7)	3.9 (.31)	6.5 (1.4)
Ca		2.30		2.40	2.34		1.83						
P		1.50		1.06	1.16		2.87						
Osm. (mosm/L)				300	281		280	–	77	100	80	157	80
P_H		7.38		7.39			7.39						
Bic. (mmol/L)		21		24			24						
PCO_2 (mm Hg)		34		40			42						
glucose (mmol/L)		4.6	5.3	5.1	4.4		5.0	neg.	neg.	neg.	neg.	neg.	neg.
NH_3-N (μmol/L)		64		61	51		54						
urea (mmol/L)		1.3		1.8	2.1		1.2	22 (1.9)	30 (1.8)	41 (3.6)	41 (4.5)	22 (1.8)	29.2 (6.3)
triglycerides (mmol/L)					1.25 1.30		1.49 1.46						
total N (mg/24 h)								84	76	104	134	–	216
α-amino-N (mg N/24 h)								5.9	13.6	13.7	16.5	–	23.0
volume (ml/24 h)								85	60	88	110	80	215
creatinine (mmol/L) (mmol/24 h)								1.06 .09	1.38 .08	1.04 .09	1.07 .12	1.45 .10	.56 .11

Table 15

PATIENT 4		BLOOD				URINE		
		INTRALIPID VAMIN ↓2 ↓5				INTRALIPID VAMIN ↓2 ↓6		
days after birth		1	2	3	4	1	2	4
Na		128	133	139	139	28 (4.9)	43 (9.0)	30 (6.3)
K		4.3	6.0	4.4	4.0	24 (4.2)	10 (2.1)	5 (1.1)
Cl	(mmol/L)	94	102	94	–	9.8 (1.7)	15 (3.2)	29 (6.1)
Ca		1.65	2.34	2.96	2.89			
P		1.98	–	–	–			
Osm. (mosm/L)		285	–	299	–	95	198	227
P_H		7.30	7.20	7.27	7.28			
Bic. (mmol/L)		30	26	36	39			
PCO_2 (mm Hg) PO_2 (mm Hg)		63 76	66 51	98 85	80 58			
glucose (mmol/L)		–	6.1	5.9	7.8	neg.	neg.	neg.
NH_3-N (μmol/L)		59	–	–	–			
urea (mmol/L)		7.5	–	9.5	–	56 (9.8)	94 (19.7)	117 (25)
triglycerides (mmol/L)		.94 .91		3.67 3.46				
total N (mg/24 h)						350	555	730
α-amino-N (mg N/24 h)						16.1	17.6	25.9
volume (ml/24 h)						175	210	210
creatinine (mmol/L) (mmol/24 h)						1.14 .20	1.14 .24	1.04 .22

Total urinary free α-amino-N was 3–12 percent of total urinary nitrogen excretion (tables 8–11).

Further data are shown in tables 12–15. Plasma glucose and ammonia concentrations and serum osmolality were within normal limits. Acid-base balance was normal, except for respiratory acidosis in the infant with respiratory distress syndrome (patient 4). Blood urea values were low in patients 1, 2 and 3, but elevated in patient 4. Serum electrolytes (Na, K, Cl) were within normal limits. Hypocalcaemia, which is usually seen in LBW infants, was corrected with calciumgluconate and parathormone.

In patients 2 and 3 plasma concentrations of triglycerides were within normal limits. In patient 4 plasma triglycerides were highly elevated on the second day of administration of Intralipid. In patient 1 plasma triglycerides were normal on days 12 and 14 (4 and 6 days after starting Intralipid), but highly elevated on day 22. It is interesting that plasma cholesterol in this patient was elevated on day 14, and also on day 29, 6 days after Intralipid administration was discontinued.

Sodium, chloride, potassium and nitrogen balances (daily intake minus urinary excretion) were highly positive in patients 1, 2 and 3, but markedly negative in patient 4.

DISCUSSION

Of the commercially available amino acid solutions Vamin is probably the best choice for infants (29). Vamin contains l-amino acids, including all essential amino acids; the concentrations of sodium and chloride are reasonably low (50 and 55 meq/l); the concentrations of potassium, calcium and magnesium are 20,5 and 3 meq/l, respectively (table 5). One disadvantage is the presence of fructose (10%) as carbohydrate. In infants fructose infusion easily leads to lactate formation. In low-birth weight infants infusion of fructose may cause accumulation of fructose-1-phosphate in the liver, and fructose-1-phosphate aldolase is a rate-limiting enzyme. Accumulation of fructose-1-phosphate is followed by loss of ATP and AMP from the liver, causing increased uric acid formation and inhibition of protein synthesis (for a review see ref. 43). Furthermore the osmolality of Vamin is very high (1275 mosm/L); P_H is 5.2. Other amino acid solutions such as Trophysan (Egic), Aminofusin (Pfrimmer), Intramin (Astra) and Steramin (Braun) are unsuitable for use in infants. On comparison with human milk protein the relative amino acid content varies considerably. In some preparations amino acids are in dl-form; some do not contain a number of amino acids. E/T ratios (table 6) are unsatisfactory. In some preparations (such as 10% Aminosol) the concentrations of sodium and chloride prohibit use in infants. Aminosol-fructose-ethanol (Vitrum) has a reasonably low electrolyte content (sodium 53 meq/l, chloride 43 meq/l). It is a protein hydrolysate; the amino acid composition is somewhat closer to that of human milk in contrast with Vamin; E/T ratio is 3.0 (table 6). It contains 15% fructose; osmolality is very high (1975 mosm./l); P_H is 5.0.

Virtually no data on plasma amino acid concentrations in LBW infants during administration of amino acid solutions (including Vamin) are available. JUERGENS and DOLIF (44) report increased plasma concentrations for several amino acids (such as methionine, phenylalanine, serine, glycine, proline) during administration of an amino acid solution in premature infants. The composition of this solution is not mentioned. STEGINK and BAKER (32) report plasma amino acid concentrations in young infants during administration of protein hydrolysate infusions (Amigen and Aminosol). Some amino acid concentrations were below normal levels, reflecting the composition of the protein hydrolysate preparation.

Conditions of amino acid imbalance, toxicity or antagonism in man have not been well-established. Most of the studies concerned animals who were fed orally; many toxic effects have been described (for a review see ref. 45).

In our opinion serious consideration should be given to the amino acid composition of commercially available preparations for use in intravenous alimentation. Our data indicate that the amino acid composition of the preparation has an important effect on the plasma amino acid concentration of the infant. It seems obvious that the preparations administered to (low-birth weight) infants should have an amino acid composition which closely resembles that of human milk.

There is not much information available on plasma triglyceride and cholesterol concentrations in low-birth weight infants during prolonged infusions of Intralipid.

WOLF (46) injected 0.5 g/kg Intralipid in 1–3 minutes in premature infants (1 and 7 days old) and measured triglyceride levels during the next 4 hours. Elimination half-time was calculated as ± 60 minutes.

On the basis of these experiments a total dose of 2 grams fat/kg/d was recommended for the first week of life (administered over a 6-hour period) and during the second week of life, 2.5–3 g/kg/d (given during 2–4-hour periods separated by an 8-hour interval).

GUSTAFSON et al. (47) (48) measured total serum lipid concentrations after rapid infusion of Intralipid in low-birth weight infants (0.1–0.5 g/kg) and calculated clearance rates. Maximum removal rate of exogenous triglycerides from the intravascular compartment in premature babies was within the range of that found in adults (corresponding to 6–8 grams fat/kg/24 hr). In small-for-date infants a lower, overall removal capacity was observed.

In newborns and infants Intralipid has been used in doses of 1–4 grams fat/kg/d without clinical side effects (27) (29). Obviously further studies must be carried out.

Although admittedly our data are very limited and patients 1, 2 and 3 were not on total parenteral alimentation, we were reassured that acid-base balance, serum electrolyte concentrations, serum osmolality and serum glucose and ammonia concentrations were within normal limits. It is very likely that the positive nitrogen and electrolyte balances in patients 1, 2 and 3 indicate net protein synthesis. During 18 days of combined oral and parenteral feeding in patient 1 (table 1) total weight increase was 540 g ($\pm$ 30 g per day). In patient 2 total weight increase between the 8th and 21st day (table 2) was 420 g ($\pm$ 30 g per day). In patient 3 average weight increase between the 4th and 10th day (table 3) was 25 grams per day.

CONCLUSION

It is concluded that currently in the routine management of low-birth weight infants parenteral nutrition should be limited to the use of 10–15% glucose solutions. Intravenous administration of such a solution should be initiated as soon as possible after birth. Oral feeding with milk (preferably by gastric drip) should start within a few hours after birth. The total amounts of fluid and calories by oral and parenteral route should be increased rapidly. When ever possible these infants should receive only oral feedings within 7 days, with a total daily intake of 200 ml/kg and 120–140 kcal/kg. On such a feeding regimen growth rates after the first or second week are normal as compared with intra-uterine growth curves.

For those infants who cannot tolerate this feeding regimen parenteral nutrition with amino acid solutions and/or fat emulsions may be considered. In our opinion intravenous alimentation of low-birth weight infants with amino acids and fats still remains within the field of clinical investigation. Commercially available amino acid solutions (including Vamin) contain unphysiological amounts of amino acids when compared with human milk. Some of these solutions are unphysiological with respect to electrolyte concentrations and the presence of fructose.

For low-birth weight infants total or partial (in combination with oral feeding) parenteral nutrition offers the possibility of optimum nutrition immediately after birth. Further studies will be necessary.

The manufacturers have to provide intravenous solutions that are more physiological for these infants.

REFERENCES

1. GOODHART, J. F., (1913) *The diseases of children*, edited and revised by G. F. Still, 10th ed., p. 36. Churchill, London.
2. HILL, L. W. and GERSTLEY, J. R., (1917) *Clinical lectures on infant feeding*, p. 56. W. B. Saunders, Philadelphia.
3. HESS, J. H., (1922) *Premature and congenitally diseased infants*, p. 179. Lea and Febiger, Philadelphia and New York.
4. Tow, A., (1937) *Diseases of the newborn*, p. 77. Oxford University Press, New York.
5. SMITH, C. A., YUDKIN, S., YOUNG, W., MINKOWSKI, A. and CUSHMAN, M., (1949) Adjustment of electrolytes and water following premature birth. *Pediatrics*, 3, 34.
6. HANSEN, J. D. L. and SMITH, C. A., (1953) Effects of withholding fluid in the immediate postnatal period. *Pediatrics*, 12, 99.
7. SMITH, C. A., (1957) Reasons for delaying the feeding of premature infants. *Ann. Paediat. Fenn.*, 3, 261.
8. YLPPÖ, A., (1954) Premature children – should they fast or be fed in the first days of life? *Ann. Paediat. Fenn.*, 1, 99.
9. SMALLPIECE, V. and DAVIES, P. A., (1964) Immediate feedings of premature infants with undiluted breast milk. *Lancet*, 1, 1349.
10. CORNBLATH, M., FORBES, A. E., PILDES, R. S., LUEBBEN, G. and GREENGARD, J., (1966) A controlled study of early fluid administration on survival of low-birth weight infants. *Pediatrics*, 38, 547.
11. AULD, P. A. M., BHANGANANDA, P. and MEHTA, S, (1966) The influence of an early caloric intake with i.v. glucose on catabolism of premature infants. *Pediatrics*, 37, 592
12. WENNBERG, R. P., SCHWARTZ, R. and SWEET, A. Y., (1966) Early versus delayed feeding of low-birth weight infants. Effects on physiologic jaundice. *J. Pediat.*, 68, 860.
13. AVERY, M. E. and HODSON, W. A., (1966) The first drink reconsidered. *J. Pediat.*, 68, 1008.

14. Wu, P. Y. K., Teilman, P., Gabler, M., Vaughan, M. and Metcoff, J., (1967) 'Early' versus 'late' feeding of low-birth weight neonates: effect on serum bilirubin, blood sugar, and responses to glucagon and epinephrine tolerance tests. *Pediatrics*, 39, 733.

15. Rabor, I. F., Oh, W., Wu, P. Y. K., Metcoff, J., Vaughan, M. and Gabler, M., (1968) The effects of early and late feeding of intra-uterine fetally malnourished (IUM) infants. *Pediatrics*, 42, 261.

16. Davies, P. A. and Davis, J. P., (1970) Very low birth weight and subsequent head growth. *Lancet*, 2, 1216.

17. Winick, M., (1969) Changes in nucleic acid and protein content of the human brain during growth. *Pediat. Res.*, 3, 181.

18. Winick, M., (1971) Cellular growth during early malnutrition. *Pediatrics*, 47, 969.

19. Winick, M., (1969) Malnutrition and brain development. *J. Pediat.*, 74, 667.

20. Dobbing, J., (1970) Undernutrition and the developing brain: the relevance of animal models to the human problem. *Am. J. Dis. Child.*, 120, 411.

21. Van Gils, J. F., (1971) Postnatal growth and development in small-for-date babies. In: G. B. A. Stoelinga and J. J. van der Werff ten Bosch (eds.), *Normal and abnormal development of brain and behaviour*, p. 53. Boerhaave Series for Post-Graduate Medical Education. Leiden University Press. Leiden.

22. Benda, G. I. M. and Babson, S. G., (1971) Peripheral intravenous alimentation of the small premature infant. *J. Pediat.*, 79, 494.

23. Driscoll, J. M. Jr., Heird, W. C., Schullinger, J. N., Gongaware, R. D. and Winters, R. W., (1972) Total intravenous alimentation in low-birth weight infants. A preliminary report. *J. Pediat.*, 81, 145.

24. Peden, V. H. and Karpel, J. T., (1972) Total parenteral nutrition in premature infants. *J. Pediat.*, 81, 137.

25. Helmuth, W. V., Adam, P. A. J. and Sweet, A. Y., (1972) The effects of protein hydrolysate-monosaccharide infusion on low-birth weight infants. *J. Pediat.*, 81, 129.

26. Wilmore, D. W., Groff, D. B., Bishop, H. C. and Dudrick, S. J., (1969) Total parenteral nutrition in infants with catastrophic gastro-intestinal anomalies. *J. Ped. Surg.*, 4, 181.

27. Borresen, H. C., Coran, A. G. and Knutrud, O., (1970) Metabolic results of parenteral feeding in neonatal surgery: a balanced parenteral feeding program based on a synthetic l-amino acid solution and a commercial fat emulsion. *Ann. Surg.*, 172, 291.

28. Hyman, C. J., Reiter, J., Rodnan, J. and Drash, A. L., (1971) Parenteral and oral alimentation in the treatment of the non-specific protracted diarrheal syndrome of infancy. *J. Pediat.*, 78, 17.

29. Harries, J. T., (1971) Intravenous feeding in infants. *Arch. Dis. Childh.*, 46, 855.

30. Heird, W. C., Nicholson, J. F., Driscoll, J. M. Jr., Schullinger, J. N. and Winters, R. W., (1972) Hyperammonemia resulting from intravenous alimentation using a mixture of synthetic l-amino acids: a preliminary report. *J. Pediat.*, 81, 162.

31. Johnson, J. D., Albritton, W. L. and Sunshine, Ph., (1972) Hyperammonemia accompanying parenteral nutrition in newborn infants. *J. Pediat.*, 81, 154.

32. Stegink, L. D. and Baker, G. L., (1971) Infusion of protein hydrolysates in the newborn infant: plasma amino acid concentrations. *J. Pediat.*, 78, 595.

33. Harries, J. T., (1972) Metabolic acidosis during intravenous feeding of infants. In: A. W. Wilkinson (ed.), *Parenteral nutrition*, p. 266. Churchill Livingstone, Edinburgh and London.

34. FISHE, C. H. and SUBBAROW, Y., (1925) Colorimetric determination of phosphorus. *J. Biol. Chem.*, 66, 375.
35. HUTCHINSON, J. H. and LABBY, D. H., (1962) New method for microdetermination of blood ammonia by use of cation exchange resin. *J. Lab. Clin. Med.*, 60, 170.
36. FAWCETT, J. K. and SCOTT, J. E., (1960) A rapid and precise method for the determination of urea. *J. Clin. Path.*, 13, 304.
37. GORTER, E. and DE GRAAF, W. C., (1955) *Klinische diagnostiek*. Stenfert Kroese, Leiden.
38. SCHMIDT, F. H. and VON DAHL, L., (1968) Zur Methode der enzymatischen Neutralfett-Bestimmung in biologischem Material. *Z. Klin. Chem. u. klin. Biochem.*, 6, 156.
39. CARR, J. J. and DREKTER, I. J., (1956) Simplified rapid technique for the extraction and determination of serum cholesterol without saponification. *Clin. Chem.*, 2, 353.
40. GOODWIN, J. F., (1968) On the measurement of urinary amino nitrogen with 1-fluoro-2, 4-dinitrobenzene. *Clin. Chim. Acta*, 21, 231.
41. GOVERDE, B. C. and VEENKAMP, F. J. N., (1972) Routine assay of total urinary hydroxyproline based on resin-catalysed hydrolysis. *Clin. Chim. Acta*, 41, 29.
42. DICKINSON, J. C., ROSENBLUM, H. and HAMILTON, P. B., (1970) Ion exchange chromatography of the free amino acids in the plasma of infants under 2500 gm at birth. *Pediatrics*, 45, 606.
43. WOODS, H. F. and ALBERTI, K. G. M. M., (1972) Dangers of intravenous fructose. *Lancet*, II, 1354.
44. JUERGENS, P. and DOLIF, D., (1972) Experimental results of parenteral nutrition with amino acids. In: A. W. Wilkinson (ed.), *Parenteral nutrition*, p. 77. Churchill Livingstone, Edinburgh and London.
45. HARPER, A. E., (1964) Amino acid toxicities and imbalances. In: H. N. Munroe and J. B. Allison (eds.), *Mammalian protein metabolism*, vol. II, p. 87. Acad. Press, New York and London.
46. WOLF, H., (1971) Metabolism of carbohydrates and fat components in premature and full-term newborn infants after infusions of triglycerides and glycerol. In: J. H. P. Jonxis, H. K. A. Visser and J. A. Troelstra (eds.), *Metabolic processes of the foetus and newborn infant*. IIIrd Nutricia Symposium, p. 269. Stenfert Kroese, Leiden.
47. GUSTAFSON, A., KJELLMER, I., OLEGARD, R. and VICTORIN, L., (1970) Intravenous fat loads in low-birth weight infants. In: *Abstracts annual meeting Eur. Soc. Ped. Res.* Stockholm, p. 16.
48. GUSTAFSON, A., KJELLMER, I., OLEGARD, R. and VICTORIN, L., (1972) Nutrition in low-birth weight infants. I Intravenous injection of fat emulsion. *Acta Paediat. Scand.*, 61, 149.

LONG-TERM PARENTERAL NUTRITION IN CHILDREN

C. RICOUR*

The use of caval catheters, whereby hyperosmolar solutions are perfused into a vein with rapid blood flow so that rapid dilution occurs, has opened up a new era in the approach to prolonged parenteral nutrition in children. Following the demonstration that dogs maintained exclusively on parenteral alimentation showed growth identical to that of control animals (1), this method of treatment was adapted to adult patients (2, 3, 4, 5, 6, 7, 8) and then to children (9, 10, 11, 12, 13, 14, 15, 16, 17, 18). This is an attempt, in the light of results obtained over a period of 3 years (19, 20), to detail the technique and to outline the indications for parenteral nutrition.

MATERIAL AND METHODS

We have used this technique in 42 children, 36 were 15 days to 16 months old with an initial weight varying from 1800 to 4500 gm and 6 were 5 to 14 years old, 58 catheters have been inserted with a mean catheter-life of 40 days (range: 8 days to 7 months). All children were seriously ill and malnutrition was life-threatening; this was due to fistulae or subtotal resection of the small intestine in 20 cases and prolonged diarrhoea in 17 cases as well as acute haemorrhagic pancreatitis, portal cavernomatosis and oesophageal perforation each in one child and severe renal insufficiency in 2 children.

The catheter we use is silastic (Dow-Corning I.D. 0.51 mm, E.D. 0.94 mm) and is well-tolerated by the venous endothelium. It floats in the superior cava vena with its distal end opening in the direction of venous flow.

It is brought into position in the operating room under general anaesthesia (rarely under local anaesthesia). Only veins draining

* Clinique des maladies du rein et du métabolisme chez l'enfant, Hôpital des Enfants-Malades, Paris, France.

into the superior vena cava are used, generally the external or internal jugular vein in infants and the humeral vein in older children. The location of the puncture is as distal as possible; the exact position of the infusion site, in the supra auricular region for maximal dilution, is always checked by radiography during insertion (fig. 1). A long subcutaneous tunnel is then made, with as little trauma as possible, so that 10–15 cm separate the cutaneous and venous entrance sites. The cutaneous exit is protected by a coating of gum silastic and covered with a wide occlusive dressing. The extracutaneous portion is surrounded by a protective tube of polyvinyl up to the antibacterial filter (Millipore – Swinnex 25–0.22 μ). A peristaltic pump (Sigmamotor) inserted between the filter and the infusion bottle ensures constant flow of the infusion.

The solution is prepared in the hospital pharmacy under rigorously aseptic conditions using Millipore filtration and laminar flow.

The solute composition is adjusted daily; the principle constituents are (table 1) water (110–130 ml/kg/24h), Na^+ and Cl^- (3 meq./kg/

Table 1. *Prolonged parenteral nutrition in children. Mean intake/kg body weight/day of water, electrolytes and nutrients.*

Water	110 – 130 ml
Electrolytes	Na Cl 3 mEq.
	K 5 mEq.
	Ca 35 mg
	P 45 mg
	Mg 10 mg
Calories	90 – 100 kcal
	Glucose 24 g
	Nitrogen $\leq$ 400 mg
+ Vitamins – Trace elements – essential fatty acids	

24 h), K^+ (5 meq./kg/24 h), Calcium (35 mg/kg/24 h), phosphorus (45 mg/kg/24 h) and magnesium (10 mg/kg/24 h). Nutrients are gradually increased at 2–3 day intervals, and by the 10th day consist of 24 g/kg/24 h glucose in 8 cases, 21 g/kg/24 h glucose with 3 g/kg/24 h fructose (in the amino acid preparation) in 34 cases. 200–400 mg/kg/24 h nitrogen are provided (Vamin) (table 2) giving a total of 90–100 calories/kg/24 h.

A multi-vitamin solution, enriched in vitamin B_{12} and folic acid, is added regularly and 5 mg vitamin K_1 is injected intramuscularly once a month (table 3). When therapy lasting several weeks is anti-

Table 2. *Prolonged parenteral nutrition in children – amino acid solutions (mg/100 mg amino acid).*

L – Isoleucine	5,6
L – Leucine	7,5
L – Valine	6,1
L – Lysine	5,5
L – Phenylalanine	7,8
L – Tyrosine	0.7
L – Cysteine	2,0
L – Methionine	2,7
L – Threonine	4,3
L – Tryptophane	1,4
L – Alanine	4,3
L – Histidine	3,4
L – Proline	11,6
L – Arginine	4,7
L – Aspartic acid	5,8
L – Glutamic acid	12,9
L – Serine	10,7
L – Glycine	3,0

Table 3. *Prolonged parenteral nutrition in children. Vitamins supplied per 24 hours.*

– Vitamin A	1250	u.i.
– Vitamin D	250	u.i.
– Vitamin E	500	μg
– Ascorbic acid	12	mg
– Thiamine	500	μg
– Riboflavine	350	μg
– Pyridoxine	500	μg
– Niacine	2,5	mg
– Vitamin B_{12}	10	γ
– Folic acid	1	mg
– Vitamin K1	5	mg/month (im)

cipated it is necessary to also provide essential fatty acids once a week (Intralipid) and trace elements (Solute Vitrum).

Careful clinical monitoring is important. Infusion flow rate, cardiac and respiratory rates, arterial blood pressure and temperature are recorded every 3 hours; body weight and volume of urinary and faecal losses are recorded every 6 hours; when there is any increase in osmotic load, urinary specific gravity and glycosuria are checked in all specimens voided. Urinary and plasma electrolytes as well as plasma Ca, P, Mg, blood glucose and haemoglobin are determined once a week.

RESULTS

Twelve out of 42 children died during the period of parenteral nutrition – 3 during the first year as a result of infections and vascular complications and 9 because of the extreme nature of their malnutrition or the irreversibility of their primary disease. In the 30 other children the initial results of treatment were very satisfactory with a mean weight gain of 150 g per week and an increase in height of 2–3 cm per month. Although discontinuation of parenteral feeding could only be temporary in 6 cases because of the shortness of the remaining bowel, in the other 24 children parenteral nutrition was discontinued gradually without incident.

A certain number of *technical complications* occurred, particularly during the first year. 10 catheters became dislodged and had to be removed. An infected haematoma, localized in the subcutaneous tunnel of the catheter, had to be excised in one child. Thrombosis in the superior vena cava occurred in one child leading to his death. Oedema of the shoulder region with the appearance of an anastomotic network of superficial veins caused concern in another child, but removal of the catheter was accompanied by an immediate regression of these symptoms.

Six instances of septicaemia occurred in 4 children, two of whom died. Two were due to Candida albicans on the 48th and 90th days and subsided rapidly within 24 hours of removal of the catheter; the blood culture was then negative. Staphylococcus aureus septicaemia was diagnosed on 3 occasions and Escherichia Coli once; one instance was on the 60th day, 48 hours after using a defective filter, and the other 3 occurred 6 and 12 days after re-using a vein which had just been catheterized.

On the 40th, 15th and 26th day, three other children showed unexplained changes in temperature without other clinical manifestations and with normal white cell counts and negative blood cultures. They reverted to normal either spontaneously or within several hours after removal of the catheter; the culture of the catheter was also sterile.

METABOLIC CHANGES

We saw no changes in plasma acid-base balance, apart from 2 cases of acidosis associated with septicaemia. Water, sodium, chloride and potassium levels were stable, although in 2 cases a transitory anti-diuresis with a hyponatraemia of 127 and 130 meq./l occurred with an increase in the osmotic load from 50 to 100 mOsm % in 24 hours; diuresis meant immediate reduction of the water load and use of a solution of half-osmolality.

Abnormalities of phosphorus and calcium metabolism were seen on 4 occasions, when the phosphorus load was less than 30 mg/kg/24 h. These were characterized by a drop in serum phosphorus to less than 20 mg/l and disappearance of urinary phosphorus; hypercalcalciuria was present though there was no change in serum calcium. In one child a serum phosphorus level of 10 mg/l was accompanied by a fine tremor of the limbs, generalized hypotonia, polypnea and impaired consiousness; these symptoms were rapidly corrected by phosphorus supplementation.

One case of a hypomagnesaemia of 6 mg/l with convulsions localized on one side regressed within hours of correction of the magnesium depletion.

One case of megaloblastic anaemia was corrected with folic acid.

Blood glucose, except in one case, was normal; the addition of fructose at the rate of 0.12–0.24 g/kg/hour in 34 cases was not accompanied by any acidosis; blood fructose levels remained <100 mg/l and no fructosuria was found.

Serum protein remained or became normal in all except one case where there was an ascitic collection.

Nitrogen retention, studied in 10 children with constant caloric intake and nitrogen loads varying from 240 to 800 mg/kg/24 h, was always >40 per cent of the nitrogen infused, and was even >80 per cent at the lowest loads; retention was 180 mg/kg/24 h (fig. 2). There was a very significant negative correlation between the percentage of nitrogen retention and the load (fig. 3).

Urinary nitrogen was essentially in the form of urea (90 per cent of total nitrogen), while ammonia nitrogen did not exceed 5 per cent save during the first few days of nutrition (4 to 10 days) when the percentage of urea nitrogen was as low as 64 per cent. Urinary creatine and uric acid were stable at 9.5 and 10 mg/kg/24 h, respectively.

No abnormalities in the urinary excretion of serine, proline, glycine, alanine, phenylalanine and histidine were found in 7 cases studied, with the exception of a constant inversion of the tyrosine/phenylalanine ratio (0.43) which was corrected at the onset of oral feeding; total

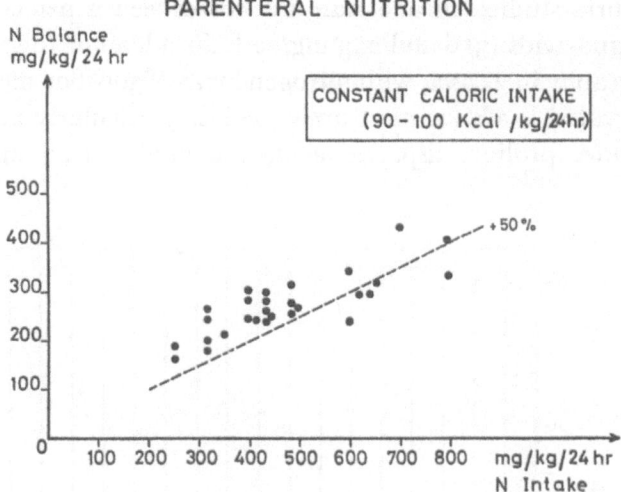

Fig. 2. Nitrogen balances in 10 children, with constant caloric intake. Each sign represents the mean value over a five-day period.

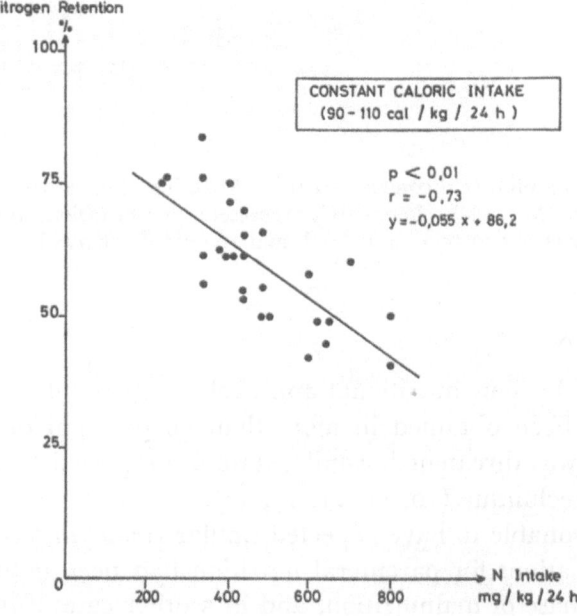

Fig. 3. Evidence of negative correlation between percentage nitrogen retention and nitrogen intake when caloric supply is constant. Each sign represents the mean value over a five-day period.

aminoaciduria studied in one case did not exceed 2 per cent of the
infused amino acids (316 and 243 mg/24 h for a load of 18 gm). Blood
chromatography in 3 cases, with nitrogen loads of 500–600 mg/kg/ 24 h,
showed elevated levels for most amino acids, particularly phenylana-
line, tyrosine, proline, aspartic acid, theonine, serine and valine
(fig. 4).

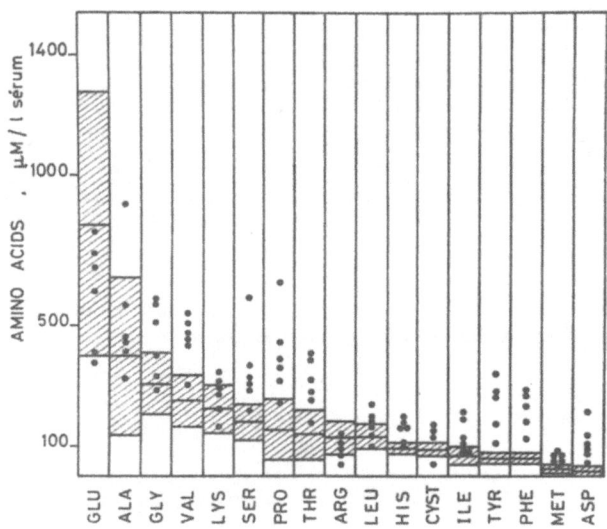

Fig. 4. Serum amino acid concentrations (μ M/l). The shaded zones correspond to
normal values (M $\pm$ 2σ); closed circles represent concentrations in 3 children with
nitrogen intakes of 500–600 mg/kg/24 h and 100 calories/kg/24 h.

DISCUSSION

Thanks to this new nutritional approach, good results with a definite
cure have been obtained in more than 50 per cent of our cases in
whom life was threatened. Similar data are reported by other groups
using this technique (10, 11, 21, 17, 22).

It is reasonable to have expected similar results in 5 other children
if the indications for parenteral nutrition had been noted before the
terminal phase of malnutrition, and in 5 other cases if infections and
vascular problems had been controlled.

Indeed, study of the *technical complications* should enable one to
prevent the majority of them. The careful fixation of the catheter at

the site of vascular insertion, in the adjacent muscle and at its cutaneous exit, and immobilization of the head or upper limb according to its position, combined with the most rigorous nursing care should prevent accidental movement of the catheter. Venous thrombosis can always be avoided if the silastic catheter is sufficiently small in calibre and adapted to the child's weight, if the site of infusion is at the point of maximum dilution and if the inferior vena cava is not used. Systematic heparin administration is then not necessary.

Infection, because of its relative frequency and severity, is the major complication; prevention requires strict aseptic conditions (23, 24). Placement of the catheter, after meticulous preparation of the skin with iodide, demands the same precautions as in vascular surgery; equally strict precautions must be taken when changing the filter and tubing every 3 days (25, 26). We believe that it is better to change the dressing as seldom as possible (once a month on the average) whereas systematic changing of the catheter, recommended by some authors (27) in the third week, seems to us to be contra-indicated for not only does it reduce the number of available veins but it also appears to be a dangerous procedure, having been responsible for 2 of our cases of septicaemia. On the other hand it is imperative that the solution be prepared by the hospital pharmacist under the conditions described above (28, 29) in a simple 24-hour bottle to keep manipulations to a minimum. No subsequent injection into the bottle or the tubing is permissible. The patient must be nursed in localities where maximum aseptic conditions can be maintained (30), and only nurses trained in this technique may care for these children.

Systematic use of antibiotics is, we believe, not indicated but if the temperature should become elevated, a blood culture is obligatory. In the event of several negative blood cultures and a good clinical state we remove the catheter only if our parenteral nutrition programme is almost completed; a positive blood culture necessitates immediate removal of the catheter and the use of antibiotics (31, 25, 32). Staphylococcus aureus, streptococci and Klebsiella have been isolated (11, 27, 21, 33); in more than 50 per cent of the cases Candida albicans (34, 11, 21) or other fungous organisms were responsible (35, 36). The use of amphotericin B or preferably 5-fluorocytosine (78) is justified only if a blood culture on the day following removal of the catheter remains positive (34).

Although infection is the major concern and fully justifies such preventive measures, major suppurative lesions which are usually peritoneal and even septicaemia which is relatively frequent in poly-perfused malnourished patients are not a contra-indications for paren-teral nutrition by caval catheter as long as antibiotic therapy is given. Six such children responded very satisfactorily to this therapy.

Analysis of the *metabolic effects* of prolonged parenteral nutrition in children is difficult because the data is, relatively speaking, frag-mented and the studies as yet short. However some statements can be made.

With regard to carbohydrates, fructose, sorbitol and xylithol have been used in adults (37, 38, 39), although more than 0.5 g/kg/hour fructose may induce hypoglycaemia (40). In children, on the other hand, the occurrence of acidosis with hyperlactic acidaemia when the rate of fructose infusions is greater than 0.30 g/kg/hour (41) limits its use considerably. For this reason we use glucose as the principle carbohydrate. Weight gain in the presence of a positive nitrogen balance (19) and, in adults, a rise in respiratory quotient (5) bear witness to its utilization. Glucose tolerance is good, as shown by normal blood glucose levels and the absence of hypoglycaemia when the infusion is discontinued (27, 41), provided the osmotic glucose load is increased or reduced by degrees and does not exceed 100 mOsm.per cent at a constant infusion rate of 1 g/kg/hour. Indeed the appearance of glycosuria usually implies an error in technique. Plasma insulin may initially reach levels of 20 to 52 μ U but becomes normal by the end of one week (42). One child only developed hyperglycae-mia and glycosuria, which required the use of insulin, at an infusion rate of less than 1 g/kg/hour; this child had an atrophic pancreas at autopsy.

As far as lipid emulsions are concerned, the filter pore size, as well as other problems (43), prevents their use by our caval catheter technique.

Our approach to protein is as follows. Because of an excess of sodium (Aminosol-Vitrum) or ammonia (Aminosol-Abbot) (44, 45, 46) and insufficiently cysteine (Amigen – Baxter) (47) in the various casein or fibrin hydrolysates, we prefer to use a mixture of crystalline L-amino acids (Vamin – Vitrum). The latter have a coefficient of utilization which is approximately twice that of the d-isomer (48, 49). Their amino acid content is similar to that of egg protein, with 18 amino acids including 12 essential or semi-essential, in particular histidine (50), alanine (51), proline (41) and cysteine (52, 53), but with a tyrosine/phenylalanine ratio <0.1 (reference protein 0.8). This probably explains the very low urinary tyrosine/phenylalanine ratio seen despite normal serum levels.

The observed increase in some (42, 44) or all amino acids (except for arginine, glutamine and lysine) reflects an excessive load (500–600 mg nitrogen/kg/24 h) which we feel should be avoided. Such a protein intake is in fact unnecessary as it has been shown in balance studies that nitrogen retention is greater than the theoretical requirement according to age when the minimum load is administered (240 mg/kg/24 h) and that there is a negative correlation between nitrogen intake and percentage retention. Moreover an excess load is not without risk (44, 54) and may be a factor in the occurrence of abnormalities of calcium and phosphorus metabolism which we (55) as well as others (56, 57, 58, 59) have seen.

Balance studies with loads of nitrogen, calcium and phosphorus varying independently or simultaneously have shown a strict correlation between these elements; when the phosphorus intake is less than 30 mg/kg/24 h hypophosphataemia with hypercalciuria, as we have observed, suggests a phosphorus deficiency. This hypothesis is confirmed by the estimation of the theoretical phosphorus requirement as a function of nitrogen and calcium retention (55).

While some suggest giving 120–130 calories/kg/24 h with 800 mg/kg/24 h nitrogen (11, 4, 60, 13, 61, 33, 14, 18), we prefer not to exceed 100 calories/kg/24 h and 400 mg/kg/24 h nitrogen with a simultaneous intake of calcium (35–40 mg/kg/24 h) and phosphorus (40–50 mg/kg/24 h) (9, 22). Otherwise serious problems may arise in highly malnourished children. In addition from the initial stages of nutritional therapy it is essential, that the protein and caloric loads be increased gradually, beginning usually with 50 calories/kg/24 h and 160 mg/kg/24 h nitrogen.

Finally, it is important to prevent deficiencies of magnesium, copper (62), zinc (63), folic acid and essential fatty acids (64, 65, 66) by periodic estimation of plasma levels and balanced intakes.

INDICATIONS

The indications for such a programme of parenteral nutrition are in theory many. In practice however because of the risks such a treatment entails, it should be used only when an adequate medico-surgical team, proper equipment and a trained nursing staff are available to provide the best guarantees of safety and against asepsis.

In general, there are two very different circumstances under which prolonged caval nutrition may be considered.

Most often, treatment is required for several weeks only (3–8 weeks). The complete cessation of gastrointestinal feeding, replaced by adequate parenteral nutrition, allows the patient to pass through an acute phase and gradual reintroduction of oral nutrients is easier.

In the young infant in particular the prognosis of acute prolonged diarrhoea, post-bacterial or otherwise, which is often aggravated by antibiotics and dietary manipulations has been changed spectacularly by such a regimen (13, 14).

Other digestive problems of diverse aetiology where enteral feeding is temporarily impossible or contra-indicated, may also be treated in this way: children with multiple trauma or extensive burns, acute pancreatitis, ulcerative colitis and regional enteritis (67) or acute malabsorption resulting from abdominal irradiation and/or chemotherapy. Other indications may be certain acute tubulopathies and in very low-birth weight babies (68, 69, 70, 71, 72, 73).

There are many opportunities for after surgery of the digestive tract especially during the neonatal period: tracheo-oesophageal fistulae, diaphragmatic hernia, omphalocele, laparoschisis, necrotizing enterocolitis and meconium ileus; fistulae of the gastrointestinal tract seem to be a particularly good indication because of the rapid and excellent results obtained (fig. 5).

The indications for *long-term parenteral nutrition* after subtotal resection of the small intestine have been discussed in a very different context. Such a resection may be due to congenital atresia or disease at any age. It would appear that until small intestinal transplantation is feasible this method, combined with other nutritional support (74, 75, 76, 78), offers the best possible chance for the patient to adapt to his remaining gut (77) and hence is the only treatment at present available.

SUMMARY

58 superior cava vena catheters, with a mean life of 40 days, were inserted in 42 children, including 36 infants, for prolonged parenteral nutrition. This new approach in nutrition produced very good results

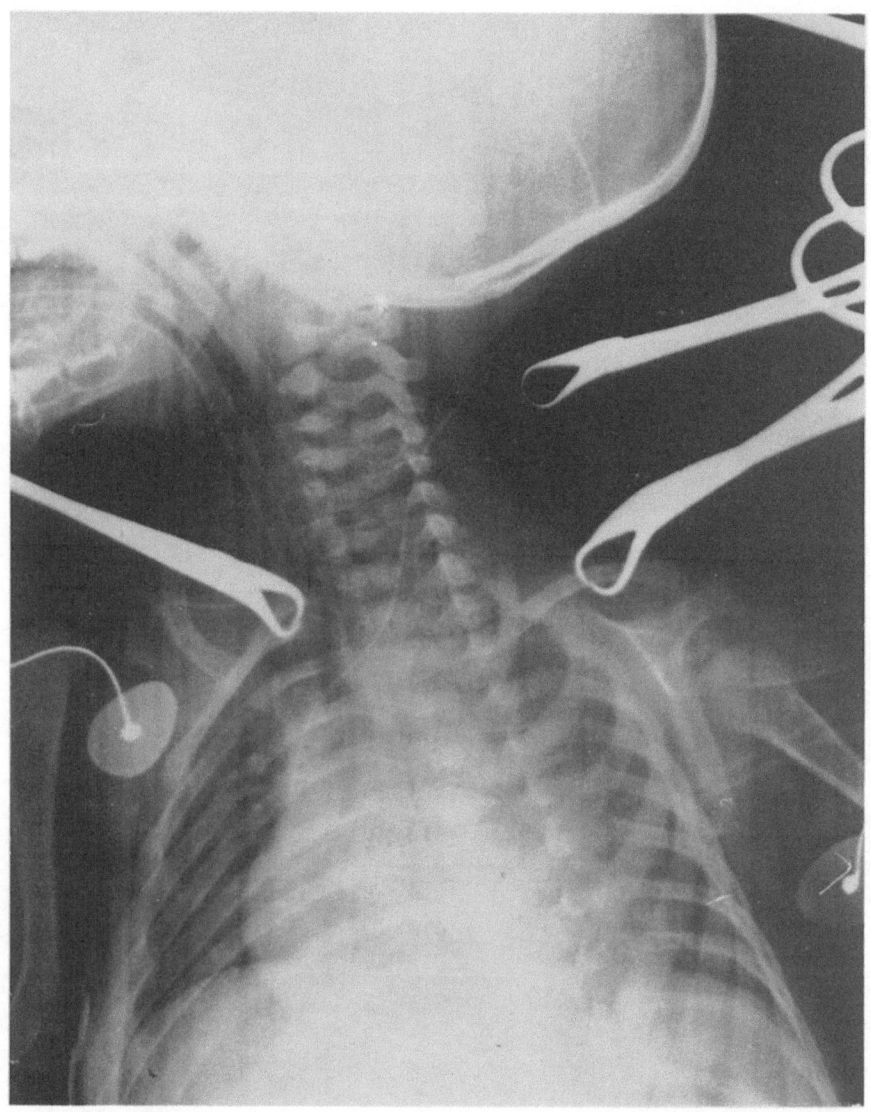

Fig. 1. Radiography during surgery to check the position on the infusion site of a superior vena cava catheter.

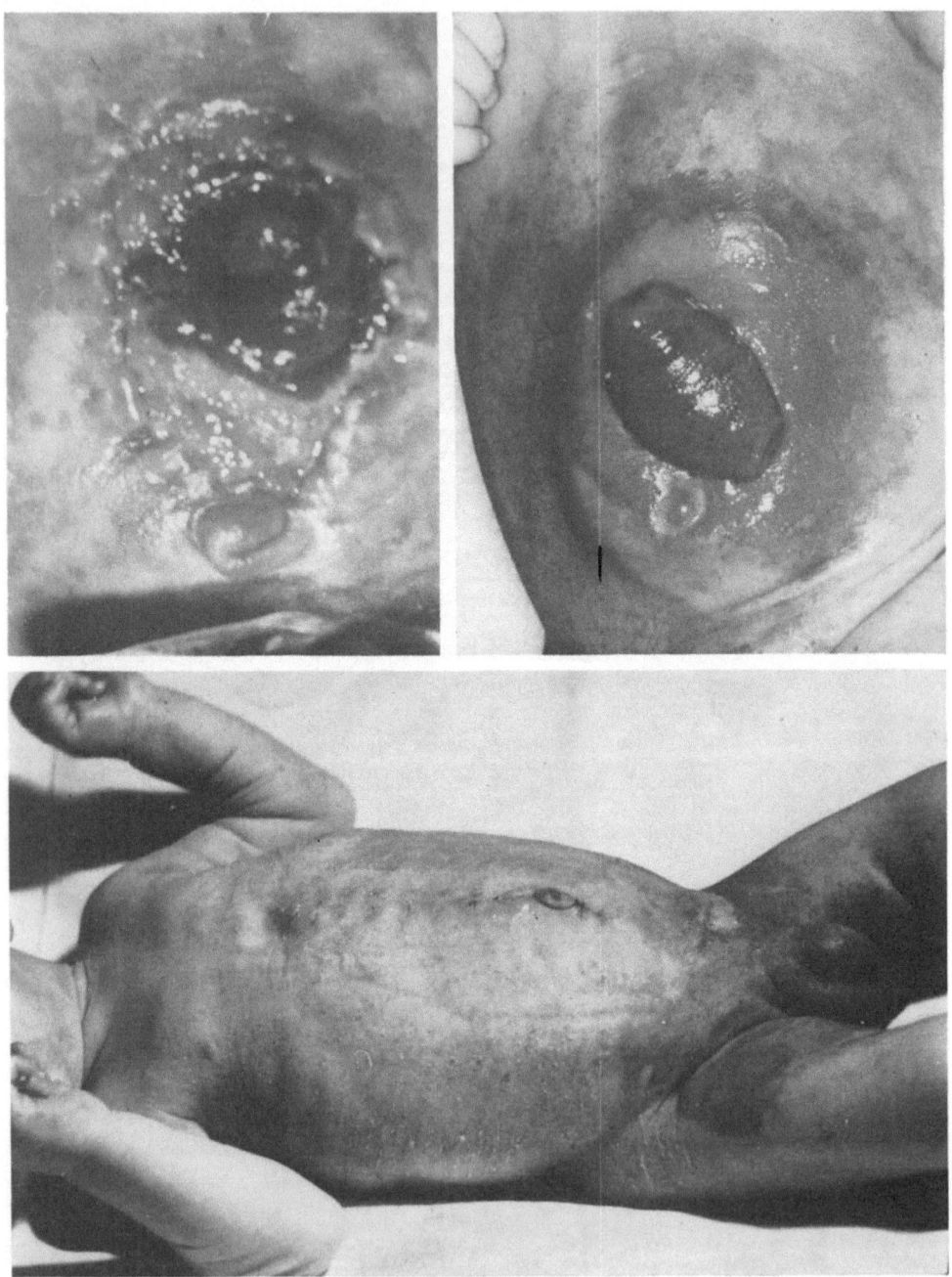

Fig. 5. Prolonged parenteral nutrition in an infant.

5a. Peritonitis, small intestinal fistula with evisceration and parietal necrosis.

5b. After 4 weeks of total parenteral nutrition, perfect cicatrization with cure of peritonitis and septicaemia.

5c. Resection of the exteriorized loop: re-establishment of jejunal continuity. Cure.

Table 4. *Prolonged parenteral nutrition in children. Trace elements required/kg body weight/ 24 hours (from* WILMORE *(22).*

Iodine	15 µg
Copper	22 µg
Zinc	40 µg
Manganese	40 µg
Cobalt	14 µg
Iron	20 µg

in more than half the cases; spectacular improvements in nutrition were obtained. A study of the technical and metabolic complications enables one to prevent most of them. In particular the prevention of infection and the risks of excessive protein and caloric intakes are stressed. Medical and surgical long-term indications are outlined.

REFERENCES

1. DUDRICK S. J., VARS H. M., RAWNSLEY H. M., and RHOADS J. E., (1966) Total intravenous feeding and growth in puppies. *Fed. Proc.*, 25, 481.
2. BITTOUN, A., RAMBAUD J. C., LOIRAT P., MODIGLIANI R., MATUCHANSKY C., DE LAGAUSIE P., DUBOST C. et BERNIER J. J., (1972) Alimentation parentérale continue pendant 16 mois chez une femme ayant subi un arrachement traumatique de la totalité du jéjuno-iléon. *Arch. Fr. Mal. App. Dig.*, 61, 392 c.
3. DUDRICK S. J., STEIGER E., LONG J. M. and RHOADS J. E., (1970) Role of parenteral hyperalimentation in management of multiple catastrophic complications. *Surg. Clin. North. Amer.*, 50, 1031.
4. GRUPPO R. A. and GRAHAM G. G., (1970) Total parenteral alimentation solution. *Hopkins Med. J.*, 127, 352.
5. NEDEY R. et LOIRAT P., (1971) Les solutés hypertoniques de glucose et acides aminés dans la nutrition parentérale exclusive et prolongée. In: *Les solutés de substitution.* Vol. I. Arnette, Paris, 441.
6. REA W. J., WYRICK W. J., MC CLELLAND R. N. and WEBB W. R., (1970) Intravenous hyperosmolar alimentation. *Arch. Surg.*, 100, 393.
7. SCHWARTZ, G. F., GREEN H. L., BENDON M. L., GRAHAM W. P. and BLACEMORE W. S., (1971) Combined parenteral hyperalimentation and chemotherapy in the treatment of disseminated solid tumors. *Amer. J. Surg.*, 121, 169.
8. SOLASSOL C., JOYEUX H., SERROU B., CALLIS A., PUJOL H., and ROMIEU C., (1972) Long term total parenteral nutrition in man: An articial gut. *Biologie et gastroenterologie*, 5, 591 c.
9. BORRESEN, H. C., CORAN A. G. and KNUTRUD O., (1970) Metabolic results of parenteral feeding in neonatal surgery. *Ann. Surg.*, 172, 291.
10. DUDRICK S. J., WILMORE D. W., VARS H. M. and RHOADS J. E., (1968) Long term total parenteral nutrition with growth, development and positive nitrogen balance. *Surgery*, 64, 134.
11. FILLER R. M., ERAKLIS A. J., RUBIN V. G. and DAS J. B., (1969) Long term parenteral nutrition in infants. *New. Engl. J. Med.*, 281, 589.

12. GROTTE G., (1971) Nutrition parentérale du nourrisson. In: *Les solutés de substitution*. Vol. I. Arnette, Paris, 509.

13. HYMAN C. J., REITER J., RODNAN J. and DRASH A. L., (1971) Parenteral and oral alimentation in the treatment of the non specific protracted diarrheal syndrome of infancy. *J. Ped.*, 78, 17.

14. MICHENER W. M. and LAW D., (1970) Parenteral nutrition: the age of the catheter. *Pediat. Clin. North.*, 17, 373.

15. RICOUR C., (1971) Nutrition parentérale prolongée chez le nourrisson: note préliminaire. In: *Les solutés de substitution*. Vol. I. Arnette Paris, 505.

16. SHERMAN J. O., EGAN T. and MACALAD F. V., (1971) Parenteral hyperalimentation. *Surg. Clin. North. Am.*, 51, 37.

17. SINCLAIR J. C., DRISCOLL J. M., HEIRD W. C. and WINTERS R. W., (1970) Supportive managements of the sick néonate. *Ped. Clin. North. Am.*, 17, 863.

18. WILMORE D. W. and DUDRICK S. J., (1968) Growth and development of an infant receiving all nutrients exclusively by vein. *J. Amer. Med. Ass.*, 203, 140.

19. RICOUR, C., NIHOUL-FEKETE C., BERTIN P., ROYER P. et PELLERIN D. (1972) Alimentation parentérale continue par cathéter intracave chez l'enfant. *Ann. Chir. Inf.*, 13, 7.

20. RICOUR C. et NIHOUL-FEKETE C., (1973) Nutrition parentérale prolongée chez l'enfant. *Arch. Fr. Ped.*, 30, 469.

21. JOHNSON D. G., (1970) Total intravenous nutrition in newborn surgical patients a three year perspective. *J. Pediat. Surg.*, 5, 601.

22. WILMORE D. W., GROFF D. B., BISHOP H. C. and DUDRICK S. J., (1969) Total parenteral nutrition in infants with catastrophic gastrointestinal anomalies. *J. Ped. Surg.* 4, 181.

23. GOLDMANN D. A., (1972) *Prevention of infection in hyperalimentation therapy*. IX International Congress of Nutrition, Mexico, 80.

24. RYAN J. A., ABEL R. M., HOPKINS C. C. and FISCHER J. E., (1972) *A prospective study of sepsis in prolonged venous hyperalimentation*. IX International Congress of Nutrition, Mexico, 80.

25. FILLER R. M. and ERAKLIS A. J., (1970) Care of critically ill child: intravenous alimentation. *Pediatrics*, 46, 456.

26. WILMORE D. W. and DUDRICK S. J., (1969) Safe long-term venous catheterization. *Arch. Surg.*, 98, 256.

27. GROFF, D. B., (1969) Complications of intravenous hyperalimentation in newborns and infants. *J. Ped. Surg.*, 4, 460.

28. FLACK H. L., GANS J. A., DUDRICK S. J. and SERLICK S. E., (1970) Current status of parenteral hyperalimentation. Presented to the first annual midyear clinical meeting of the American Society of Hospital Pharmacits.

29. SERLICK S. E., DUDRICK S. J., and FLACK H. L., (1968) Nutritional intravenous feeding. A contribution by the hospital pharmacits. Presented to the third annual midyear meeting. American Society of hospital Pharmacits.

30. GLUCK L., (1970) Design of a perinatal center. *Ped. Clin. North. Amer.*, 17, 777.

31. BANKS D. C., YATES D. B., CAWDREY H. M., HARRIES M. G. and KIDNER P. H., (1970) Infection from intravenous catheters. *Lancet*, 1, 443.

32. SMITS H. and FREEDMAN L. R., (1967) Prolonged venous catheterization as a cause of sepsis. *New. Engl. J. Med.*, 276, 1 229.

33. KAPLAN, M. S., MARES A., QUINTANA P., STRAUSS J., HUXTABLE R. F., BRENNAN P. and HAYS D. M., (1969) High-caloric glucose nitrogen infusions. *Arch. Surg.* 99, 567.

34. ASHCRAFT K. W. and LEAPE L. L., (1970) Candida sepsis complicating parenteral feeding. *Amer. Med. Ass.*, 212, 454.

35. Curry O. R. and Quie P. G., (1971) Fungal septicemia in patients receiving parenteral hyperalimentation. *N. Engl. J. Med.*, 285, 1221.

36. Rodrigues R. J., Shinya H., Wolff W. I. and Puttlitz D., (1971) Torulopsis Glabrata fungemia during prolonged intravenous alimentation therapy. *New. Engl. J. Med.*, 284, 540.

37. Mehnert H., Forster H., Geser C. A., Haslbeck M. and Dehmel K. H., (1970) Clinical use of carbohydrates in parenteral nutrition. In: *Parenteral nutrition.* vol. I. Charles Thomas, Springfield, 112.

38. Meng H. C. and Anderson G. E., (1972) The use of sorbitol in parenteral nutrition. *Fed. Proc.*, 31, 670 (Abs).

39. Schumer W., (1971) Adverse effects of xylitol in parenteral alimentation. *Metabolism*, 20, 345.

40. Sahebjami H. and Scalettar R., (1971) Effects of fructose infusion on lactate and uric acid metabolism. *Lancet*, I, 366.

41. Harries J. T., (1971) Intravenous feeding in infants. *Arch. Dis. Child.*, 46, 855.

42. Das J. B., Filler R. M., Rubin V. G. and Eraklis A. J., (1970) Intravenous dextrose. Amino-acid feeding: the metabolic response in the surgical neonate. *J. Ped. Surg.*, 5, 127.

43. Amris C., Brockner J. and Larsen., (1964) Changes in the coagulability of blood during the infusion of intralipid. *Acta Chir. Scand. suppt.*, 325, 70.

44. Ghadimi H., Abaci F., Kumar S. and Rathi M., (1971) Biochemical aspects of intravenous alimentation. *Pediatrics*, 48, 955.

45. Heird W. C., Nicholson J. F., Driscoll J. M., Schullinger J. N. and Winters R. W., (1972) Hyperammonemia resulting from intravenous alimentation using a mixture of synthetic L-amino-acids. A preliminary report. *J. Ped.*, 81, 162.

46. Johnson G. D., Albritton W. L. and Sunshine P., (1972) Hyperammonemia accompanying parenteral nutrition in newborn infants. *J. Ped.*, 81, 154.

47. Stegink L. D. and Baker G. L., (1971) Infusion of protein hydrolysates in the newborn infant: Plasma aminoacid concentrations. *J. Ped.* 78, 595.

48. Heller L., (1970) *Problems of complete parenteral nutrition. Parenteral nutrition* vol. I Charles Thomas, Springfield. 516.

49. Jarnums S., Jeejeebhoy K. N., Borker A. V. and Westergaard H., (1962) Nitrogen balance during parenteral administration of racemic and L-isomeric aminoacids. *Scand. J. Gastroenterology*, 4 supplt 3, 35.

50. Holt (Jr) L. E. and Snyderman S. E., (1965) Protein and aminoacid requirements of infants and children. *Nutrition abstracts and reviews* 35, I.

51. Jurgens P. and Dolif D., (1968) Die bedentung nichtessentieller aminoseuren fur den stichstoffhaushalt des meuschen unter parenteraler ernahrung. *Klinische Wochenschrift*, 46, 131.

52. Besten L. D. and Stegink L. D., (1972) Effect of parenteral alimentation mixtures on plasma aminoacid levels in adult subjects: comparaison of the rate of administration. *Fed. Proc.*, 31, 732 (Abs).

53. Sturman J. A., Gaull G. and Raiha N. C. R., (1970) Absence of cystathionase in human fetal liver: is cystine essential. *Science* 169, 74.

54. Silvis S. E., and Paragas P. V., (1971) Fatal hyperalimentation syndrome animal studies. *J. Lab. Clin. Med.*, 78, 918.

55. Ricour C., and Balsans S., (1972) *Phosphorus in long term parenteral nutrition in infants.* IX International Congress of Nutrition Mexico, 145

56. Metzger R., Burke P., Thompson A., Lordon R. and Frimpter G. W., (1971) Hypophosphatemia and hypouricemia during hyperalimentation with an aminoacid glucose preparation. *J. Clin. Inv.*, 50, 65 a.

57. SCHULTIS K. and BEISBARTH H., (1972) *Changes in serum phosphate and related parameters caused by parenteral administration of carbohydrate.* IX International Congress of Nutrition Mexico, 144.

58. SILVIS S. E., and PARAGAS P. V., Jr. (1972) Paresthesias weakness seizures and hypophosphotemia in patients receiving hyperalimentation. *Gastroenterology*, 62, 513.

59. TRAVIS S. F., SUGERMA H. J., RUBERG R. L., DUDRICK S. J., DELIVORIA-PAPADOPOULOS M., MILLER L. D. and OSKI F. A., (1971) Alterations of red-cell glycolytic intermediates and oxygen transport as a consequence of hypophosphatemia in patients receiving intravenous hyperalimentation. *New Engl. J. Med.*, 285, 763.

60. HAYS D. M., KAPLAN M. S., MAHOUR G. H., STRAUSS J. and HUXTABLE R. F., (1972) High-calorie infusion therapy following surgery in low-birth-weight infants: metabolic problems encountered. *Surgery*, 71, 834.

61. JEAN R., BONNET H., RIEU D., REY J. M., ALQUIER V. and BRANDY M., (1972) Balance azotée du nourrisson normal et malade. *Ann. Pediat.*, 19, 401.

62. KARPEL J. T. and PEDEN V. H., (1972) Copper déficiency in long term parenteral nutrition. *J. Ped.*, 80, 32.

63. AHNEFELD, F. W. and FODOR L., (1972) *Metabolism of zinc in the postoperative phase.* IX International Congress of Nutrition, Mexico, 146.

64. CALDWELL M. and JONSSON H., (1972) *Severe essential fatty acid deficiency in man: occurence, manifestations and corrections during prolonged total parenteral alimentation.* IX International Congress of Nutrition, Mexico, 197.

65. MAYNARD A. T., DUDRICK S. J., MAC FADYEN B. V. JR and RUBERG R. L., (1972) Essential fatty acid deficiency with intravenous hyperalimentation. *Fed. Proc.*, 31, 717 (Abs).

66. WILMORE D. W., HELMKAMP G. M. JR, MOYLAND J. A. JR. and PRUITT B. A., JR. (1972) *Influence of parenteral diet on serum and red-cell fatty acid composition following thermal injury.* IX International Congress of Nutrition Mexico, 198.

67. FISCHER, J. E., FOSTER G. S., ABEL R. M., ABBOTT W. M. and RYAN J. A., (1972) *Intravenous hyperalimentation as a primary therapy for inflammatory bowel disease.* IX International Congress of Nutrition. Mexico, 15.

68. DRISCOLL J. M., HEIRD W. C., SCHULLINGER J. N., GONGAWARE R. D. and WINTERS R. W., (1972) Total intravenous alimentation in low-birth weight infant: a preliminary report. *J. Ped*, 81, 145.

69. HEIRD W. C. and DRISCOLL J. M., (1972) Intravenous alimentation in pediatric patients. *J. Ped*, 80, 351.

70. HELMUTH W. V., ADAM P. E. J. and SWEET A. Y., (1972) The effects of protein hydrolysate-mono saccharide infusion on low-birth-weight infants. *J. Ped.*, 81, 129.

71. JURGENS P., DOLIF D., PANTELIADIS C. and HOFERT C., (1972) *Complete parenteral nutrition of prematures. The role of aminoacid composition.* IX International Congress of Nutrition, Mexico, 17.

72. PEDEN V. H. and KARPEL J. T., (1972) Total parenteral nutrition in premature infants. *J. Ped.*, 81, 137.

73. SCHREIER K., (1972) *The influence of aminoacid infusion on the development of premature infants.* IX International Congress of Nutrition Mexico, 18.

74. BELIN R. T., KOSTER J. K. JR., BRYANT L. J. and GRIFFEN W. O. JR., (1972) Implantable subcutaneous feeding chamber for non continuous central venous alimentation. *Surgery*, 134, 491.

75. SCRIBNER B. H., COLE J. J., CHRISTOFER G., VIZZO J. E., ATKINS R. C. and BLAGG C. R., (1970) Long term total parenteral nutrition. *J. Amer. Med. Ass.*, 212, 457.

76. SHILS M. E., WRIGHT W. L., TURNBULL A. and BRESCIA F., (1970) Long term parenteral nutrition through an arteriovenous shunt. *New Engl. J. Med.*, 283, 341.
77. WILMORE D. W., DUDRICK S. J., DALY J. M. and VARS H. M., (1971) The role of nutrition in the adaption of the small intestine after massive resection. *Surg. Gynec. Obst.*, 132, 673.
78. FASS R. J. and PERKINS R. L., (1971) 5 Fluorocytosine in the treatment of cryptococcal and candida mycoses. *Ann. Int. Med.*, 74, 535.

SUPPLEMENTARY PARENTERAL NUTRITION IN INTERNAL MEDICINE. ITS EFFECT ON CALORIC AND NITROGEN BALANCE

N. ZÖLLNER*

The course of many chronic diseases, malignant or non-malignant, is characterized by wasting. Loss of weight may occur early in patients with cancer; it also accompanies chronic polyarthritis or the advanced stages of chronic bronchitis. The attending physician may care little about what seems to be a symptom; all of his endeavours may be directed by the answer to the question of whether the therapy considered will cure. However next to cure, comfort and well-being, i.e. a state of relative health, are very important objectives toward which measures must be taken. For a patient doomed to die, every day of fitness during his remaining months is obviously important, but the same is also true for patients with non-fatal but crippling and wasting diseases.

Wasting in chronic diseases as seen to-day is rarely a consequence of excessive use of energy but is instead nearly always due to reduced food uptake. At first it also seemed reasonable to assume that undernutrition is one of the major causes of the loss of strength in chronically ill patients, since improving nutrition in a number of cases led to improved vigour. Early experiments to test this hypothesis were carried out around the turn of the century and again in the twenties. They did not meet with much success, mainly because of the difficulty of regulating the patients' food uptake according to the experimental design. Efforts to increase oral food uptake very often fail in chronically ill persons, notably in patients with cancer.

When the means of increasing the total uptake of all or single nutrients by the intravenous route became available, experiments became less dependent on the patients' ability to cooperate. At that time we decided to re-investigate some aspects of the question whether adequate nutrition influences the course of chronic diseases. To-day

* Polyclinic, Dept. of Internal medicine, University of Munich, W.-Germany.

I shall concern myself with caloric (weight) and nitrogen balances. I shall also offer a few comments on clinical observations.

METHODS

The report concerns patients who were able to eat more than 1000 kcal per day, taking up between 5.0 and 17.6 g N per day. Most of them were either underweight or losing weight when they joined the study. The majority had proven malignancies. There were a number of patients with other chronic diseases: polyarthritis, various forms of malabsorption and chronic disorders of the liver.

All patients were hospitalized. Those in whom nitrogen balance studies were planned were confined to a single room and attended to by a team of a physician and a dietitian. On the basis of the dietary history, a diet containing constant amounts of nitrogen and calories was planned, the amounts being adjusted in such a way that the patient would in all probability eat all he would get. During earlier studies, second portions of equal size were analyzed. These analyses showed that the differences between food tables and analytical results eventually equal out with surprising accuracy. In our best experiment, calculated nitrogen uptake was 326.05 g, nitrogen uptake as determined 325.64 g. (This is the sum of 36 experimental days. The largest deviation on a single day was 1.65 g, i.e. the calculated intake surpassed the determined intake by 21 per cent.)

Nitrogen excretion in urine and faeces was determined in daily samples. Nitrogen losses through skin and hair were not taken into account.

After a first balance period of 6–8 days, oral feeding was supplemented by a daily infusion of 800 kcal. in the form of a fat emulsion. After several days on the supplement regime, there was another control period. Usually several control and supplement periods followed. All patients received a conventional vitamin preparation, covering but not greatly exceeding the recommendations of the Deutsche Gesellschaft für Ernährung.

RESULTS
Caloric balance

If given enough fat emulsion, all patients could be made to gain weight or the rate of weight loss could be decreased. This statement is based on the results in 65 patients, 35 of whom were reported on earlier (ZÖLLNER and SCHUMACHER, 1962). If the number of extra calories is related to the weight gain of these patients, one might conclude from the ratio (2.9 kcal/g weight gain) that extra calories lead to the formation of lean body tissue. However closer scrutiny of those cases where caloric balance was studied more carefully shows that if caloric balance is compared with the product of the change in weight and the caloric value of adipose tissue (6 kcal/g), the results

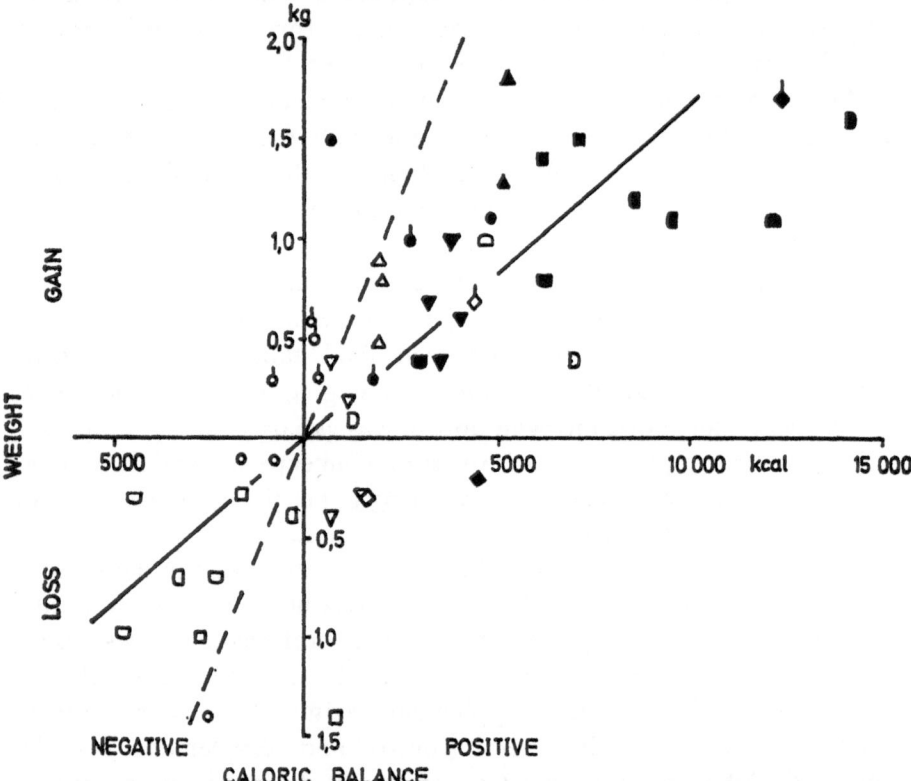

Fig. 1. Plot of weight change versus the difference between caloric intake and calculated caloric requirements. Data from 12 unpublished experiments. Open symbols denote periods without, closed symbols with supplementary intravenous nutrition. Each symbol represents the result of a balance period of four to fourteen days. Predicted weight changes are indicated by the heavy line if extra calories are deposited as adipose tissue, broken line if deposited as lean tissue. Points of case 5 (∇) run parallel to the line for lean tissue. In this case nitrogen balance was persistently positive. Points of case 2 (□), the female of tables 1 and 2 and figure 4 with cancer of the uterus, run parallel to the line for adipose tissue. In this case nitrogen balance was persistently negative.

Table 1. *Comparison of caloric balances calculated as the difference between caloric intake and caloric requirement (Column B – C) with the balances calculated as the product of the change in body weight and the caloric values of adipose and lean tissue, respectively.*

Patient	Estimated caloric requirement A (kcal/day)	Period	Caloric intake B (kcal/day)	Calculated balance of calories B-C (kcal per period)	Body weight end of period (kg)	Change in weight (kg)	Caloric balance per period calculated for caloric value of adipose tissue (kcal)	lean mass (kcal)
Female 69 years old 1.47 m	1380	Control	1474	+ 846	36.5	− 1.4	− 8400	2800
		Fat infusion	1092+800	+ 6144	37.9	+ 1.4	+ 8400	2800
		Control	1175	− 2870	36.9	− 1.0	− 6000	2000
		Fat infusion	1176+800	+ 7152	38.4	+ 1.5	+ 9000	3000
		Control	1233	− 1764	38.1	− 0.3	− 1800	600
Male 62 years old 1.66 m	2095	Control	2573	+ 1912	60.5	+ 0.5	+ 3000	1000
		Fat infusion	2567+800	+ 5088	62.3	+ 1.8	+10800	3600
		Control	2580	+ 1940	63.2	+ 0.9	+ 5400	1800
		Fat infusion	2560+800	+ 5060	64.5	+ 1.3	+ 7800	2600
		Control	2590	+ 1980	65.3	+ 0.8	+ 4800	1600

Table 2. *Calculation of energy requirement for weight gain by comparison of supplemented and unsupplemented periods. Data from table 1, length of periods from original records.*

Patient	Female, 69 years old 1.47 m		Male, 63 years old 1.66 m	
Periods compared	3	4	3	4
Length of periods (days)	14	12	4	4
Extra calories (kcal)		9600		3200
Change in weight (kg)	— 1.0	+ 1.5	+ 0.9	+ 1.3
adjusted for equal length of period	— 0.9			
Weight gain during supplemented period (Difference between periods 4 and 3) (kg)		2.4		0.4
Extra calories per unit weight gain (kcal/g)		4		8

fit better than when the caloric value of lean tissue (2 kcal/g) is used (table 1, figure 1). The results show that the energy contained in the newly gained substance lies between the energy content of lean and adipose tissue.

The weak point in such calculations is the estimation of caloric requirement. However if one recalculates from another assumption, i.e. that the energy required during the supplemented and non-supplemented periods is the same per day, one arrives at basically the same conclusion (table 2).

It has not been possibile so far to decide from our data whether part of the fat emulsion is deposited in the adipose tissue or whether some of its energy content is used to form lean tissue. Interpretation of nitrogen balance would favour the idea that both possibilities exist.

CLINICAL OBSERVATIONS

It was mentioned that the weight gain of patients *not under the conditions of the balance experiment* was one gram per 2.9 kcal supplementary calories. However closer scrutiny showed that once adequate nutrition was established parenterally, the patients started to eat more. Indeed when questioned, 25 per cent of the patients mentioned increased appetite while six per cent complained about a decrease. In most cases, no change in appetite was noted. This means that in more than 90% of the cases supplementary intravenous nutrition with a fat emulsion does not produce a feeling of satiety, i.e. that one does not risk a further restriction of the already restricted oral food uptake.

Indeed we observed several patients who, once improved, increased oral food uptake and continued to gain weight on oral food alone, although they had continuously lost weight before supplementary nutrition. This reminds me of the nutritional breakthrough mentioned earlier at this meeting by Professor JONXIS.

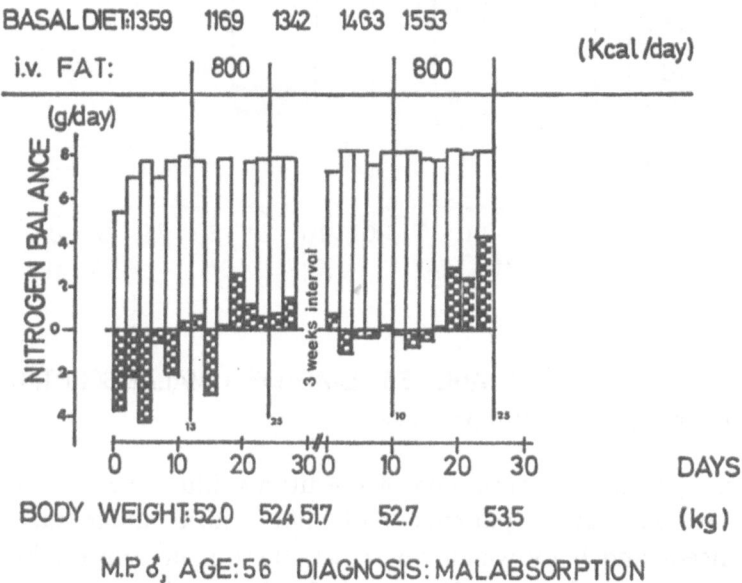

Fig. 2. Influence of supplementary intravenous nutrition with fat on nitrogen balance in a 56-year-old male patient with a malabsorption syndrome of long standing after subtotal gastric resection (BILLROTH II).

NITROGEN BALANCE

Figure 2 shows what one would expect. If the administration of calories is increased from a level below the estimated requirement of 1900 kcal per day to slightly above that value, nitrogen balance becomes positive. However this does not occur immediately but only after a period of several days; it is seen twice in this patient and also in several other patients in whom nitrogen balance could be influenced by administration of fat.

Figure 3 shows that the same data plotted in another, although conventional way, averaging periods to obtain smoothness, are much less informative and even partly misleading.

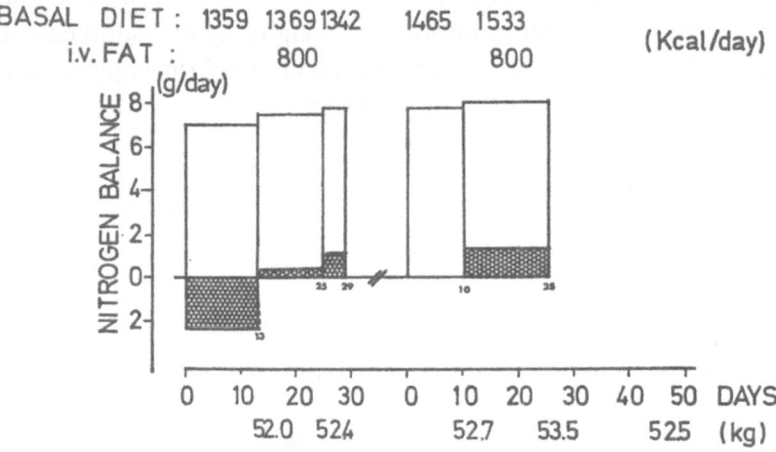

M.P ♂ AGE: 56   DIAGNOSIS: MALABSORPTION

Fig. 3. Data of figure 2, plotted per period.

Figure 4, a case of carcinoma of the uterus, illustrates the typical finding in our cancer patients. Although caloric intake surpasses caloric needs and body weight increases, there is no appreciable influence on nitrogen balance. If, on the other hand, nitrogen balance is positive in non-malignant disease because the diet is already sufficient, additional calories do not promote further nitrogen deposition (figure 5).

Our data for chronically ill patients may be summarized as follows: If caloric balance is rendered positive by supplementary intravenous administration of calories, improvement of nitrogen balance is not a necessary consequence in spite of adequate nitrogen intake. This is contrary to the results found in experimental animals as well as acutely ill human beings, e.g. postoperatively or post-traumatically. Furthermore it is not a reversal of the process during fasting. Possibly

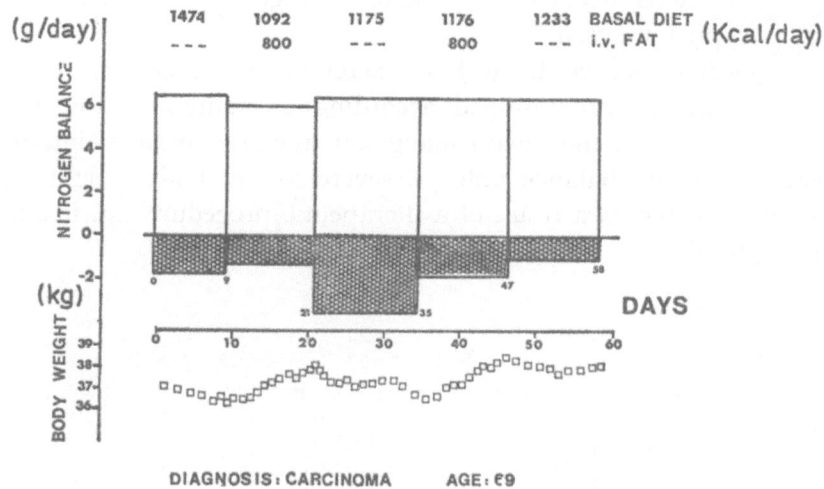

Fig. 4. Lack of influence of supplementary intravenous nutrition with fat on nitrogen balance in a 69-year-old patient with carcinoma of the uterus.

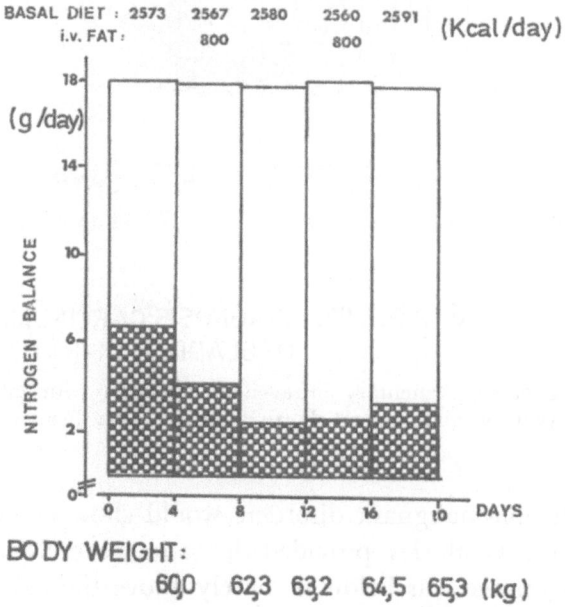

Fig. 5. Lack of influence of supplementary intravenous nutrition with fat on nitrogen balance in a 63-year-old male patient with portal hypertension.

the caloric excess necessary to produce nitrogen rentention is larger than that which we used.

It is possible that we should have exercised our patients.

If the patients are grouped according to malignant and non-malignant diseases, those with malignant diseases would maintain a negative nitrogen balance unless a severe loss in body weight had recently occurred as a result of a therapeutic procedure e.g. irradiation (figure 6).

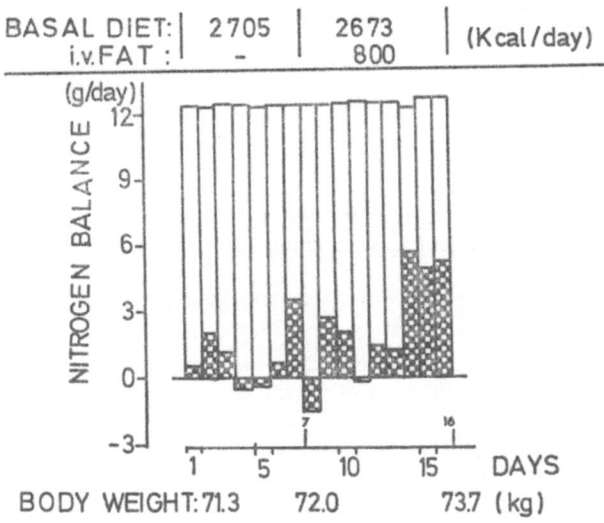

δ, AGE: 67, DIAGNOSIS:CARCINOMA
OF BLADDER (X-RAY)

Fig. 6. Influence of supplementary intravenous nutrition with fat on nitrogen balance in a 67-year-old male patient shortly after radiation therapy for carcinoma of the bladder.

Those with non-malignant disorders would show the influence of the supplementary calories, provided they were severely underweight *and* oral food uptake was below or barely above the caloric requirement. In this group even a balance which is already slightly positive could be further improved. On the other hand, in patients of normal body weight who are already sufficiently well-fed, a positive nitrogen balance could not be increased by additional calories. This of course makes sense.

DISCUSSION AND CLOSING COMMENT

Interpretation of experiments with chronically ill patients is difficult. I leave it open to speculation as to whether the particular insensitivity to extra calories of the nitrogen retaining mechanism is due to the disease. The clinician caring for patients in the late stages of cancer has certainly seen many starve to death and would therefore like the situation to be otherwise. Certainly more efforts might be made for this group of patients. Probably amino acids should be provided parenterally together with the calories. Possibly our results indicate that once again the nitrogen requirement during our lifetime is elevated and cannot be satisfied orally. And hopefully better nutrition at life's end may make this end more bearable.

REFERENCES

For a review of the literature on intravenous nutrition see Supplement to *Nutr. Metabol.*, 14 (1972).
Some of the experimental material presented has been published; see
GLUNZ, K. und ZÖLLNER, N., (1963), Über den Einfluß intravenöser Fettzufuhr auf die Stickstoffbilanz bei chronischen internen Leiden. *Verh. dtsch. Ges. inn. Med.*, 69, 404.
ZÖLLNER, N. und SCHUMACHER, H., (1962), Klinische Beobachtungen bei der parenteralen Zufuhr von Fettemulsionen. *Med. Welt*, 2669.

DISCUSSION

PAPER OF PROF. WRETLIND

Prof. Hegsted: It seems to me as well as many others that histidine should really be considered an essential amino acid regardless of age. The evidence that it is non-essential is just too inadequate to support that assumption. Would you agree?

Prof. Wretlind: Yes, I agree.

Prof. Bickel: We have had some experience with the treatment of histidinaemia. Even at the age of 5 or 6 children seem to respond to a diet free of histidine which also shows that it must still be an essential amino acid. Otherwise they would produce it themselves.

Dr. Ricour: What is the mechanism of blood clearance of this fat emulsion? What is the difference in structure between chylomicrons and artificial fat emulsions like intralipid?

Prof. Wretlind: From a chemical and physical point of view, there is only a slight difference between chylomicrons and the fat droplets in intralipid. Both contain about the same amount of phospholipids; they contain some cholesterol. The main difference is that normal chylomicrons are covered by a layer of proteins, which is not found in artificial fat emulsions.

The clearance of artificial fat droplets and chylomicrons is exactly the same. So far studies have been done in dogs and in man. If the emulsifying agents are changed, even very slightly, there will be a change in the elimination rate. However it is very hard to know whether this is an advantage or disadvantage. We think that natural chylomicrons give the optimum elimination rate.

Dr. Ricour: Is it dangerous to start fat emulsions intravenously in children with undernutrition and sepsis?

Prof. Wretlind: As far as we know it is not dangerous. There is one condition in which you should be careful. That is in septic shock or if the patient has demonstrated allergic reactions to something else. Under these conditions some complications have been observed. Fat emulsions are also contra-indicated for patients with liver damage.

Whether or not it is an advantage to give complete intravenous feeding is as yet not known. I think however that you should be careful in patients with liver damage.

Prof. Visser: Do you recommend fat emulsions and amino acid solutions continuously or intermittently?

Prof. Wretlind: Our general approach is to give them only during the day or only during the night. The main reason is to leave 12 hours free during which the patient can move around. From a nutritional point of view, there is no convincing evidence that it matters whether you give the nutrients during 12 or 24 hours a day. From a physiological point of view, it may be better to give the nutrients when you normally eat but we certainly don't know very much about this. In our animal investigations we have found no difference. The body seems to be able to store the nutrients, a well-known fact for many years.

Prof. Muller: The normal requirements of energy are about 25 to 30 kcal/kg/day for an adult person. In intensive care patients after surgery, we very often have patients with high fever or sepsis. Do you have any rule of thumb as to what the extra energy requirements are?

Prof. Wretlind: Yes. We have several limits. First of all we have the 30 kcal/day. In these cases our fat dosage is between 4 and 5 g/kg/day. For carbohydrates, it is 4,5 or 6 g/kg/day. We increase the amino acid supply to about 2 g/kg/day. In some cases, where there seems to be a very high energy requirement, the amount has been increased to as much as 12 g of fat per kg per day. But I would not recommend such a high dose of fat. It is better to give 4 or 5 g of fat per kg per day, until we know more about it. This type of investigation cannot unfortunately be performed in animals.

22

Dr. de Leeuw: Is there a need for heparin when you give fat intra-venously?

Prof. Wretlind: It is obvious that when you give heparin, you have a much more rapid clearing of fat from the blood. Whether this is an advantage is difficult to say. Some people give heparin, others don't. It does not hurt to give heparin. However heparin does have a place in paediatrics, that is in small-for-date infants. It has been shown that small-for-date infants can tolerate higher amounts of fat if heparin is given. It is not only a question of the liberation of lipoprotein lipase, but it is also in some way related to the production of the enzyme.

Prof. Zöllner: I'm interested in your report that severe liver damage is a contra-indication. We have always used intravenous fat emulsions in patients with liver disease and ascites and quite advanced cirrhosis. We have never seen any evidence that it would harm the patient. A second question would be, does this modern emulsion still show breakage. This makes us a little bit uneasy. The emulsion looks like milk and you cannot guess if it is still stable.

Prof. Wretlind: We have never seen any problem when fat emulsions were given to patients with reversible liver damage. The only reason why I mentioned it is from a theoretical point of view. With regard to the breakage of the emulsions, it seems that the fat emulsions nowadays are very stable. The reason why I'm not afraid of this breakage is that it does not matter if you infuse an oil containing phospholipid. The oil will be emulsified in the blood immediately, as long as phospholipids are present.

PAPER OF DR. STAUFFER

Dr. Cortens: It is said that the capacity for intestinal hypertrophy is much greater in young children than in adults. In your last patient there is only 21 cm of small intestine left. The patient died after 68 weeks of parenteral nutrition. Did you find at autopsy evidence of hypertrophy of the remaining small intestine?

Dr. Stauffer: The intestine was larger, but not markedly increased in length. However the length of the gut is difficult to assess, especially when you compare autopsy findings and intra-operative measurements. The fact that the intestine was larger might be due to partial obstruction at the site of the anastomosis and is not a certain sign of hypertrophy. At histological examination, there were considerable chronic inflammatory changes with partial atrophy of the villi which could explain the poor outcome of this case. As you see, this was not a very good case for studies of signs of compensatory hypertrophy.

However experimental work, especially in rats, provides evidence of such a compensatory hypertrophy of the residual gut. According to Loran, Weser, Skala and others, the residual intestine becomes larger, the villi longer and arborized and, in addition, there is a marked hyperplasia of the mucosal cells. These changes result in an increased total absorption capacity of the residual bowel. This work was, as I mentioned, done in rats. Whether the same anatomical adaptation occurs in man is not certain. Recently Bell and co-workers described an increase in number and length of the villi in a 17-month-old child with only a few inches of small bowel left after volvulus in the neonatal period. This is however in contradiction to the findings of Porus (1965) for two adult patients with 27 and 52 cm of small intestine left; he found only hyperplasia of the mucosa and no other signs of hypertrophy. More research has to be done in man to clear up this very important problem. This is however only possible with exact morphometric measurements in suction biopsies which are difficult to get in man for different reasons.

Prof. McCance: I think I can give you an answer to your question. In our experience if you bypass the whole jejunum and half of the ileum in pigs, the blind part of the gut shows perfectly normal growth in length. If you kill the animal you will find the whole length of the small intestine almost normal. We have never found any evidence of microscopic hypertrophy in the remaining part of the intestine, unless there is an obstruction. Then it will be very striking. We have gone through this quite carefully in various ways. We have studied cross sections and measured them against controls. We have weighed them. We have weighed the ileum very carefully and weighing the ileum requires a certain amount of care because the terminal 15 cm of ileum in the pig is considerably heavier than the other 100 cm. If you include that part you may get false evidence of hypertrophy. You have to compare the exact same part of the intestine if you work on a weight basis.

Dr. Stauffer: I completely agree. We do extensive intestinal resections in guinea pigs now and have obtained the same results.

Dr. Ricour: Is it not sufficient to give 100 kcal/kg/day in parenteral nutrition, because you bypass intestinal absorption?
    What do you do with the lymphatic vessels in transplantation of the intestine?

Dr. Stauffer: We do not reconstruct the lymphatic vessels at present. However reconstruction of the lymphatics would be technically feasible with the operating microscope and was suggested recently by the Russian authors Maximkowa and Lumba at the International Congress on Gastroenterology in Paris in 1972. On the other hand, Goott and Lillehei already showed in 1959 that in the reimplanted whole small intestine in the dog, the lymphatics regenerate promptly and resume full functional capacity. The regeneration in these auto-transplants began at the end of the second week after transplantation and were almost completed after 6–8 weeks. This has been shown by injecting sky blue dye into the lymph nodes of the transplant, which appeared within minutes in the lymphatic channels around the portal vein as well as in the thoracic duct. These observations were confirmed by injecting renographin into the lymphatic channels. In small intestinal allotransplants the regeneration of lymphatics seems to be strikingly retarded. Ruiz from the Lillehei group did not find any signs of regeneration of the lymphatics in small intestinal allotransplants within 3 weeks. The same lack of regeneration of lymphatics has been reported by Olivier in Paris in his patient with a small intestinal allotransplantation, who died 26 days after surgery. Survival time in small intestinal transplantation is however as yet too short with a few exceptions for these studies and there is no definite answer to this problem today.

Dr. Shmerling: It has been shown on the slide that the amount of calories given is not 140 kcal/kg/day but 100 to 140. It depends on the child, the age, the condition and the treatment whether you give more or less. Usually we try to work with a minimum and then increase as it is demanded.

Prof. Schretlen: Your first two patients received parenteral nutrition for about 7 to 12 weeks. After that you stopped. What kind of food do they get at this moment.

Dr. Shmerling: For both of these patients, there was of course a transitional period of nutrition, starting with an elementary diet, a homemade diet, changing very slowly to normal oral feeding. Both children now eat absolutely normal food. They usually avoid sugar, simply because it does not suit them very well. But they have no other restrictions in their diet. Growth and psychological development are absolutely normal.

PAPER OF DR. SHAW

Prof. Schretlen: You use aminosol as a protein source. Do you have an idea of the amino acid levels in the blood?

Dr. Shaw: Yes. We have not done systematic studies, but we have studied two infants more or less intensively. Two colleagues of mine have compared periods of amino acid infusion with equivalent periods when only dextrose was given. They found that the levels of some amino acids actually fell upon the administration of the amino acid mixture. This was interpreted as being a rise in amino acid level due to starvation. I don't know. That was one case.

In the case I have studied myself, amino acid levels were within normal limits.

Dr. Ricour: Your phosphorus intake was 22 mg/kg/day. What was the phosphorus level in the blood in your patients?

How is the mineralization?

Dr. Shaw: The phosphorus and calcium levels in the blood are normal. With respect to mineralization I can't tell you. We have done calcium balance studies in infants fed orally, but we have not yet performed calcium balances in infants on parenteral nutrition. Probably the period is really too short. But I would suggest from my knowledge of the rate of accumulation of calcium by the foetus in the uterus that mineralization is definitely not as good as it should be.

Dr. Steendijk: I would like to continue on this point a little bit. What do you call a normal phosphorus level in the blood of very small infants?

Dr. Shaw: I don't know.

Dr. Steendijk: I think that's the point. It might well be lower than it would have been in the uterus. Therefore mineralization may slow down and you might even get rickets in these children.

Dr. Shaw: We see high phosphorus levels in the blood of infants fed with cow's milk. The point is that the amount of calcium we administer is substantially lower than what the child would accumulate in the uterus. The reason we do not give larger amounts is that I have no idea whether they would be able to accomodate it. Even if they could accommodate it, the effect on acid-base metabolism would not be to their advantage because all of these infants are ill.

Dr. Steendijk: I quite agree.

Dr. Wilson: I noticed that you give your vitamin D in the form of cholecalciferol. Does hydroxylation proceed at a normal rate in these low birth weight infants?

Dr. Shaw: I am afraid we have not measured hydroxycholecalciferol. But this is something we plan to do. It was not until recently that the method became available to us.

PAPER OF PROF. VISSER

Dr. Steendijk: I would like to make a short comment on the growth data of Prof. Visser. There are now several studies which show that the skull, the head circumference, catches up more rapidly than either length or weight in these children. We have found the same results as you have. I would suggest that whenever you give a small-for-date infant enough food in whatever way to start growing, the skull will grow faster. It is simply the pattern of growth of that child. But you have to give enough food.

Prof. Visser: Yes, I agree.

Prof. Bickel: You showed a normal increment of head circumference in prematurely born infants. What is your reference.

Prof. Visser: The increments of head circumference in our patients were compared with the normal intra-uterine growth curves.

In prematurely born infants there is no catch-up growth for head circumference. You only see this phenomenon in small-for-date infants, who are undernourished in the uterus.

Prof. Bickel: Prematurely born infants never fall above those intra-uterine curves?

Prof. Visser: No, they don't.

Dr. de Leeuw: What do you think is less desirable in the case of parenteral nutrition of low birth weight infants: to have elevated serum amino acid levels or to give no amino acid levels at all for a relatively long period.

Prof. Visser: I cannot answer this question. I really don't know what they mean, these elevated amino acid plasma levels. It might be completely harmless, although on the other hand some of these levels are very high. When we think of the phenylalanine concentration, they are even more than 6 mg/100 ml, which really may be too high.

Dr. Widdowson: Why do you choose the amino acid pattern of human milk as your standard? This is after all not the physiological food of the foetus of this age. The foetus is infused with the amino acids from the mother's plasma. Why not choose for example the amino acid pattern in the body of the developing foetus.

Prof. Visser: You are quite right. This is the other possibility, but I have no data to compare with.

Dr. Valaes: I wonder if you have any experience with the synthetic diet in the very tiny premature baby who does not tolerate oral feeding. Do you see any advantage in this?

Prof. Visser: I have no personal experience with the synthetic diet by the oral route in prematurely born babies. I'm not sure that if they won't accept oral milk feedings they will accept synthetic diets orally. In some cases there is diarrhoea. It could be worthwhile to try.

Dr. Valaes: Do you think it would be dangerous to give intralipid when the baby has hyperbilirubinaemia? The intralipid would affect the bilirubin-binding capacity.

Prof. Visser: I cannot answer this question. We have not studied the bilirubin-binding capacity in our patients.

Dr. Hekkens: I should like to have your comment on the E/T ratio. This has been used very often commercially. You can have a good E/T ratio and still have bad utilization of essential amino acids.

How long does it take before there is adaptation to the type of amino acid mixture you have been using.

Prof. Visser: Only a limited number of studies have been done. We are increasing them now. As far as I can see the period of adaptation is variable but may take one or two weeks. This is acceptable in view of adaptive enzyme processes. Your question on E/T ratio is a very difficult one. The E/T ratio only gives the total amount of essential amino acids per 16 g of nitrogen.

Dr. Hekkens: That doesn't say everything about the quality of the protein you are using.

Prof. Visser: No, but this is why I presented the slide with all the individual amino acids in the amino acid solution as compared with egg protein and human milk. They are comparable except for some differences. I really don't know why a solution like vamin differs as far as a number of the amino acids is concerned. That we have to ask the manufacturer.

Dr. Fernandes: I just have a remark on the question of intralipid and hyperbilirubinaemia. The most important point is the level of free fatty acids. This is more important than the level of triglycerides in regard to the binding of bilirubin to plasma albumin.

Dr. Eggermont: Is the route of administration of vamin important for plasma amino acid levels. For instance peripheral vein, umbilical vein or umbilical artery?

Prof. Visser: We give our amino acid solution by peripheral vein since we try to follow a set routine. I would guess that it would make no difference, but I'm not sure.

Dr. Hommes: May I come back to the problem posed by Dr. Widdowson. I don't have an answer but perhaps I can describe the problem a little bit more accurately. This may also provide a clue to the increased levels of plasma amino acids you have observed. That is that not only human milk should be taken as a reference but the pattern should also be related to developmental aspects of specific enzymes in the catabolism of different amino acids. This is a problem. I can't give an answer.

Prof. Hegsted: It seems to me that the physiological parameter would be the rate of deposition of various amino acids. That may have nothing to do with plasma amino acid levels. We certainly get increases in amino acids after meals, for example. I think you could follow the theoretical pattern of amino acids that have to be deposited. I wonder if there are any data on rates or on efficiency of utilization.

Prof. McCance: This is a problem that obviously can be settled experimentally. Take the foetus out of an animal. We know the composition of its body; feed it an assortment of amino acids and see how they go.

Dr. Widdowson: I would like to say that we are at present making analyses of the composition of amino acids in foetuses in great detail. So we will have this information very shortly.

PAPER OF DR. RICOUR

Dr. Steendijk: I was impressed by the figure for calcium excretion in the urine, which at first was 24 mg and then went down to 12 mg/kg/day. Those figures are very high. Votre patron, monsieur Royer, said many years ago that values above 5 mg/kg/day are too high. Do you see any nephrocalcinosis or nephrolithiasis as a result of this hypercalciuria?

Dr. Ricour: We have not observed renal stones in our patients.

PAPER OF PROF. ZÖLLNER

Dr. Fernandes: I would like to make some remarks on fat utilization. It is known that the clearing capacity has rather wide ranges. It is fairly small in premature babies and rather high in older children and adults. In order to profit from the clearing capacity it is important to know the amount that can be given. Therefore monitoring of the fat levels is essential. We have two methods. One is by rather crude estimate: you have to stop the fat infusion and look at the serum turbidity one hour later. Another more accurate estimation is to measure triglyceride levels during the infusion. Then we can see that there are children who tolerate only 1 g of fat per kg per day and others who tolerate 10 g or more.

A second question has already been mentioned. What is our position with regard to heparin. The dose of heparin given during the fat infusion is far below the dose used for estimation of the lipoprotein activity of the patient. Maybe it has something to do with sparing the vessels or increasing the clearing capacity. However we don't know. Perhaps it might be better to abandon heparin.

Prof. Zöllner: We feel that it really is not very important what level the infused lipids reach during the infusion as long as it has returned to the pre-infusion level before we start the next infusion, i. e. usually from one morning to the next. In a way we feel that the blood acts as a fat reservoir. High levels of neutral fats are not at all harmful to the patient. As a matter of fact when we tried to make the infusions last several hours, many of our patients turned the rate of infusion higher in order to get it over. They still had disposed of all that fat by the next morning. With regard to heparin I have little to say. We think that the clearing of fat is very rapid. We never use heparin routinely.

Prof. Wretlind: I would like to discuss your statement that a positive nitrogen balance is not possible in patients with carcinoma or malignant disease. I just wonder if that statement is correct. You gave your patients 6 or 8 g of nitrogen. What would happen if you gave larger amounts of nitrogen?

I would also like to mention physical activity. Dr. Solassol et al in Montpellier have used total or supplementary intravenous feeding in cancer patients. It is quite obvious to anyone who has seen these patients that they are kept in perfect nutritional condition for several months, even with very severe carcinoma. I just wonder if their results might depend on the fact that they give their infusion solution during 12 hours at night. During the day, the patient performs exercises. This physical activity is a very important anabolic factor. It would be very interesting to carry out control investigations with and without physical activity. As soon as you put a patient in bed and give him more energy than he needs, there is an increase in body weight but at the same time a decrease in the lean body mass. But if the patient is physically active, the lean body mass will increase again. I just wonder if you have any comment on this question.

Prof. Zöllner: All of our patients had a nitrogen uptake ranging between 6 and 17.6 g/day. Our results are applicable only within this range of nitrogen uptake. As a matter of fact the nitrogen uptake of most of our patients was between 6 and 10 g, which is close to the minimum nitrogen requirement. Orally we could not raise it. This was all they would take. So our hands were bound, and we did not want to spoil our experiment. But of course the experiments could be repeated, since very good amino acid solutions are now available.

All of our patients were ambulatory within their room. So no patient was really bed-ridden. But the room was rather small, it was a sort of metabolic cage.

The patients with non-malignant nutritional disorders, mainly those with malabsorption after Billroth II operations, retained nitrogen under the same experimental conditions. So I feel rather certain that although excercise may be necessary, it is not the whole story. The disease in itself may have some influence on nitrogen retention.

Prof. Eekels: Well, ladies and gentlemen, before closing this session, I think it is my duty to say on behalf of all participants how very grateful we are to Prof. Jonxis, the organizer and spiritual father of this congress, which was very successful indeed. Thank you very much.

INDEX OF SUBJECTS